Simulation in Radiology

SIMULATION IN RADIOLOGY

EDITORS

HUGH J. F. ROBERTSON, MD, DMR, FRCPC, FRCR, FACR

PROFESSOR OF CLINICAL RADIOLOGY
LOUISIANA STATE UNIVERSITY SCHOOL OF MEDICINE
AND
CLINICAL PROFESSOR OF RADIOLOGY
TULANE UNIVERSITY MEDICAL CENTER
NEW ORLEANS, LOUISIANA

JOHN T. PAIGE, MD

ASSOCIATE PROFESSOR OF CLINICAL SURGERY
DIRECTOR, APPLIED SURGICAL SIMULATION
LOUISIANA STATE UNIVERSITY SCHOOL OF MEDICINE
NEW ORLEANS, LOUISIANA

LEONARD R. BOK, MD, MBA, JD

PROFESSOR OF RADIOLOGY
CHAIRMAN DEPARTMENT OF RADIOLOGY
LOUISIANA STATE UNIVERSITY SCHOOL OF MEDICINE
NEW ORLEANS, LOUISIANA

OXFORD
UNIVERSITY PRESS

OXFORD
UNIVERSITY PRESS

Oxford University Press, Inc., publishes works that further
Oxford University's objective of excellence
in research, scholarship, and education.

Oxford New York
Auckland Cape Town Dar es Salaam Hong Kong Karachi
Kuala Lumpur Madrid Melbourne Mexico City Nairobi
New Delhi Shanghai Taipei Toronto

With offices in
Argentina Austria Brazil Chile Czech Republic France Greece
Guatemala Hungary Italy Japan Poland Portugal Singapore
South Korea Switzerland Thailand Turkey Ukraine Vietnam

Published by Oxford University Press, Inc.
198 Madison Avenue, New York, New York 10016
www.oup.com

Library of Congress Cataloging-in-Publication Data
Simulation in radiology / edited by Hugh J. Robertson, John T. Paige, Leonard Bok.
p. ; cm.
Includes bibliographical references and index.
ISBN 978–0–19–976462–4 (pbk. : alk. paper)
I. Robertson, Hugh J. II. Paige, John T. III. Bok, Leonard. [DNLM: 1. Computer Simulation.
2. Radiology—education. WN 18]
616.07'572—dc232012006844

9 8 7 6 5 4 3 2 1

Printed in

on acid-free paper

This book is dedicated to the patients of Charity Hospital of New Orleans. Since 1736, they have inspired the health professionals with whom they have entrusted their care to provide the best medical care possible through research, innovation, and clinical excellence.

Contents

Contributors

Charles N. Aprill, MD
Clinical Associate Professor of Radiology
Louisiana State University School of Medicine
New Orleans, Louisiana

Nabeel A. Arain, MD, MBA
Fellow, Minimally Invasive/Advanced Laparoscopic Surgery and Robotic Surgery
Southwestern Center for Minimally Invasive Surgery
University of Texas Southwestern Medical Center
Dallas, Texas

Veronica Crisostomo Ayala, DVM, PhD
Endoluminal Therapy and Diagnosis Department
Jesus Uson Minimally Invasive Surgery Centre
Caceres, Spain

Paul Babyn, MD, CM, FRCPC
Professor and Head, Department of Medical Imaging
University of Saskatchewan and Saskatoon Health Region
Royal University Hospital
Saskatoon, SK, Canada

Kendra Barrier, MSN, RN
Instructor of Nursing
Louisiana State University School of Nursing
New Orleans, Louisiana

Laura Bonanno, DNP, CRNA
Assistant Professor of Nursing
Program Director, Nurse Anesthesia Program
Louisiana State University School of Nursing
New Orleans, Louisiana

John W. Bonnett, MD
Assistant Professor of Clinical Radiology
Wayne State University School of Medicine
Detroit, Michigan

Stephanie Casey, MD
Assistant Professor of Clinical Radiology
Louisiana State University School of Medicine
New Orleans, Louisiana

Sheila W. Chauvin, PhD, MEd
Director, Office of Medical Education Research and Development (OMERAD), School of Medicine
Director, Academy for the Advancement of Educational Scholarship
Professor of Internal Medicine
Professor, School of Public Health
Louisiana State University
New Orleans, Louisiana

Robert Dawson, MD
Clinical Professor of Neurosurgery
Clinical Professor of Radiology
Louisiana State University School of Medicine
New Orleans, Louisiana

Chiraag V. Dharia, MD
Radiology Resident (Radiologist In-Training)
Henry Ford Hospital
Detroit, Michigan

Gladys L. Fernandez, MD
Manager, Baystate Simulation Center
Baystate Medical Center
Assistant Professor of Surgery
Tufts University School of Medicine
Springfield, Massachusetts

Hector Ferral, MD
Professor of Radiology
Section Chief, Interventional Radiology
Rush University Medical Center
Chicago, Illinois

Roque Ferreyro, MD
Associate Professor of Clinical Radiology
Louisiana State University School of Medicine
New Orleans, Louisiana

Richard Fremaux, MD
Assistant Professor of Clinical Radiology
Louisiana State University School of Medicine
New Orleans, Louisiana

Deborah Garbee, PhD, APRN, ACNS-BC
Associate Dean Undergraduate Nursing Programs
Adult Health CNS Program Director
Assistant Professor of Nursing
Louisiana State University School of Nursing
New Orleans, Louisiana

Frederick D. Grant, MD
Staff Physician, Nuclear Medicine and Molecular Imaging
Instructor of Radiology
Harvard Medical School
Boston, Massachusetts

Jan Grund-Pederson, MArch
Director of US Operations
Mentice Inc.
Evanston, Illinois

Brad J. Hymel, MD
Senior Resident, Department of Anesthesiology
Louisiana State University School of Medicine
New Orleans, Louisiana

Francine Jacobson, MD, MPH
Assistant Professor of Radiology
Harvard Medical School
Boston, Massachusetts

Alan David Kaye, MD, PhD, DABPM
Professor and Chairman,
Department of Anesthesia
Louisiana State University School of Medicine
New Orleans, Louisiana

Valeriy V. Kozmenko, MD
Assistant Professor of Clinical Anesthesiology
Director of Simulation, Department of Anesthesiology
Louisiana State University School of Medicine
New Orleans, Louisiana

Michael Maristany, MD
Assistant Professor of Clinical Radiology
Louisiana State University School of Medicine
New Orleans, Louisiana

Winter Melancon, MBA
Business Manager
Department of Radiology
Louisiana State University School of Medicine
New Orleans, Louisiana

Mishal Mendiratta-Lala, MD
Assistant Professor of Clinical Radiology
Wayne State University School of Medicine
Detroit, Michigan

Thea Moran, MD
Assistant Professor of Clinical Radiology
Louisiana State University School of Medicine
New Orleans, Louisiana

Mignonne Beaudoin Morrell, MD
Radiology Chief Resident
Louisiana State University School of Medicine
New Orleans, Louisiana

Rocio Perez-Johnston, MD
Fellow, Abdominal Imaging and Intervention
Massachusetts General Hospital
Boston, Massachusetts

James Riopelle, MD
Professor of Clinical Anesthesiology
Louisiana State University School of Medicine
New Orleans, Louisiana

Frank J. Rybicki, MD, PhD
Director, Cardiac CT and Vascular CT/MRI
Director, Applied Imaging Science Laboratory
Associate Professor of Clinical Radiology,
Harvard Medical School
Boston, Massachusetts

Gauravi Sabharwal, MD
Assistant Professor of Clinical Radiology
Associate Director, Radiology Residency Program
Wayne State University
Detroit, Michigan

Daniel J. Scott, MD, FACS
Associate Professor of Surgery
Director, Southwestern Center for Minimally Invasive Surgery
University of Texas Southwestern Medical Center
Dallas, Texas

Luis F. Serrano, MD
Associate Professor of Clinical Radiology
Louisiana State University School of Medicine
New Orleans, Louisiana

Neal E. Seymour, MD
Chief, Department of Surgery
Baystate Medical Center
Professor of Surgery
Tufts University School of Medicine
Springfield, Massachusetts

Malachi G. Sheahan III, MD
Associate Professor of Surgery
Director, Vascular Surgery Fellowship
Louisiana State University School of Medicine
New Orleans, Louisiana

Robert S. Sitarz, MD
Fellow, MR Imaging
University of Maryland
Baltimore, Maryland

David L. Smith, MD
Assistant Professor of Clinical Radiology
Louisiana State University School of Medicine
New Orleans, Louisiana

Michael L. Steigner, MD
Instructor of Radiology
Harvard Medical School
Boston, Massachusetts

Jennifer Stimec, MD, FRCPC
Hospital for Sick Children
Toronto, Ontario, Canada

William J. Swartz, PhD
Professor of Cell Biology and Anatomy
Louisiana State University School of Medicine
New Orleans, Louisiana

Aran Toshav, MD
Assistant Professor of Clinical Radiology
Director, Radiology Residency Program
Louisiana State University School of Medicine
New Orleans, Louisiana

S. Ted Treves, MD
Professor of Radiology
Harvard Medical School
Boston, Massachusetts

Christopher Vargo, MD
Assistant Professor of Clinical Radiology
University of Nebraska Medical Center
Omaha, Nebraska

Richard H. Whitworth, Jr., PhD
Associate Professor of Cell Biology and Anatomy
Louisiana State University School of Medicine
New Orleans, Louisiana

Todd R. Williams, MD
Clinical Associate Professor of Radiology
Wayne State University School of Medicine
Detroit, Michigan

Joan C. Wojak, MD
Clinical Associate Professor of Radiology
Louisiana State University School of Medicine
New Orleans, Louisiana
Medical Director of Radiology
Our Lady of Lourdes Regional Medical Center
Lafayette, Louisiana

Shirley Yodzis, MD
Associate Professor of Clinical Radiology
Louisiana State University School of Medicine
New Orleans, Louisiana

Foreword

SIMULATION IS fast becoming a key component of the professional development of health care providers across the entire continuum of their career. I have had the good fortune of witnessing the impact of this transformation here at Louisiana State University in New Orleans. In 2000, we redesigned the undergraduate curriculum at the School of Medicine in which simulation-based training in education was incorporated from day one. Today, medical students at our institution regularly practice skills, treat simulated patients, and learn the art of medicine using simulation-based techniques at the Isidore Cohn, Jr. MD Student Learning Center.

Over the decade, simulation-based training has expanded from its undergraduate beginnings to incorporate both graduate medical education of multiple specialties and practicing physicians. Today, we occupy a 30,000 square-foot facility extending over two floors, providing simulation-based education and training to multiple medical specialties and learner groups. In the process, we have striven to be a leader in innovative simulation-based education and research.

Simulation in Radiology is an example of such leadership. It is the first such textbook addressing simulation-based training and education in the field of radiology. The editors have combined their various expertise and backgrounds in simulation-based education and training, diagnostic and interventional radiology, and residency education to create a reference for individuals interested in incorporating simulation-based training into any subspecialty of radiology. They have focused not only on the role of simulation in radiology, but they have also addressed key issues related to basic general principles and the incorporation of simulation into an effective educational program. A particular strength is their use of experts from diverse backgrounds (i.e., education, surgery, anatomy, computer technology) to create a concise, yet comprehensive work. I am confident that this textbook will become an essential reference for medical educators wanting to incorporate simulation into radiology.

Charles Hilton, MD
Associate Dean for Academic Affairs
ACGME Designated Institutional Official
Louisiana State University School of Medicine
New Orleans, Louisiana

Preface

GRADUATE MEDICAL education (GME) has undergone a transformation of epic proportions over the last decade. The traditional apprenticeship model of training is being transformed by an objectives-driven, educational model founded on adult learning principles. In today's highly dynamic, complex health care environment, the competencies of professionalism, interpersonal skills and communication, practice-based learning and improvement, and systems-based practice are becoming as important to learn as medical knowledge, technical skills, and patient care. Trainee work hour restrictions, changing modes and technologies in clinical practice, and an emphasis on patient safety have limited direct patient educational opportunities for residents. In response to these multiple trends, medical educators have adopted new educational tools and techniques to continue to provide the highest quality GME possible.

One of the most effective educational tools embraced by medical educators for this new paradigm in GME has been simulation-based training (SBT). The advantages of SBT are manifold: standardization of the educational experience; the ability to teach low-frequency, high-risk events; the opportunity for deliberate practice; the enhancement of safety; and immersive, team-based learning are some examples. In fact, these advantages have long been recognized by other high-risk, dynamic industries such as aviation and nuclear energy that have employed SBT for years. In medicine, the specialty of anesthesiology was an innovator in the use of SBT in GME and other aspects of professional development. Emergency medicine, surgery, obstetrics and gynecology actively use SBT in GME. Research on SBT in these medical specialties has successfully demonstrated its usefulness in cognitive and technical skills acquisition, as well as in improvement in team functional dynamics.

This book developed from our recognition of the utility and need for SBT incorporation into all of the subspecialty service areas of radiology. It is divided into three sections focusing on key aspects of SBT. The first section includes considerations related to using simulation in training, including general principles, ethical considerations and regulations in cadaveric use, an overview of computer-based simulation, and some available simulation devices. The second section provides an overview of educational principles and testing necessary to the understanding and implementation of SBT, integration of SBT into GME, and considerations in the development and operation of a simulation center. The third section presents a summary review of the scientific literature and current work being done in SBT in radiology, including the acquisition of required basic skills, team training and crisis management, and specific work related to the subspecialty areas of radiology. The format of the chapters is intended to provide a concise overview but not an all-inclusive review of the subject matter. We hope that this book will be of interest and assistance to all involved in diagnostic imaging and interventional radiological procedures.

Hugh J. F. Robertson
John T. Paige
Leonard R. Bok

Acknowledgments

WE WISH to recognize Winter Melancon for her tireless and dedicated assistance in bringing this book to fruition. Her keen attention to detail and constant encouragement were invaluable. We thank our families for their patience and support during the rewarding yet time-consuming process of bringing this work to publication.

SECTION 1

SIMULATION: TECHNICAL CONSIDERATIONS

1

Principles of Simulation

JOHN T. PAIGE

WHAT IS *simulation*? Such a query is an appropriate starting point for a book dedicated to simulation in radiology. Arising from the Latin noun *simulatio,* meaning "an imitating, feigning," the term first appeared in the English language around the mid-14th century in the context of "a false show, false profession."[1] This definition has evolved to include other more recent, germane uses. According to the Merriam-Webster Online Dictionary, it can now also be defined as "the imitative representation of the functioning of one system or process by means of the functioning of another."[2] Such usage dates from 1954. Interestingly, the verb *simulate* has more recent roots, first showing up in the English language in the 1620s, as a derivative of the Latin verb *simulare* meaning "to imitate." Its use in the context of "imitative for the purposes of experiment or training" first occurred in 1966.[1] Thus, the term *simulation* as it is used in the context of medical education and training today is a relatively recent one, reflecting the recent technological advancements of the computer age.

In medicine, simulation has been defined several ways. McGaghie describes it as "a person, device, or set of conditions which attempts to present [education and] evaluation problems authentically. The student or trainee is required to respond to the problem as he or she would under natural circumstances. Frequently the trainee receives performance feedback as if he or she were in the real situation."[3] For Gaba, simulation is "a technique—not a technology—to replace or amplify real experiences with guided experiences that evoke or replicate substantial aspects of the real world in a fully interactive manner."[4] It is, therefore, "an instructional process that substitutes real patient encounters with artificial models, live actors, or virtual reality patients."[5] Andreatta et al[6] provide perhaps the most succinct definition, explaining that "[t]he term simulation in medical education refers to instruction that makes use of facsimiles of clinical contexts wherein learners interact to acquire knowledge, skills, and affective elements that will ultimately transfer to the real clinical context."

Whatever definition one prefers, simulation encompasses a broad variety of formats in medicine, ranging from simple table-top question-and-answer sessions to fully immersive interactions with a computerized mannequin; from suturing a banana peel to performing a procedure on a cadaver; or from reviewing images in a film library to performing a virtual computed tomography colonoscopy reconstruction and read from start to finish. In fact, simulation has been a part of medicine education and training much longer than the word used to describe it. Galen dissected animals to learn about anatomy. Vesalius focused on cadaveric anatomical studies. Even birthing mannequins date to the late 17th century in France.[7]

No matter how old the lineage of simulation in medicine, its use has dramatically increased over the last decade, prompting a proliferation of research, applications, and texts such as this book. The reason for this growth in simulation-based training (SBT) and education is manifold. Issenberg et al[8] identified five contributing factors. First, the move to a more outpatient-based, cost-effective model of care has decreased learning opportunities for students and residents alike in the clinical setting. Second, the development of new technologies (e.g., endoscopy and minimally invasive surgery) has required physicians to learn new skill sets. Third, the Accreditation Council for Graduate Medical Education's (ACGME) introduction of the six core competencies has driven educators to find a reliable means for their assessment. Fourth, the patient safety movement has underlined deficiencies in physician training, such as the effective use of team-based competencies. Finally, the introduction of educational concepts such as deliberate practice has highlighted the need for the structured training of physicians outside of the clinical environment.

This chapter attempts to provide a framework for approaching and understanding simulation in medical education and training through an overview of key principles related to its application. First, it will review useful nomenclature, concepts, and classifications related to simulation formats and simulators. Next, it will provide representative examples of potential uses and applications of simulation in medicine, and it will discuss important considerations for its use in training. It will then provide a targeted review of how to measure its impact, and it will close with some points related to its successful implementation. In the process, it will hopefully provide the reader with a strong foundation for understanding the chapters to follow and applying simulation in radiology.

HELPFUL NOMENCLATURE, CONCEPTS, AND CLASSIFICATIONS

As with any field of study, simulation science has its own specific nomenclature, concepts, and classifications. Having a familiarity with them is particularly useful for a novice interested in applying simulation in training or education. To begin, a *simulator* is defined as a device that attempts to mimic aspects of the real world.[9] As Gaba notes, in health care, such a device typically "presents a simulated patient (or part of a patient) and interacts appropriately with the actions taken by the simulation participant."[4] For every simulator, a *simuland* and *referent* exist. A simuland is "the system being simulated by a simulation," whereas the referent is the "codified body of knowledge about a thing being simulated."[10] For example, the simuland for a computerized mannequin simulator is an actual patient. In this case, the referent would include current understanding regarding physiology and pharmacology.

Simulators can be classified according to a variety of methods based on such characteristics as fidelity (see below), capability, cost, or user feedback.[11] Meller[12] developed a typology of simulators based on elements of the clinical experience and how they interact with the user. Clinical components included the patient/disease process (P1); the procedure, diagnostic test, or equipment in use (P2); the physician/paraprofessional (P3); and the professor/expert (P4). Possible interactions with these four elements include passive (p), active (a), and interactive (i). With this system, each element can be rated according to its interaction with the user, allowing for a codified language related to simulator functionality.

A key concept related to simulation and simulators is that of *fidelity*. In simulation, fidelity is defined as the degree to which a simulator or simulation replicates reality. Hence, a low-fidelity simulator (i.e., a piece of rubber tubing with a slit in it for practicing simple interrupted suturing) poorly replicates what it is supposed to represent, whereas a high-fidelity simulator (i.e., a virtual reality endovascular trainer housed within an exact replica of an endovascular suite) is very true to life. As Beaubien and Baker[9] have pointed out, however, care must be taken to avoid adopting a unidimensional view of simulation fidelity, since it oversimplifies the interaction that occurs on multiple levels between the simulation/simulator and the learner.

Rehmann et al's[13] three-dimensional (3-D) approach to fidelity helps tease out such intricacies. In their schemata, simulation fidelity is assessed on three levels: *equipment fidelity* (i.e., the degree to which the simulator looks like the real setting), *environment fidelity* (i.e., the degree to which the simulator acts like the real setting), and *psychological fidelity* (i.e., the degree to which the simulator makes the learner feel that he or she is in the real setting). Using this framework, a simulator could provide varying levels of fidelity for each dimension. Other authors have proposed similar models of simulation fidelity, with categories roughly corresponding to Rehmann et al's (Table 1.1).[13–15] Fidelity is important in simulation-based training and education because of the positive correlation between increasing fidelity and the likelihood of learning transfer to clinical practice.[6]

In addition to avoiding a unidimensional approach to fidelity, Andreatta et al[6] have pointed out that care also must be taken to differentiate fidelity from *technology*. Often, these concepts are used synonymously. They are, however, not the same. Thus, a low-technology simulator need not always be low-fidelity and vice versa. The context of the training is important. For example, a sophisticated computerized mannequin (i.e., a high-technology simulator) might be true to life regarding its physiological responses related to drug administration and disease state (i.e., have high environment fidelity), but, used in the context of practicing physical exam skills, it might not lead to a "suspension of disbelief" among learners (i.e., have high psychological fidelity).

Function (i.e., capability) is also an important concept related to simulators and simulation. Simulation-based training can run the gamut of experiences, from teaching a specific skill set or task to teaching a complex, interactive behavioral response. Simulators, therefore, can be designed to serve a particular purpose along this continuum of training. *Part-task simulators* mimic all or part of a particular skill, task, or procedure. Examples include a box trainer used to learn basic minimally invasive surgical skills, an airway model for intubation, or a knot-tying board. Other more technologically advanced examples include virtual reality machines for laparoscopic, endoscopic, and endovascular training. Such part-task devices that mimic an entire procedure are referred to as *procedural trainers*.

Full simulators mimic an entire process or system. Sophisticated computerized mannequins capable of producing true-to-life physiological responses and mimicking heartbeats, pulses, and breathing are the most well-known example. These total simulators can be used in so-called *immersive simulation*, SBT environments designed to immerse the learner(s) in a realistic simulation experience mimicking real life to such a degree that suspension of disbelief (i.e., high psychological fidelity) is achieved. Such immersive SBT can take place within a specialized simulation center or in the actual clinical environment itself. In this setting, high equipment and environment fidelity is naturally achieved, since the actual clinical space is involved. When conducted in the actual clinical space, the simulation experience is referred to as *in situ*, *point of care*, or *situated training*.

Hybrid simulation involves the combination of one or more types of simulators or forms of simulation in a SBT experience. For example, a part-task model could be combined with an actor to allow for a more comprehensive training experience.[16] Alternatively, a part-task model could be used in conjunction with a computerized mannequin to expand the capabilities of the training experience. Hybrid training is increasing in popularity.

Certain physical characteristics of simulators can serve as useful classifiers. *Organic simulators* originate from living organisms. Examples include cadavers or live animals. *Animate simulators* consist of living animal models (e.g., a porcine model for learning how to conduct a laparoscopic fundoplication), whereas *inanimate simulators* are lifeless. *Computer-based*

Table 1.1 Models of Simulation Fidelity

DIMENSION OF FIDELITY	REHMANN ET AL.[13]	DIECKMANN ET AL.[14]	RUDOLPH ET AL.[15]
Real-life look	Equipment fidelity	Physical fidelity	Physical fidelity
Real-life action	Environment fidelity	Semantical fidelity	Conceptual fidelity
Real-life feel	Psychological fidelity	Phenomenal fidelity	Emotional fidelity

simulators rely on software applications for function. Among this category, *virtual reality simulators* use sophisticated programming to create a virtual representation of a procedure, person, or situation. *Mannequin-based simulators* use mannequins, in one form or another, to simulate a patient. Such physical classifications, when used in describing a simulator, assist in quickly conveying operational and constitutional aspects of its use. For example, describing a simulator as a computer-based mannequin conveys the fact that it could be used for immersive simulation. On the other hand, an inanimate box trainer is more suited for skill training.

One final format of simulation that has had a long history of use in medicine is the *standardized patient* (SP). First introduced in 1964 at the University of Southern California,[17] SPs have been used extensively in medical education. Defined as "a normal person who has been carefully coached to accurately portray the characteristics of a specific patient," an SP is able to present learners with a consistent set of symptoms, signs, or issues, thus allowing for standardization of teaching and assessment.[18] They have been demonstrated to impact positively the acquisition of knowledge, skills, and attitudes, but evidence showing that they can cause actual behavioral change in learners is still sparse.[18] As mentioned above, SPs are now being employed in combination with part-task trainers to create hybrid teaching[16] and assessment[19] simulation experiences for learners.

USES AND APPLICATIONS OF SIMULATION IN HEALTH CARE

Simulation has many uses in health care, each of which has several potential applications (Table 1.2).[20–32] They range from simple basic skills training[20,21,33,34] to complex computer simulations looking at the implications of national health care policy.[32] An understanding of this diversity of applications of simulation in medicine will help inform an individual's decisions regarding the best manner in which to integrate simulation into the work and educational environment. Five key uses of simulation in particular are worth mentioning: SBT for technical skills acquisition, SBT for cognitive skills enhancement, SBT for team-based training, simulation as a tool for error proofing, and simulation as an instrument for modeling.

One of the most high-profile uses of simulation in health care today is as a means to promote and accelerate technical skills acquisition outside of the actual clinical environment. Applications are manifold and include SBT in basic skills, bedside tasks, and procedures. The field of surgery has been a leader in this domain of simulation, having developed a comprehensive national technical skills curriculum sponsored by the Association of Program Directors in Surgery (APDS) and the American College of Surgeons (ACS).[35] Additionally, the technical skills component of the Fundamentals of Laparoscopic

Table 1.2 Uses and Applications of Simulation in Health Care

USE	POTENTIAL APPLICATIONS	REPRESENTATIVE EXAMPLE(S)
Technical skills training	Basic skills acquisition	Fundamentals of laparoscopic surgery (FLS)[20,21]
	Task training	Endotracheal intubation[22]
	Procedural training	Carotid stent placement[23]
Cognitive training	Diagnostic reasoning	Computerized virtual patients[24]
	Algorithm training	Advanced Cardiac Life Support (ACLS)[25]
Team training	Crew-based training	Anesthesia Crew Resource Management (ACRM)[26]
	Interprofessional training	In situ operating room team training[27]
Error proofing	New worker/work environment testing	Orientation of code teams to new facility[28]
	Identification of latent conditions	Latent condition identification in new facility[29]
Modeling	Work flow analysis	Surgical flow modeling[30]
	Cost-effectiveness analysis	Interventions to enhance mammography use[31]
	Health care policy analysis	Health care policy modeling[32]

Surgery (FLS) certification program arose from the development and validation of a basic laparoscopic skills training curriculum originating at McGill University in Montreal.[36–38] Currently, proficiency-based curricula exist for SBT in several skills, tasks, and procedures in surgery, including both open[33,34] and laparoscopic[20,21] basic skills, as well as central line placement[39] and virtual reality cholecystectomy.[40] Such curricula can serve as a model for developing effective SBT strategies in disciplines just beginning to integrate simulation into training and education.

Cognitive skill enhancement is another key use of simulation in health care. One important application of such simulation is in the domain of diagnostic reasoning. Often, such SBT is conducted using computer-based scenarios, although evidence of their effectiveness in transferring cognitive skill to actual clinical practice has been mixed.[41,42] Another application is in teaching essential algorithms, such as in Advanced Cardiac Life Support (ACLS).[25] Simulation-based training in this setting provides a safe environment for learning algorithms with application in the clinical setting.

In addition to technical skills acquisition and cognitive skill enhancement, simulation is also being increasingly used for team training of health professionals. First developed in anesthesia by Gaba and colleagues,[43,44] team-based training has expanded to include other dynamic, high-risk fields of medicine, including emergency medicine,[45] surgery,[27,46] and obstetrics/gynecology.[47] It typically focuses on teaching key team-based competencies known to improve the effectiveness and reliability of a team. An example of content taught during such SBT includes Salas et al's[48] Big Five competencies (i.e., team leadership, mutual performance monitoring, backup behavior, adaptability, and team orientation) and their three coordinating mechanisms (i.e., shared mental model, mutual trust, and open communication). Simulation-based training of such team-based competencies is often immersive in character, involving high-fidelity mannequins and environments. It can involve only members from one discipline (i.e., *crew-based* training) or a complete interprofessional team (i.e., true *team-based* training). Chapter 12 (Interprofessional Team-Based Training) offers a more comprehensive review of team-based training.

In addition to training, simulation in health care can also be used for other purposes. Error proofing is an example. Also known as *poka-yoke*, it involves creating fail-safe mechanisms within a system in order to prevent mistakes from occurring.[49] One application is in testing a facility for hidden or *latent conditions* that, if unrecognized, could lead to catastrophic sentinel events (e.g., performing the wrong procedure on a patient).[29] If identified before a sentinel event, however, such conditions can then be corrected through interventions, thereby mitigating or removing the possible threat. Another poka-yoke application with simulation is testing new facilities (e.g., a new hospital wing or outpatient surgery center) or health care teams (e.g., residents starting on code blue teams) to ensure familiarity with an environment and to identify unanticipated latent conditions.[28]

Finally, simulation can be used in computer modeling in health care. Applications include the creation of models for work flow analysis,[30] cost-effectiveness analysis,[31] and determining the consequences of health policy decisions.[32] Such simulation modeling provides the opportunity to evaluate complex interactions and interrelations in an attempt to improve patient care, cost, and/or safety. Its use will likely grow in popularity with increasing computing power and pressures to streamline costs and efficiency within the industry.

Many of the above-mentioned uses and applications of simulation in health care can be applied to simulation in radiology and, in fact, are addressed in this book. For example, using simulation to teach knot tying, a basic technical skill, is discussed in chapter 10 (Basic Skills: Knot-Tying). Management of contrast reactions via high-fidelity simulation—a team-based topic—is covered in chapter 13 (Team Training and Crisis Management: Contrast Reaction Management). The use of SBT to teach and evaluate cognitive skills in nuclear medicine is reviewed in chapter 26 (Simulation in Nuclear Medicine Education). Such examples, along with others in the chapters to follow, give a sample of the wide range of applications of simulation in the field of radiology.

THE ROLE OF SIMULATION IN TRAINING AND EVALUATION

As demonstrated in the previous section, simulation can play a crucial role in the education, training, and evaluation of health care students and professionals (e.g., technical skills acquisition, cognitive skills enhancement, team-based training). It cannot, however, be implemented in a vacuum. To achieve its maximal impact, it must be embedded in a well-constructed curricular structure founded on sound educational principles and theories. Without this educational framework, its usefulness is lost. The same logic is true regarding its use as an evaluative tool. Without sound and rigorous validity and reliability testing, worthwhile formative and summative feedback and evaluation based on simulation-based assessment instruments and their metrics are difficult, if not impossible. Thus, simply using simulation in itself does not equate to having formed a curriculum or developed an evaluation instrument. Simulation is merely a tool, a "technique,"[4] in the armamentarium of the educator to enhance curricula and evaluative methods. Chapter 5 (Educational Principles in Simulation) and chapter 6 (Assessment in Simulation) provide excellent reviews of educational and assessment principles needed to integrate successfully simulation into training and evaluation. Additionally, chapter 7 (Building and Incorporating Simulation into a Radiology Residency Program Curriculum) provides a framework for how these principles can be applied to simulation in radiology. Several important concepts deserve mention here: the principles and theories related to skills acquisition and the development of expertise, the characteristics of effective high-fidelity SBT, and useful approaches for the development of metrics and instruments in SBT.

ADULT LEARNING, SKILLS ACQUISITION, AND EXPERTISE

Whenever it is applied in health care, simulation-based education must be founded on principles of adult learning, also known as *andragogy*. First described by Malcolm Knowles in his seminal work, *The Adult Learner*,[50] andragogy is based on the belief that adults learn in a fundamentally different way than children do because of the manner in which they approach gaining new knowledge. For Knowles, adult learners are motivated to solve problems, want to control their learning experience, and seek to apply immediately any new knowledge or skills they acquire. In addition, they like to collaborate with others, as well as engage in self-appraisal of their performance. As a result, educational programs targeting adults should attempt to tailor themselves to accommodate these traits for maximal learning.

In addition to Knowles' theory of adult learning, two other concepts related to learning are important to know when applying simulation in health care. The first is Ericsson's *Theory of Expertise*.[51,52] It is founded on the premise that expertise in competitive professional domains such as music, chess, and sports is attained through a process known as *deliberate practice*. This form of practice is characterized by several specific features. First, it involves focused, repeated practice of specific skills or tasks targeted for improvement by a coach or teacher. Second, it must entail immediate, detailed feedback on performances. Finally, such practice must allow ample opportunity to perform the drill or task selected for improvement. By incorporating deliberate practice into their regimen, learners are able to push their limits, helping to gain expertise after approximately 10,000 hours.

The second concept is the Fitts-Posner *Three-Stage Theory of Motor Acquisition*.[53,54] Developed in the late 1960s, this theory posited three distinct stages of development in the acquisition of a motor skill: *cognition*, *integration*, and *automation*. In cognition, the learner attempts to understand the skill at hand, requires explanation and demonstration of the skill to be learned, and can only perform it in distinct, often erratic steps. In integration of the skill, the learner starts to comprehend the skill and focuses on its mechanics. He or she begins to engage in deliberate practice of the skill with feedback and is able to perform it in a more fluid, less erratic manner. With automation, the learner focuses on skill precision and speed. The skill is now automated, and practice focuses on refinement. In addition, the skill can now be performed fluidly, with any necessary adaptive maneuvers.

Taken together, Ericsson's Theory of Expertise and the Fitts-Posner Three-Stage Theory of Motor Acquisition reveal important points related to simulation-based educational endeavors for skill acquisition. First, training should be focused, deliberate, and repeated. Second, it should aim for integration/automation of skill and must include timely feedback on performance. The recent development of proficiency-driven, simulation-based technical skills curricula in surgery, designed to give learners exposure to drills over several discrete time periods (i.e., *distributed training*) rather than in one prolonged setting (i.e., *massed training*), reflects incorporation of these concepts into simulation-based education in health care.[20,21,33,34,39,40,55]

CHARACTERISTICS OF EFFECTIVE SIMULATION

In 2005, Issenberg et al[8] published a Best Evidence in Medical Education (BEME) systematic review outlining ten key features for effective learning using high-fidelity simulation. Providing feedback during simulation-based learning experiences, repetitive practice of skills by the learner, and integration of simulation into the overall curriculum were all identified as important features. Additionally, increasing levels of practice difficulty for the learner, adaptation of the simulator for multiple learning strategies, and the provision of a variety of clinical cases by the simulator were also noted to be crucial. Furthermore, the use of a controlled environment, clearly defined benchmarks and objectives, and individualized learning were found to be essential. Finally, ensuring that the simulator was a valid learning tool was deemed key. Adhering to these ten items will help in the development of an effective high-fidelity simulation-based educational program.

In their review, Issenberg et al noted that providing feedback was the most often cited feature for effective learning in high-fidelity medical simulation.[8] Often, in such a setting, it manifests itself as a debriefing following the simulation experience. If the simulation provides the psychological fidelity needed to draw the learner into the educational experience, the debriefing is the catalyst for learning. In it, the learning objectives are reviewed and instilled in the learner. Rudolph et al[56] have described three distinct phases of the debriefing process. The *reactions phase* is characterized by a discussion of the initial emotional reactions of the learners to the simulation-based experience. In the ensuing *analysis phase,* an investigation (i.e., analysis) of the experience occurs, with identification of performance gaps. The debriefing then finishes in the *summary phase,* in which a distillation of the lessons learned during the experience occurs.

Fernandez et al[57] have pointed out that a key aspect to any debriefing is that the facilitator keeps the focus on "what is right" over "who is right." Although a facilitator should aim to be only a resource for the participants involved in the debriefing, he or she may have to serve more as their guide or director.[58] For any debriefing, a facilitator has three main duties regarding learning: making it safe, making it stick, and making it last. These duties correspond to key concepts related to ensuring an effective debriefing experience (Table 1.3).[56–60] Finally, many debriefing techniques exist for ensuring effective learning (e.g., +/Δ[58] or advocacy and inquiry[56]), thus providing the facilitator with a variety of strategies.

METRICS AND INSTRUMENT DEVELOPMENT

As in other fields, a measurement made during a SBT experience is only as good as the metric chosen and the instrument utilized. For example, as Gallagher et al[55] point out, the use of time as a metric to measure the ability to tie a laparoscopic knot is rather crude, since it cannot provide any insight into the quality of the knot created (e.g., how secure, how strong). Hence, care must be taken in choosing what is to be measured and even how it is to be measured.

Once an appropriate metric is chosen, further care must be taken in developing the instrument used to measure it. Such development must be focused, methodical, and scientific. Before any instrument can be employed in any useful manner for either formative or summative feedback, its validity, as well as its reliability, needs to be well established. As mentioned above, chapter 6 (Assessment in Simulation) addresses both concepts thoroughly. Two brief points should be mentioned here. First, validation of any tool is an ongoing process wherein its ability to measure what it purports to measure is demonstrated in various situations (e.g., training in a simulation center versus training in situ) among different learners (e.g., medical students, residents, practicing physicians). Through such cumulative evidence, confidence in the instrument's ability to measure what it claims to measure is gained. In addition, validity has many facets, making the nomenclature surrounding it confusing, especially since concepts related to it have evolved over time.[61]

Table 1.3 Key Concepts Related to Effective Debriefing and Corresponding Facilitator Duties

DEBRIEFING CONCEPT	FACILITATOR DUTY
Create a safe learning environment[56,57,58]	Make it safe
Encourage reflective practice[56,57,60]	Make it stick
Elicit commitment to change[56,59]	Make it last

Second, for an instrument to be worthwhile, it must be reliable, as well as valid. For example, if two different raters cannot consistently give similar scores for the same performance in a repeatable fashion, then the instrument cannot be effectively used for evaluative purposes. Hence, in each circumstance that a tool is employed, its validity and reliability should be adequately demonstrated.

MEASURING THE IMPACT OF SIMULATION-BASED TRAINING

As mentioned above, SBT can be used to help teach a variety of skills (e.g., technical, cognitive, team-based) in health care. Measuring the effectiveness (i.e., the impact) of such training in a standardized, systematic fashion is a critical part of curricular evaluation and crucial in improving and refining any program. Kirkpatrick's Four Levels[62] and MacGaghie's Translational Phases[63] are two such models for measuring training effectiveness (Table 1.4). Each rates the effectiveness of a particular training program based on its escalating impact from the learner level to clinical outcomes.

In Kirkpatrick's model, four levels of training effectiveness are noted. Level 1 is devoted to measuring the reaction of the learner to the training activity (i.e., whether the learner liked the experience). Level 2 focuses on measuring evidence of learning (i.e., the acquisition of new knowledge, skills, and/or attitudes by learners). Level 3 measures actual behavioral change (i.e., translation of learning to the clinical environment), and Level 4 captures improvement in outcomes (i.e., better patient results). The Translational Phases theory has three categories of training effectiveness. The T1 phase measures improvements observed in the educational setting (i.e., at the site of training). The T2 phase captures improvements in patient care practices (i.e., behavioral changes), and the T3 phase measures improvements in patient and public health outcomes. Using either system, an educator can evaluate the effectiveness of a training intervention, thus allowing for refinement and improvement of curricula.

Needless to say, Level 4/T3 phase evidence of training effectiveness is the ultimate goal of any SBT intervention. Currently, evidence in the literature supporting such an impact is sparse. Noteworthy examples, however, do exist. Barsuk et al[64] have demonstrated decreases in central line infection rates in the intensive care unit after implementing an SBT protocol. Draycott et al[65,66] have improved brachial plexus injury rates from shoulder dystocia, as well as hypoxic-ischemic encephalopathy rates in neonates through SBT. Finally, Rogers et al[67] decreased complication rates in cataract surgery with a structured SBT curriculum for residents. Level 3/T2 phase evidence is more frequently reported compared to Level 4/T3 phase evidence, but it is still relatively uncommon. A few examples are worth mentioning. Korndorffer et al[68] demonstrated that proficiency-based training in laparoscopic suturing improved operative performance. Seymour et al[69] were one of the first groups to show a translation of laparoscopic skills learned during virtual reality training to actual performance in the operating room. Sroka et al[70] has recently shown that FLS training improves operative performance in cholecystectomy. Finally, Wayne et al[71] demonstrated that real-time clinical compliance to ACLS protocols was greater after SBT. Clearly, SBT does have a positive impact on learners that translates to both improved patient care and outcomes. Educators should continue to strive to show evidence of such Level 4/T3 phase improvements to strengthen SBT incorporation into curricula.

Table 1.4 Measuring Simulation-Based Training Effectiveness

KIRKPATRICK LEVELS[62]	MEASUREMENT	TRANSLATIONAL PHASES[63]	MEASUREMENT
1	Reaction (positive response)	1	Change in educational laboratory
2	Learning (change in knowledge, skills, attitudes)		
3	Performance (behavioral change)	2	Improved patient care practices
4	Impact (improved outcomes)	3	Improved patient and public health

IMPLEMENTATION

To a novice, implementation of SBT into an educational program might seem a daunting task. It is more feasible when a systematic approach is used. The author has developed such an approach for in situ high-fidelity team training.[72] Its use, however, is possible for other SBT endeavors. The approach groups potential challenges to implementation into five major categories, known as the "5Ps": finding a *patron,* developing a *plan,* locating a *place,* assembling the appropriate *people,* and choosing the right *products.*[72] Each category can then be approached from a strategic (i.e., planning) and/or tactical (i.e., operational) standpoint to help with successful implementation. For example, strategic aspects of finding a patron would involve identifying and getting the support of a well-placed person or persons to assist in funding, protected time, and institutional support for the SBT endeavor. Strategic aspects of developing a plan would involve creating a curriculum for the SBT founded on sound educational principles. Tactical aspects of finding a place would include locating an actual spot for training. Tactical aspects of assembling the appropriate people would include identifying the learners for the training activity. In this systematic manner, an SBT activity or program can be implemented with relatively little headache, since key planning and logistical issues are addressed.

The 5P approach to implementation is one of many ways to integrate simulation into educational curricula in a systematic manner. Chapter 7 (Building and Incorporating Simulation into a Radiology Residency Program Curriculum) and chapter 8 (Development and Operation of a Simulation Laboratory at a Major Medical Center) provide excellent overviews of other approaches to this challenge. No matter which one is chosen, success is often based on a methodical attention to detail and planning.

CONCLUSION

Simulation is a powerful tool with a variety of applications in medical education and training. It cannot, however, be implemented in a vacuum. For maximal benefit, it must be integrated into a curriculum based on sound educational principles and utilizing assessment instruments that are both valid and reliable. In addition, its effectiveness should be measured using an established model such as Kirkpatrick's Four Levels or MacGaghie's Transitional Phases. When employed in this manner, simulation has the potential of positively impacting patient care, attaining Level 4/T3 evidence. Finally, although implementation may at first seem a challenge, using a systematic approach to it will help.

This chapter has served as an introduction to key concepts related to the use of simulation in health care. In the pages that follow, these concepts will be applied, in order to demonstrate the potential and promise of integrating simulation into radiology. Enjoy!

REFERENCES

1. Online Etymology Dictionary. Accessed June 29, 2011, at http://www.etymonline.com/index.php?search=simulation&searchmode=none

2. Free Merriam-Webster Dictionary. Accessed June 29, 2011, at http://www.merriam-webster.com/dictionary/simulation

3. McGaghie WC. Simulation in professional competence assessment: basic considerations. In: Tekian A, McGuire CH, McGaghie WC, eds. *Innovative Simulations for Assessing Professional Competence.* Chicago: Department of Medical Education, University of Illinois at Chicago; 1999:7–22.

4. Gaba DM. The future vision of simulation in health care. *Qual Saf Health Care.* 2004;13:i2-i10.

5. Okuda Y, Bryson EO, Demaria S Jr, et al. The utility of simulation in medical education: what is the evidence? *Mt Sinai J Med.* 2009;76:330–343.

6. Andreatta PB, Bullough AS, Marzano D. Simulation and team training. *Clin Obstet Gynecol.* 2010;53:532–544.

7. McGaghie WC, Issenberg SB, Petrusa ER, et al. A critical review of simulation-based medical education research: 2003–2009. *Med Educ.* 2010;44:50–63.

8. Issenberg SB, McGaghie WC, Petrusa ER, et al. Features and uses of high-fidelity medical simulations that lead to effective learning: a BEME systematic review. *Med Teach.* 2005;27:10–28.

9. Beaubien JM, Baker DP. The use of simulation for training teamwork skills in health care: how low can you go? *Qual Saf Health Care.* 2004;13:i51–i56.

10. Lampotang S. Medium and high integration mannequin patient simulators. In: Riley RH ed. *Manual of Simulation in Healthcare.* Oxford, UK. Oxford University Press; 2008:51–64.

11. Clark EAS, Fisher J, Arafeh J, et al. Team training/simulation. *Clin Obstet Gynecol.* 2010;53:265–277.

12. Meller, G. A typology of simulators for medical education. *J Digit Imaging.* 1997;10:i194–i196.

13. Rehmann A, Mitman R, Reynolds M. *A Handbook of Flight Simulation Fidelity Requirements for Human Factors Research*. Technical Report No. DOT/FAA/CT-TN95/46. Wright-Patterson AFB, OH: Crew Systems Ergonomics Information Analysis Center; 1995.

14. Dieckmann P, Gaba D, Rall M. Deepening the theoretical foundations of patient simulation as social practice. *Simul Healthc.* 2007;2:183–193.

15. Rudolph JW, Simon R, Raemer DB. Which reality matters? Questions on the path to high engagement in healthcare simulation. *Simul Healthc.* 2007;2:161–163.

16. Moulton CA, Tabak D, Kneebone R, et al. Teaching communication skills using the integrated procedural performance instrument (IPPI): a randomized control trial. *Am J Surg.* 2009;197: 113–118.

17. Barrows HS, Abrahamson S. The programmed patient: a technique for appraising student performance in clinical neurology. *J Med Educ.* 1964;39:802–805.

18. May W, Park JH, Lee JP. A ten-year review of the literature on the use of standardized patients in teaching and learning: 1996-2005. *Med Teach.* 2009;31:487–492.

19. Boulet JR. Summative assessment in medicine: the promise of simulation for high-stakes evaluation. *Acad Emerg Med.* 2008;15:1017–1024.

20. Ritter EM and Scott DJ. Design of a proficiency-based skills training curriculum for the fundamentals of laparoscopic surgery. *Surg Innov.* 2007;14:107–112.

21. Scott DJ, Ritter EM, Tesfay ST, et al. Certification pass rate of 100% for fundamentals of laparoscopic surgery skills after proficiency-based training. *Surg Endosc.* 2008;22:1887–1893.

22. Sprick C, Owen H, Hein C, et al. A new part task trainer for teaching and learning confirmation of endotracheal intubation. *Stud Health Technol Inform.* 2011;163:611–615.

23. Berry M, Reznik R, Lystig T, et al. The use of virtual reality training in carotid artery stenting: a construct validation study. *Acta Radiol.* 2008;49: 801-805.

24. Cook DA, Erwin PJ, Triola MM. Computerized virtual patients health professions education: a systematic review and meta-analysis. *Acad Med.* 2010;85:1589–1602.

25. Wayne DB, Siddall VJ, Fudala MJ, et al. Simulation-based training of internal medicine residents in advanced cardiac life support protocols: a randomized trial. *Teach Learn Med.* 2005;17:210–216.

26. Gaba DM, Howard SK, Fish KJ, et al. Simulation-based training in anesthesia crisis resource management (ACRM): a decade of experience. *Simul Gaming.* 2001;32:175–193.

27. Paige JT, Kozmenko V, Yang T, et al. High-fidelity, simulation-based, interdisciplinary operating room team training at the point of care. *Surgery.* 2009;145:138–146.

28. Villamaria FJ, Pliego JF, Wehbe-Janek H, et al. Using simulation to orient code blue teams to a new hospital facility. *Simul Healthc.* 2008;3:209–216.

29. Geis GL, Pio B, Pendergrass TL, et al. Simulation to assess the safety of new healthcare teams and new facilities. *Simul Healthc.* 2011;6:125–133.

30. Sobolev BG, Sanchez V, Vasilakis C. Systematic review of the use of computer simulation modeling of patient flow in surgical care. *J Med Syst.* 2011;35:1–16.

31. Wu JH, Fung MC, Chan W, et al. Cost-effectiveness analysis of interventions to enhance mammography compliance using computer modeling (CAN*TROL). *Value Health.* 2004;7:175–185.

32. Glied S, Tilipman N. Simulation modeling of health care policy. *Annu Rev Public Health.* 2010;31:439–455.

33. Scott DJ, Goova MT, Tesfay ST. A cost-effective proficiency-based knot-tying and suturing curriculum for residency programs. *J Surg Res.* 2007;141:7–15.

34. Goova MT, Hollett LA, Tesfay ST, et al. Implementation, construct validity, and benefit of a proficiency-based knot-tying and suturing curriculum. *J Surg Educ.* 2008;56:309–315.

35. Scott DJ, Dunnington DL. The new ACS/APDS Curriculum: moving the learning curve out of the operating room. *J Gastrointest Surg.* 2008;12:213–221.

36. Derossis AM, Fried GM, Abrahamowicz M, et al. Development of a model for training and evaluation of laparoscopic skills. *Am J Surg.* 1998;175:482–487.

37. Fraser SA, Klassen DR, Feldman LS, et al. Evaluating laparoscopic skills: setting the pass/fail for MISTELS system. *Surg Endosc.* 2003;17:964–967.

38. Swanstrom LL, Fried GM, Hoffman KI, et al. Beta test results of a new system assessing competence in laparoscopic surgery. *J Am Coll Surg.* 2006;202:62–69.

39. Barsuk JH, McGaghie WC, Cohen ER, et al. Use of simulation-based mastery learning to improve the quality of central venous catheter placement in a medical intensive care unit. *J Hosp Med.* 2009;4:397–403.

40. Aggarwal R, Ward J, Balasundaram I, et al. Proving the effectiveness of virtual reality simulation for training in laparoscopic surgery. *Ann Surg.* 2007;246:771–779.

41. Jerant AF, Azari R. Validity of scores generated by a web-based multimedia simulated patient case software: a pilot study. *Acad Med.* 2004;79:805–811.

42. Shokar GS, Burdine RL, Callaway M, et al. Relating student performance on a family medicine clerkship with completion of web cases. *Fam Med.* 2005;37:620–622.

43. Gaba DM, DeAnda A. A comprehensive anesthesia simulation environment: re-creating the operating room for research and training. *Anesthesiology.* 1988;69:387–394.

44. Howard SK, Gaba DM, Fish KJ, et al. Anesthesia crisis resource management training: teaching anesthesiologists to handle critical incidents. *Aviat Space Environ Med.* 1992;63:763–770.

45. Reznek M, Smith-Coggins R, Howard S, et al. Emergency Medicine Crisis Resource Management (EMCRM): pilot study of a simulation-based crisis management course for emergency medicine. *Acad Emerg Med.* 2003;10:386–389.

46. Moorthy K, Munz Y, Adams S, et al. A human factors analysis of technical and team skills among surgical trainees during procedural simulations in a simulated operating theatre. *Ann Surg.* 2005;242: 631–639.

47. Merién AER, van de Ven J, Mol BW, et al. Multidisciplinary team training in a simulation setting for acute obstetric emergencies: a systematic review. *Obstet Gynecol.* 2010;115:1021–1031.

48. Salas E, Sims DE, Burke CS. Is there a big five in teamwork? *Small Group Res.* 2005;36:555–599.

49. MoreStream.com. Error-proofing (poka-yoke). Accessed July 8, 2011, at http://www.moresteam.com/toolbox/t412.cfm

50. Knowles MS, Holton III EF, Swanson RA. *The Adult Learner,* 5th edition. Woburn, MA: Butterworth-Heinemann; 1998.

51. Ericsson KA. Deliberate practice and the acquisition and maintenance of expert performance in medicine and related domains. *Acad Med.* 2004;79(Suppl 10):S70–S81.

52. Crochet P, Aggarwal R, Dubb SS, et al. Deliberate practice on a virtual reality laparoscopic simulator enhances the quality of surgical technical skills. *Ann Surg.* 2011;253:1216–1222.

53. Fitts PM, Posner MI. *Human Performance.* Belmont, CA: Brooks/Cole; 1967.

54. Reznick RK, MacRae H. Teaching surgical skills—changes in the wind. *N Engl J Med.* 2006;335:2664–2669.

55. Gallagher AG, Ritter EM, Champion H, et al. Virtual reality simulation for the operating room: proficiency-based training as a paradigm shift in surgical skills training. *Ann Surg.* 2005;241:364–372.

56. Rudolph JW, Simon R, Raemer DB, et al. Debriefing as formative assessment: closing performance gaps in medical education. *Acad Emerg Med.* 2008;15:1010–1016.

57. Fernandez R, Vozenilek JA, Hegarty CB, et al. Developing expert medical teams: toward an evidence-based approach. *Acad Emerg Med.* 2008;15:1025–1036.

58. Fanning RM, Gaba DM. The role of debriefing in simulation-based learning. *Simul Healthc.* 2007;2:115–125.

59. Gururaja RP, Yang T, Paige JT, et al. Examining the effectiveness of debriefing at the point of care in simulation-based operating room team training. In: Henriksen K, Battles JB, Keyes MA, Grady ML, eds. *Advances in Patient Safety: New Directions and Alternative Approaches* (Vol. 3: Performance and Tools). Rockville, MD: Agency for Healthcare Research and Quality; 2008. Accessed December 24, 2011, at http://www.ncbi.nlm.nih.gov/books/NBK43676/pdf/

60. Dreifuerst KT. The essentials of debriefing in simulation learning: a concept analysis. *Nurs Educ Perspect.* 2009;30:109–114.

61. Korndorffer JR Jr, Kasten SJ, Downing SM. A call for utilization of consensus standards in the surgical education literature. *Am J Surg.* 2010;199: 99–104.

62. Kirkpatrick DI. *Evaluating Training Programs: The Four Levels,* 2nd edition. San Francisco, CA: Berrett-Koehler; 1998.

63. MacGaghie WC, Draycott TJ, Dunn WF, et al. Evaluating the impact of simulation on translational patient outcomes. *Simul Healthc.* June 23, 2011. [Epub ahead of print.]

64. Barsuk JH, Cohen ER, Feinglass J, et al. Use of simulation-based education to reduce catheter-related bloodstream infections. *Arch Intern Med.* 2009;169:1420–1423.

65. Draycott TJ, Crofts JF, Ash JP, et al. Improving neonatal outcome through practical shoulder dystocia training. *Obstet Gynecol.* 2008;112:14–20.

66. Draycott TJ, Sibanda T, Owen L, et al. Does training in obstetric emergencies improve neonatal outcome? *BJOG.* 2006;113:177–182.

67. Rogers GM, Oetting TA, Lee AG, et al. Impact of a structured surgical curriculum on ophthalmic resident cataract surgery complication rates. *J Cataract Refract Surg.* 2009;35:1956–1960.

68. Korndorffer JR, Dunne JB, Sierra R, et al. Simulator training for laparoscopic suturing using performance goals translates to the operating room. *J Am Coll Surg.* 2005;201:23–29.

69. Seymour NE, Gallagher AG, Roman SA, et al. Virtual reality training improves operating room performance: results of a randomized, double-blinded study. *Ann Surg.* 2002;236:458–464.

70. Sroka G, Feldman LS, Vassiliou MC, et al. Fundamentals of laparoscopic surgery simulator

training to proficiency improves laparoscopic performance in the operating room—a randomized controlled trial. *Am J Surg*. 2010;199:115–120.

71. Wayne DB, Didwania A, Feinglass J, et al. Simulation-based education improves quality of care during cardiac arrest team responses at an academic teaching hospital: a case control study. *Chest.* 2008;133:56–61.

72. Paige JT, Team training at the point of care. In: Tsuda S, Scott DJ, Jones DB, eds. *Textbook of Simulation, Surgical Skills, and Team Training.* Woodbury, CT: Cine-Med, Inc; in press.

2

Ethics and Regulations of Cadaver Use in Simulation

RICHARD H. WHITWORTH, JR. AND WILLIAM J. SWARTZ

FRESH, UNEMBALMED cadavers have been used for many years to simulate the performance of various clinical procedures that are routinely done on living patients in the operating room or physicians' offices. Current trends emphasize the use of highly sophisticated computerized mannequins as the basis for advanced simulation-based training (SBT). Nothing developed and employed to date, however, will ever replace the fresh, unembalmed cadaver as the ideal anatomic model for SBT of invasive clinical procedures.

The use of unembalmed cadavers has distinct advantages over the use of commercially manufactured high-fidelity, part-task, or virtual reality simulators. The high-fidelity computerized mannequins have been able to mimic some normal human physiologic responses and are, in many instances, able to accurately represent human anatomy. At present, however, these mannequins are not designed to exhibit the individual variations in normal anatomy found in fresh, unembalmed cadavers. Mannequins and part-task trainers also cannot accurately simulate the distinctive feel and tactile feedback provided by actual human tissues.

SIMULATION-BASED TRAINING USING CADAVERS

Surgeons perform surgical approaches on cadavers to test new techniques or instrumentation, often with the participation and support of medical equipment companies and/or physician organizations. Using cadavers, surgeons can perform and practice operations outside of the operating room, thus assisting them in remaining current with the latest innovations and methods in their areas of expertise. Such methods are not limited to surgical procedures. Paramedical and Emergency Medical Services personnel benefit from being able to practice life-saving emergency techniques on fresh, unembalmed cadaver specimens, thus providing a high degree of anatomic realism to their training programs. In addition, other health care professionals, such as student and practicing nurses and physician assistants, benefit markedly by utilizing unembalmed cadavers in their training programs. The patient probably benefits most from health care professionals receiving procedural SBT using anatomically accurate, fresh, unembalmed cadavers.

Cahill and Freeland[1] proposed a series of standards that can serve as guidelines to the utilization and study of unembalmed human cadaver specimens. These standards address "procurement and screening, processing, transportation, record keeping, the concept of borrowing, and final disposition" of unembalmed human cadaver specimens. These same basic standards govern the use of unembalmed cadaver specimens today.

PROCUREMENT OF CADAVERIC MATERIAL

All unembalmed cadaveric specimens *must* be obtained from reputable body donor programs that have procured their specimens in accordance with all applicable federal, state, and local regulations. Although the Uniform Anatomical Gift Act (UAGA) was enacted primarily with reference to donation of organs for transplantation, many of its components also apply to whole-body donations for medical education or medical research purposes. The original UAGA, promulgated in 1968, was adopted by all 50 U.S. states.[2] It established the right of a donor to bequeath his or her body to medical science for education. Anatomical gifts can be made for the purposes of transplantation, therapy, research, or education.

The first revision intended to update the UAGA took place in1987, but it was adopted by only 26 states. Subsequent amendments by individual state governments eliminated the uniformity of state and federal laws that was one of the goals of updating the federal UAGA. In 2006, the UAGA again underwent a major revision in an attempt to address some problems and to make the donation process uniform in all 50 states. The major changes and their legal implications were thoroughly reviewed by Kurtz et al.[3] Louisiana recently became a signatory by enacting Louisiana HB 1123, which became state law in 2010.

Unclaimed bodies are another potential source of unembalmed human anatomical specimens, and this is allowed by the laws of many states. Locally, we have elected not to accept or utilize unclaimed bodies because of the lack of social or medical history. Such unclaimed bodies are more likely to present problems with blood-borne pathogens.

ROLE OF STATE ANATOMICAL BOARDS

Most states normally have one or more "anatomical boards," established by state governments and frequently associated with departments of anatomy in medical schools or medical centers. Many departments of anatomy have established *willed body programs* that oversee and regulate the procurement and preparation of cadavers for medical education and research purposes. In Louisiana, the Bureau of Anatomical Services was established by the state government to oversee the procurement, distribution, and utilization of cadavers.

The American Association of Anatomists recently approved guidelines for body donation programs to regulate their accepting donation of bodies for medical education and biomedical research. These guidelines were developed as minimum requirements that should be established by any willed body program.

The guidelines for donation of bodies for medical education and biomedical research as suggested by the American Association of Anatomists denote several specific requirements to meet the minimal standards. The donation of bodies must follow all state and local laws and statutes. Institutional willed body programs may introduce more stringent requirements but should not have fewer requirements than those included in the state and local laws. It is recommended that institutions establish an institutional oversight committee that will have the responsibility of overseeing the body donation program. Such committees have the responsibility of establishing rules that clearly define the use of cadavers at the institution for educational and research needs and procedures for reviewing the utilization of cadavers on a regular basis. Strict attention must be paid to policies of the state anatomical board and institution where SBT using cadavers is to take place.

ROLE OF ADMINISTRATIVE STAFF

The institutional oversight committee, as recommended by the American Association of Anatomists, should appoint an individual to oversee and to assume the responsibility for the daily operation of the body donation program. A qualified administrative staff is essential in carrying out these duties. This individual and the support staff have the responsibility for accepting body donation requests; keeping accurate records; maintaining a database of registered donors, with all pertinent information; and tracking specimens, to include the source, current location, where and how each specimen is utilized, and its final disposition.

HANDLING OF DONATED SPECIMENS FOLLOWING DEATH

Willed body programs have established varying arrangements for the pick-up and delivery of the bodies of deceased donors to their facilities. In the case of the Louisiana Bureau of Anatomical Services, a contract has been established with a licensed funeral home for delivery of the cadaver from the place of death to our facility. The funeral home must be able to respond 24 hours per day, have adequate personnel and equipment to make multiple simultaneous pickups, and be able to deliver the body within an appropriate timeframe as soon as possible after death, in compliance with all state and local regulations. Of prime importance is the ability of funeral home personnel to communicate adequately and respectfully with the relatives of the deceased donor and to conduct all of their activities with utmost courtesy and understanding. In addition, the funeral home must be able to obtain the necessary burial transit permit and complete and file an official death certificate with the appropriate state agencies. Funeral home personnel, frequently in consultation with willed body program personnel, must be able to evaluate the acceptability of the donated body for its use in medical education or research with reference to established criteria. Bodies to be donated must be preregistered with the willed body program, must not have any prior embalming or autopsy procedures performed, and must not have any indication of infectious diseases, such as human immunodeficiency virus (HIV) or hepatitis B or C.

Upon arrival at our facility, each cadaver is immediately placed in the walk-in morgue cold box by funeral home personnel to maintain the remains in as pristine a condition as possible. The morgue facility must have strict security and be safe from unauthorized access. All activities involving the transfer or preparation of donated cadavers must be conducted free of public observation.

Upon delivery to the morgue facility, each cadaver must be logged into the receipt log, with the name of the deceased, date, and time of the delivery accurately recorded in the register, along with the name of the individual who delivered the cadaver. At the time of the entry, an accession number is assigned to the body as a means of tracking that cadaver, or specimens derived from it, up until its final disposition. This accession number must be maintained for every specimen derived from that donation. It is imperative that accurate records be kept of every donation, its utilization, and final disposition. Throughout the process, the identity of the donor must be kept confidential.

TREATMENT OF BODIES ON ARRIVAL AT SITE

Morgue personnel must attend to the cadaver as soon as possible after delivery, in order to properly process it. Experience of morgue personnel is essential. Formal training, as well as years of experience, is critical to preparing ideal cadavers or cadaver specimens for SBT procedures.

The donated bodies are initially examined by morgue personnel to determine whether they would be best used as embalmed cadavers for teaching gross anatomy courses or as unembalmed specimens for SBT, resident training, continuing medical education, or postgraduate medical education courses. This decision is based on need and other criteria, such as size and specific specimen needs. Based on the evaluation of the morgue personnel, acceptable donated cadavers are assigned for usage either as a fresh specimen or as an embalmed specimen. Those bodies that are jaundiced, or those that have been inadvertently accepted prior to confirmed documentation of positive serology for HIV or hepatitis, are immediately cremated.

PREPARATION AND HANDLING OF BODIES FOR USAGE AS FRESH UNEMBALMED SPECIMENS

For those donations selected to be used as fresh, unembalmed specimens for SBT or postgraduate education courses, several tubes of serum are harvested for subsequent serology testing. The serum samples are tested for HIV and hepatitis A, B, and C. The majority of the population routinely tests positive for hepatitis A. A positive serology test result for hepatitis A, therefore, does not preclude a body's utilization as an unembalmed cadaver. If, at any time, a serology test is returned positive for either HIV, hepatitis B, or hepatitis C, the cadaver or all specimens obtained from that cadaver are removed from the freezer and immediately cremated.

Depending on the surgical or interventional procedures selected for SBT, unembalmed cadavers are used as whole intact cadavers or as dismembered body parts to allow the greatest utilization of the donation. Donations selected to be used as intact, fresh, unembalmed specimens, as well as those consisting of body parts, are washed thoroughly and frozen below 4°C. Both cadaver formats are harvested and labeled with the appropriate accession number. The donor individuals gave their bodies after death for the betterment of mankind. Philosophically, it is our responsibility to ensure that each and every donation is utilized to its best advantage for the training of the residents, physicians, or other health care professionals for whom we are providing specimens for SBT in continuing or postgraduate education programs. To maximize the use of every donation, specimens are frequently harvested and customized to meet specific criteria to optimize them for specific specialized courses. For example, pelves with lower extremities work well for courses dealing with various surgical approaches to total hip or total knee replacement.

Specimens to be used in a simulation-based course must have negative serology tests for HIV and hepatitis B and C. Specimens must be properly thawed, cleaned, and prepared for use in specific simulation-based courses. We have found that strict control of the thawing process is of paramount importance. Simply removing the specimens from the freezer and allowing them to thaw destroys tissue integrity. Depending on the type of specimen and any special modifications that are needed, it normally requires 5–6 days to carry out the thawing procedures. The specimens are removed from the freezer and thawed at room temperature for a period of 8–10 hours, washed thoroughly several times during that time period, and then returned to the cold box overnight. This process is repeated each day for 5–6 days, until the specimens are totally thawed and meticulously cleaned. Joints should be freely movable. Tissues should have a texture as close to that of the living as possible. Some laboratories thaw specimens quickly by placing them in warm water. This process causes tissues to absorb large amounts of water, thus rendering the tissues "mushy" and inappropriate for SBT.

During a course utilizing fresh, unembalmed cadaver specimens, participants should be gloved and gowned, and should be required to follow all universal fluid barrier precautions in the event that a falsely negative serology result was reported. Universal fluid barrier precautions were established by the Centers for Disease Control (CDC) to help prevent the transmission of blood-borne pathogens such as HIV or hepatitis B.[4] These precautions include the use of gloves and gowns at a minimum, and masks and protective eyewear in any course in which there is the potential for the generation of splashed body fluids.

Unembalmed cadaver specimens should be utilized only in secure facilities specifically designed to accommodate fresh, unembalmed cadaver specimens. The facility must be constructed so that all surfaces that come into contact with the cadaver specimens or body fluids can be thoroughly disinfected. These facilities must have the capability for proper disposal of "sharps" instruments, cleaning of surgical instruments and equipment, and biohazardous waste disposal. All cadaver specimens must be properly prepared, oriented, and draped.

Upon completion of fresh cadaver courses, proper clean-up procedures must be followed. All sharps must be placed in proper containers for disposal. Any surface that was intentionally or inadvertently touched by a participant must be wiped and disinfected. The floors in the facility must be mopped and disinfected. All instrumentation must be appropriately washed and disinfected. In addition to instruments being soaked in Cidex, chlorine bleach, or a similar surgical disinfectant, they are cycled through washers/disinfectors designed for such cleaning. All contaminated gloves, gowns, surgical drapes, etc. must be disposed of in accordance with existing biohazardous waste disposal regulations. Finally, all unembalmed cadaver specimens must be cremated. Disposal of cadaveric remains should be documented, and must follow all state and local regulations and requirements.

PREPARATION AND HANDLING OF BODIES TO BE EMBALMED

If it is determined that a received donation is best utilized in an embalmed state, after the assignment of an accession number, various embalming procedures are followed. Serology tests are normally not conducted on cadavers destined to be embalmed. The embalming process, when properly employed, uses a combination of fixatives (including formaldehyde, phenol, etc.) that is believed to inactivate HIV and hepatitis viruses.

Cadavers to be embalmed are washed thoroughly and then embalmed by cannulating the internal carotid artery with one cannula oriented superiorly and another cannula pointed inferiorly. Unlike embalming that takes place in funeral homes, the blood is not drained from these cadavers during the embalming process. The embalming fluid contains specific percentages of formalin, phenol, alcohol, glycerine, thymol, and water. The cadavers are embalmed under pressure until embalming of all body parts is deemed satisfactory. Adequate embalming is determined based on appearance, palpation, and other criteria by morgue personnel. If necessary, the femoral artery may also be cannulated, and the use of a trocar inserted into body tissues can be employed to achieve complete embalming.

The embalmed cadavers are placed in large plastic bags and stored on shelves in the cold boxes until they are needed. Embalmed cadavers are ideal for long-term studies, such as training students in the basic gross anatomy of the human body. They may be used for long periods of time by multiple users, if necessary, thus maximizing the use of each and every donation. Although the exposure to infectious diseases is markedly reduced or eliminated when using embalmed cadavers, precautions should be taken during usage in order to prevent injury and excessive exposure to formaldehyde. It has been stated that "the risk of postmortem transmission of HIV is greatly decreased by delaying embalming procedures for at least 24 hours after death and waiting even longer to dissect unembalmed, refrigerated bodies."[5] This conclusion is based on a study performed by Bankowski et al,[6] in which HIV recovery from blood samples drawn at different times after death "correlated inversely with time elapsed since death." Probably the best approach is to treat all cadaveric tissue, whether embalmed or fresh and unembalmed, as though it were potentially infectious.

FRESH VERSUS EMBALMED SPECIMEN USAGE IN SIMULATION-BASED TRAINING

Fresh, unembalmed cadaveric tissues and embalmed cadavers both have advantages and disadvantages. The embalming process has the effect of long-term preservation of the body tissues for extended studies. Embalmed cadavers are probably the best for learning basic anatomy, when such training is going to require extended periods of time for the study to be completed. Embalming also reduces or eliminates the potential for exposure to infectious disease. The embalming process reduces the value of embalmed cadavers for SBT for residents and for postgraduate education simulation courses. The embalming process leaves tissues relatively stiff and rigid, joints that are immovable, and tissues that lack natural texture and color.

Fresh, unembalmed cadaveric tissues are best for SBT and for teaching surgical approaches and procedures, particularly for residents and practicing clinicians. Fresh, unembalmed cadavers have been used successfully in the training of medical students in performing procedural[7] and invasive skills.[8,9] Contrary to some reports that "freezing harms their texture,"[10] we have found that when specimens are prepared according to our thawing protocol, fresh, unembalmed cadaver tissues have a characteristic feel and texture that is as close as possible to living human tissues. This fact makes them ideal as organic simulators for practicing surgical approaches or training clinical personnel in performing surgical or interventional procedures.

Fresh, unembalmed cadaver specimens used in our postgraduate education programs are routinely tested for HIV, hepatitis A, B, and C. Although serology testing on cadaver serum samples may not be 100% reliable, it represents a best effort to ensure the safety of those program participants who use fresh cadaveric specimens. Programs that use lightly embalmed specimens[10] do not perform serology tests for blood-borne pathogens. This fact could lead to some unforeseen infectious consequences.

Fresh, unembalmed cadavers are optimal for teaching basic suturing techniques, as well as invasive procedures such as lumbar puncture, endotracheal intubation, cricothyroidotomy, thoracostomy tube placement, and Foley catheterization to junior medical students.[9] Senior medical students and residents benefit from using fresh, unembalmed cadavers to practice such procedures as central line placement, basic open and laparoscopic surgical skills, and advanced suturing techniques. Clinical faculty and residency directors utilize fresh, unembalmed cadaver specimens to give their residents valuable experience in performing surgical approaches routinely used in the operating room. For arthroscopic orthopedic training, properly prepared fresh, unembalmed cadaver joint specimens are freely movable and look essentially identical to living joint specimens. Unembalmed cadavers are ideal for training in laparoscopic abdominal or thoracic surgery, in that the internal organs maintain a life-like texture and mobility. Fresh, unembalmed cadaver specimens have been shown to be ideal for craniomaxillofacial surgical training, including plastic surgery procedures, procedures for fracture repair, and neurosurgical procedures.

Fresh, unembalmed cadavers would be the perfect model for training radiology residents in a variety of venues. Fresh cadavers could be used as an ideal platform to teach residents normal radiologic anatomy. Using actual human specimens would serve to demonstrate the normal anatomic variations seen in living patients. Unembalmed cadavers could be used to train radiology residents to identify pathology present in the cadavers. Interventional radiological procedures could be demonstrated and practiced. Radiologically guided invasive procedures could be perfected by residents in the cadaver, before they are required to perform such procedures on living patients.

The only disadvantage of fresh tissues is the relatively short time that they remain in prime condition for use after thawing and final preparation. Some laboratories have utilized "lightly embalmed" cadaver specimens, which work well in their programs.[11] The advantage of lightly embalmed specimens is that they last for a longer period of time than do fresh, unembalmed specimens, thus allowing their use by a series of small groups over a period of approximately 2 weeks. Usually, the lightly embalmed cadaver is left intact and stored in a small laboratory, allowing groups of physicians or residents from different medical specialties to utilize the cadaver for scheduled periods of time. Lightly embalmed cadavers have been reported to be "kept in a cooler for up to 6 weeks before use with negligible loss of tissue quality and color."[10] It is obvious, however, that considering the molecular nature of the embalming process, even light embalming changes the characteristics of the tissues.

DISPOSAL OF CADAVER SPECIMENS FOLLOWING COMPLETION OF COURSES

Following completion of the use of the cadavers for research, education, or SBT purposes, the cadaver specimens should be disposed of following all applicable state and federal guidelines. Under normal circumstances, both embalmed and fresh, unembalmed specimens are cremated after use. Following the cremation of a cadaver, the ashes must be recovered and returned to the family, if the family has so requested. Ashes of those for whom no request for return was received are buried in a local cemetery, in a designated area marked by a monument in their honor.

TRAFFICKING OF CADAVERS ACROSS STATE LINES

Due to the fact that some medical facilities in the country do not have an adequate supply of cadavers to support their needs, it is sometimes necessary to ship cadavers or cadaver specimens across state lines. When this is necessary, all appropriate federal, state, and local regulations must be followed. The transfer of cadavers or cadaveric specimens should be between reputable willed body programs affiliated with established medical institutions. It is also recommended that, if such transfer to another institution is anticipated, potential donors are informed before donation that their bodies may be transferred to another medical school or educational institution, if the need arises. The American Association of Anatomists also recommends that shipment of cadavers must follow all state and local requirements.

Selling of specimens to third-party brokers, who are in business for profit, is discouraged. Utilization of specimens sold to third-party brokers in a manner and location not intended by the donors has led to major litigation directed toward the selling institution. The authors strongly recommend not utilizing third-party body brokers as a source of cadaveric specimens unless no other alternative is available. Although some of these brokers have documentation indicating approval of regulatory oversight organizations, questionable practices may lead to litigation or, at a minimum, adverse publicity that could have a negative impact on institutional cadaver donation programs throughout the country. Solicited legal opinions concerning the transfer of cadavers or cadaver specimens indicate that one may not make a profit from the sale of cadaveric material but may recover the costs of providing that material for medical education and research.

COSTS

The costs of providing embalmed cadavers for regular gross anatomy courses or fresh, unembalmed cadaver specimens for continuing medical education for residents or practicing physicians vary widely throughout the United States. Major expenditures are directed toward salaries for highly qualified office and morgue personnel. Office personnel must be competent to oversee the maintenance of the body program by processing donations and keeping accurate records of the donors. Highly qualified morgue personnel are responsible for the preparation of both embalmed and fresh specimens for the different uses at student, resident, or postgraduate levels. Other costs deemed necessary include costs for the contract with the funeral home to pick up and deliver the bodies of donors to the morgue facility. This contract includes paying the funeral home's personnel and their administrative costs for filing death certificates. Budget allowances must also be made for ancillary items, such as telephone bills, postage, computer maintenance, and the like.

Everyone dealing with cadaveric specimens should be familiar with the UAGA.[12] This act does not directly address the buying or selling of cadaver tissues for medical education or research. It does address the sale of organs for transplantation purposes as follows:

> SECTION 10. SALE OR PURCHASE OF PARTS PROHIBITED.
>
> (a) A person may not knowingly, for valuable consideration, purchase or sell a part for transplantation or therapy, if removal of the part is intended to occur after the death of the decedent.
>
> (b) Valuable consideration does not include reasonable payment for the removal, processing, disposal, preservation, quality control, storage, transportation, or implantation of a part.
>
> (c) A person who violates this section is guilty of a [felony] and upon conviction is subject to a fine not exceeding [$50,000] or imprisonment not exceeding [five] years, or both.

Some state statutes (e.g., Michigan) have statements that specifically address profiting from cadaver specimens for medical education and research, whereas other states' regulations do not. Our solicited legal opinions from Louisiana state legal personnel concerning charges for cadavers or cadaver specimens indicate that one may not make a profit from the sale of cadaveric material but may recover the costs of providing that material for medical education and research.

CONCLUSION

An increasing emphasis is being placed on using simulation-based techniques to train medical students, residents, physicians, and other health care professionals. We definitely agree that manufactured simulation devices and mannequins have a place in the training of medical professionals. They are especially useful in training individuals in emergency situations, in which such simulators can respond in a manner similar to a live patient.

The use of cadaver material is also an essential component of SBT. When cadavers are required to be used for an extended period of time, embalmed specimens are the appropriate choice. When considering training students, residents, and physicians for surgical approaches and interventional procedures, however, the use of fresh, unembalmed specimens is optimal. Such tissues, when frozen and then thawed properly, closely simulate living tissues with regard to feel, texture, and joint movability. This fact provides the health care professional with a subject as close to the living patient as possible. In order for a facility to be successful in developing and carrying out such a program, however, strict adherence must be paid to all federal, state, and local regulations. Qualified administrative and morgue personnel are essential. With these requisites in place, a successful fresh cadaveric SBT program can be achieved.

REFERENCES

1. Cahill DR, Freeland AE. Standards for the study of unembalmed human cadaveric material. *Clin Anat.* 1992;5:145–150.

2. Sadler AM Jr, Sadler B, Stasson EB. The Uniform Anatomical Gift Act: a model for reform. *JAMA.* 1968; 206:2501–2506.

3. Kurtz SF, Strong CW, Gerasimow D, The 2006 Revised Uniform Anatomical Gift Act—A Law to Save Lives. *Health Law Analysis.* 2007;11:44–49.

4. CDC Update. Universal precautions for prevention of transmission of human immunodeficiency virus, hepatitis B virus, and other blood borne pathogens in healthcare settings. *MMWR.* 1988;37:377–388.

5. Marks, SC. Jr. Editorial. *Clin Anat.* 1993;6:255.

6. Bankowski MJ, Landay AL, Staes B, et al. Postmortem recovery of human immunodeficiency virus type 1 from plasma and mononuclear cells. *Arch Pathol Lab Med.* 1992;116:1124–1127.

7. Ocel, JJ, Natt N, Tiegs RD, et al. Formal procedural skills training using a fresh frozen cadaver model: a pilot study. *Clin Anat.* 2006;19: 142–146.

8. Tabes, JA, Rosenson J, Price DD, et al. A comprehensive, unembalmed cadaver-based course in advanced emergency procedures for medical students. *Acad Emerg Med.* 2005;12:782–785.

9. Whitworth, RH. Jr. At LSU Health Sciences Center, fresh is best. *FASEB J.* 2009;23:8.4.

10. Anderson SD. Practical light embalming technique for use in the surgical fresh tissue dissection laboratory. *Clin Anat.* 2006;19:8–11.

11. Levine RL, Kives S, Cathey G, et al. The use of lightly embalmed (fresh tissue) cadavers for resident laparoscopic training. *J Minimally Invasive Gynecol.* 2006;12:451–456.

12. Dalley II AF, Driscoll RE, Settles, HE. The uniform anatomical gift act: what every clinical anatomist should know. *Clin Anat.* 1993;6:247–254.

3

An Overview of Computer Use in Simulation

JAN GRUND-PEDERSON

A SIMULATOR does not need to be technically complex or consist of high-tech components. An effective simulator could be an orange used for the purpose of training suturing, using real needles and thread. In laparoscopy, pegboards and similar arrangements have been used with success to train psychomotor skills. So, what benefits over other types of simulation does the use of computer-based simulation provide? Why increase the technical complexity in a simulator that will be used for training purposes? This chapter addresses these important questions.

ADVANTAGES OF COMPUTER-BASED SIMULATION

One of the most obvious benefits of using computers in a simulated training environment is that objective information about the trainee's performance can be collected and stored. This information can be used to compare the trainee's results over time, thereby tracking progress. The information can consist of anything that can be measured by the computer and software. For example, some specific objective measurements that can be collected during a fluoroscopic simulation include the total time spent to complete a task, total X-ray fluoroscopy time, and the amount of contrast used during the task. The number of measurements multiplies, however, when computer-based simulation is used: overall "economy of movement" (i.e., the amount of catheter/wire combined rotation), catheter movement without guidewire leading, and total distance traveled in the "vessel," can also be tracked, to name just a few. But, although the computer can track and store large amounts of data, it is important to keep in mind that no inherent assessment system is present in the data. Most may agree that a low total amount of time spent on a task is preferable, but a low number in itself does not guarantee that the task was performed well. An assessment system needs to be built to utilize the data that have been collected. The foundation for such an assessment system is, however, the objective data that the computer can collect. Without this, all tasks need to be subjectively assessed by an observer. This is one of the major advantages of the use of computer-based simulation—it allows the observer to collect data objectively and then assess the performance of the trainee. Such collection and assessment can be done without an instructor having to be present at the time of a selected training/ practice session.

In a traditional simulator that does not use computers, what is seen directly is basically all that the trainee observes and thereby learns. For example, in plastic simulators for arthroscopy, a real arthroscope is inserted to examine visually the joint structures present. Using a computer to generate some or all of the visuals vastly expands the potential learning possibilities. Different disease states or anatomical variations can be computer generated for visualization and to create multiple patient case scenarios. Such variety cannot be created with a plastic model without actually changing the model. Computer use thus creates possibilities for providing broader training content since the recorded variations are stored on the computer and can be accessed when needed.

Using a computer, anatomical structures that are difficult to see in a real clinical situation can be enhanced visually. Performing a cardiac transseptal puncture (i.e., puncturing the fossa ovalis with a catheter-based needle) in actual clinical practice depends on secondary visual cues. The operator cannot directly see the fossa ovalis; instead, he has to decide correct catheter placement by observing the movements of the catheter. In a computer-enhanced model, the fossa ovalis can be rendered visible for the trainee. This visualization can then be shown with decreasing clarity as the trainee progresses in his or her learning and requires less assistance from the simulation system. Structures can also be removed by the computer during the simulation to facilitate "looking around the corner." Even invisible objects and forces can be visualized on the monitor by the trainee, in order to improve the learning experience. For example, the forces acting on a device can be demonstrated to the learner on the monitor and thus reinforce learning objectives. In many endovascular procedures, the success of the procedure depends on a stable position of the guiding catheter/sheath. The computer can visualize the forces acting on the wire guide and catheter, and this feedback gives the trainee the ability to experiment with different catheter shapes and different positions of the guiding catheter/sheath to find more stable constellations, thus allowing the trainee to see on the computer screen how the forces change. Such computer-based simulation can give the trainee a deeper understanding of the vascular catheterization procedure.

Many training scenarios can be built around the management of unexpected events, the so-called "what if" situation. A computer-assisted system can be programmed to trigger complications and force the trainee to take action to meet the situation. This adaptability is difficult to accomplish in a more traditional simulator setup in which the physical scenario usually is fixed during the training exercise. This fact exemplifies another advantage of a computer-based simulation system: the content can be much more flexible and adapted to the current need of the trainee. This allows more complex scripted case scenarios to be built, in which successive steps depend on the trainee's responses and actions to the current situation. If the trainee does not react properly, or if the wrong drug is administered, what will happen? If the trainees' response to the new situation is not optimal, what should then happen? Thus, the same basic exercise varies for different trainees or even for the same trainee, depending on the actions taken. The content can be adapted to the skill level of the current trainee, so that it allows for more complex scenarios to build as training progresses.

AN EXAMPLE OF COMPUTER USE IN SIMULATION: THE ENDOVASCULAR SIMULATOR

Several endovascular computer-based simulators are commercially available, each with some inherent differences (Figure 3.1). Many common features and parts, however, make up an endovascular simulator, in addition to the computer itself, which is a vital part of the system. These features include the interface device through which the learner manipulates the simulator, the reconstruction of the anatomical and physiological features of the virtual patient, and the user interface providing communication between the simulator and the learning process. A description of each of these components follows in figure 3.1.

The Interface Device: The Physical Model

For a vascular simulator to be effective, a way must be provided for the trainee to insert and manipulate interventional devices, such as sheaths, catheters, guidewires, dilatation catheters with balloons, and stents. In clinical practice, these devices are

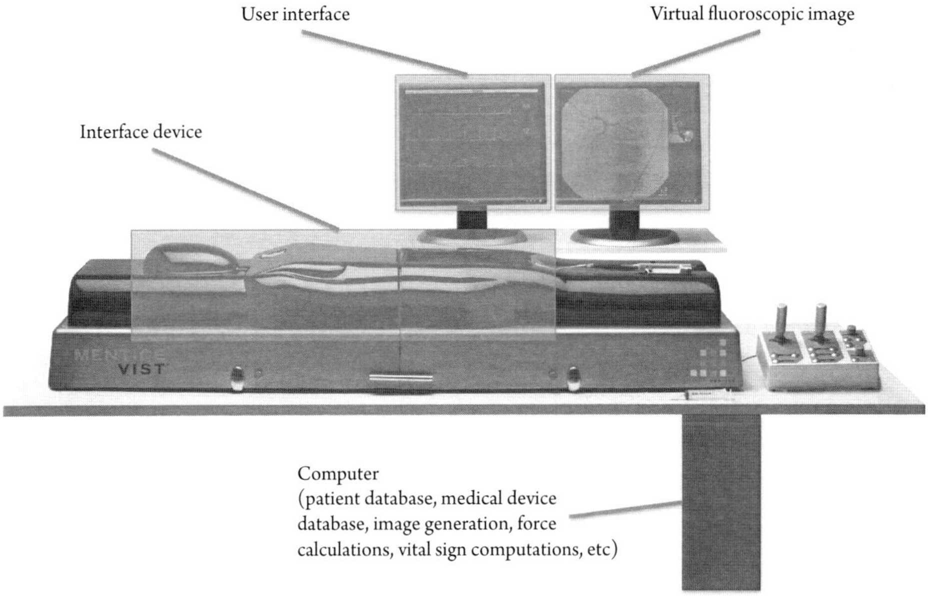

FIGURE 3.1 Example of an endovascular simulator system with its components. Reproduced with permission of Mentice, Inc.

inserted into the patient's blood vessels, usually through an arterial or venous puncture in the groin or arm. A simulator utilizes an interface device as the entry point for the interventional procedural devices. The interface device then tracks the movements of the interventional devices and communicates these motions to the computer. Typically, the interface device only communicates the positions and rotations of the interventional devices to the computer. The communication between the computer and the interface device can be through a USB portal connection or some other communication protocol.

The interface device uses different types of sensors to track the movement and rotation of the medical interventional devices. Sensors can, for instance, be mechanical (e.g., wheels) or optical. Most endovascular simulators can handle several nested (i.e., concentric) tools. Such monitoring is a relatively complicated task since it is difficult to track a tool when it is inside another. In many instances, this difficulty is resolved by not tracking the inner tools until they are completely outside of the outer tool(s) (Figure 3.2).

For training purposes, this ability to handle nested tools is very important since the manual manipulation of multiple interventional devices is a relevant task to master in order to be safe and effective in the patient interventional setting.

To track multiple tools of different sizes, some types of sensor detect which type of tool is inserted into the interface device. This type of monitoring is important since the order in which the trainee inserts devices can vary; thus, a way of knowing what physical device is actually inserted must be present. A simulator can use specifically prepared interventional devices that contain some form of identification information, thus allowing the interface device to detect what type of medical device is inserted. The interface device must then contain some form of identity reader. Alternatively, the interface device can contain some form of optical detector that can detect different sizes of interventional devices. In general, the more accurate the sensor, the larger the variety of actual interventional devices that can be used with the simulator. In this way, the realism of the simulated procedure is enhanced, and the subsequent handling of real interventional devices is facilitated.

Tracking the medical devices is an important task of the interface device. The computer can then calculate where in the virtual anatomy the medical devices are currently located. Since only tracking devices are present inside the interface device, the forces acting upon the medical devices will always be the same, even if a simulated complete blockage of the virtual blood vessel is present on the computer monitor or the virtual anatomy depicted consists of

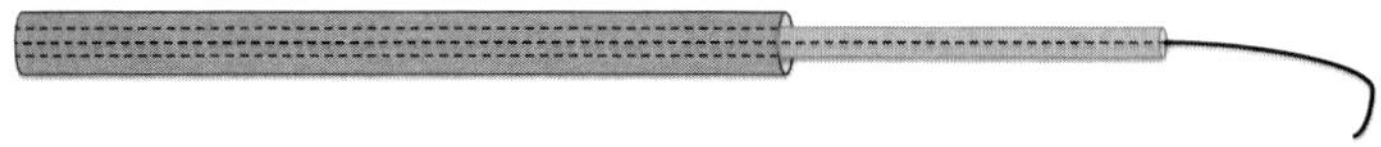

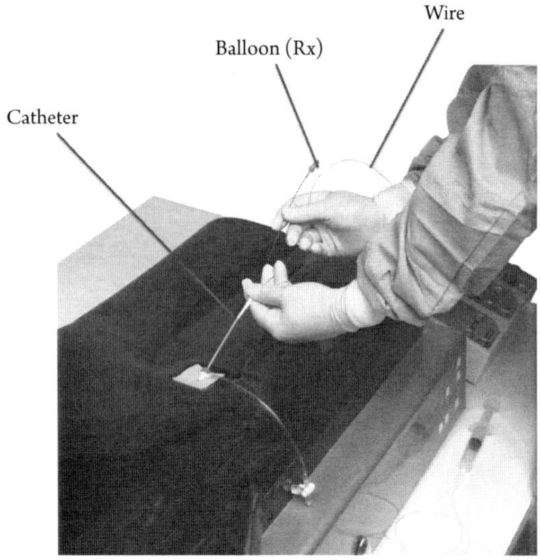

FIGURE 3.2 An example of three nested tools. The outermost guide catheter with an angioplasty balloon catheter within it and an innermost guidewire in the balloon catheter. Reproduced with permission of Mentice, Inc.

very tortuous vessels. Since the computer knows the position of the devices and also holds the information about the virtual anatomy, the software is able to compute forces that restrict the motion of the interventional devices. Some interface devices have the capability to not only track the medical devices but also interact with them, so that the trainee is able to feel resistance to manual catheter movements, thus providing so-called *haptic feedback*.

Haptic feedback can be more or less refined, depending both on the design of the interface device itself and on the computer software that calculates the restrictive forces. Different approaches to providing haptic feedback exist. One is passive, in which the interface device can only hinder the movements of the medical devices. The interface device basically applies pressure on the medical device, so that the trainee feels resistance. This passive approach results in an inability to distinguish between translational and rotational haptic feedback. If the interface device hinders the movements of the medical device, then both translation and rotation are typically affected. Such a restriction is a drawback since, in real clinical situations, these forms of haptic feedback are separate. If a catheter with a shaped tip is moved through a vessel, it may be much more difficult to rotate the catheter than it is to push or pull it. Likewise, when using a needle to puncture a structure, it will be difficult to push the needle. The rotation of the needle and the ability to pull it back, however, will not be restricted.

In active haptic feedback, the interventional devices are not only restricted in movement, but can also be pushed or pulled by the interface device. Such pushing or pulling can never be achieved with passive feedback. A typical example of when push or pull by the interface device is needed is during the interaction between individual nested interventional devices. If the trainee pulls back a wire with a filter attachment (intentionally or unintentionally) into a catheter, the catheter also moves. Such dual movement can only be achieved with an active approach to haptic feedback, in which larger forces can be transferred. Typically, such active feedback is needed for larger interventional devices (e.g., pacemaker leads, vena cava filters, or abdominal aortic aneurysm grafts). The active haptic feedback itself does not necessarily uncouple the translational and rotational feedback, but the technical solutions used to achieve this typically do.

One important aspect of simulation training for endovascular procedures is the ability to find the appropriate anatomical angiographic views. To do so, controls exist for the simulated rotation and tilting of the C-arm fluoroscopy device, for moving of the table, and for moving the image intensifier and other equipment. Some simulators contain this functionality in a separate control box, which then communicates with the computer. The control box only sends information to the computer regarding which buttons are pressed, what levers are moved, and similar information. The computer software then translates this information into virtual movements of the C-arm or other objects, so that the virtual X-ray image can be displayed correctly for simulation procedure performance.

Other equipment can be integrated with the simulation, and thus the handling of this equipment can also be trained (e.g., power contrast medium injector, intravascular ultrasound, fractional flow reserve, etc.). This integration is not currently typical for an endovascular simulator, but it could be an important future step that will allow personnel to train with the complete range of medical devices needed in more complex interventional procedures.

The Virtual Patient: Constructing an Anatomical and Physiological Representation

To be able to interpret the movements of medical devices into something meaningful, a computer representation of the virtual patient is required. Typically, this representation is a three-dimensional (3-D) display of at least the blood vessels, since they are the anatomical structures that the vascular interventional devices will navigate. Other structures need to be represented in some procedures, such as the chambers of the heart. Inside the virtual vessels, the virtual medical devices move, based on the data that the interface device sends to the computer. The virtual vessel anatomy, therefore, is the foundation upon which the simulation scenario is built.

The virtual anatomy/vessels can be constructed de novo using a computer-assisted design (CAD) package. Because the modeler requires input from someone or somewhere to be able to design a credible virtual anatomy, anatomy books, drawings, angiographic images, and the like are used to assist in the creation of the virtual vessels using a CAD approach.

Another approach to vessel construction is to utilize the 3-D data sources that exist in computerized tomographic (CT) or magnetic resonance (MR) images. These images are, in essence, a large number of two-dimensional image slices that, when stacked together, create a 3-D anatomy. The CT/MR images can be used to extract the structure of vessels, which then are stored on the computer. This extraction requires that the CT or MR images be segmented. The process of segmentation entails identifying and marking the vessel(s) present in each CT or MR image slice. Such work can be a tedious process, but today many automatic and semi-automatic algorithms exist that can be used to reduce the time needed for segmentation. The resulting vessel anatomy can be used directly in the simulation, or it can be altered to fit the training needs for specific procedures and/or devices. A combination of the more automatic conversion of CT/MR and the manual construction of "CAD anatomy" can also be employed in vessel construction.

Regardless of the technique chosen for constructing virtual vessels for the simulator, computer software allows for versatility in training. For example, one basic anatomy can be used to create several training case scenarios (i.e., vessel stenoses, aneurysms, tortuosity, etc.). These scenarios can be added to or subtracted from a training regimen to create cases that fit specific learning objectives.

The virtual patient also needs to be visualized. In clinical practice, such "visualization" is often done using fluoroscopy. Hence, virtual X-rays can be created to mimic the actual clinical experience. In this case, a more comprehensive 3-D representation of the anatomy (i.e., bone, kidneys, etc.) is required, in addition to vessel structure. The location of the virtual X-ray tube is the basis for the computations of the virtual X-ray picture. Such a flexible approach attempts to mimic fluoroscopy, so that virtual anatomy can be visualized from any angle. An initial drawback to this approach was that the virtual X-ray images were not always sufficiently realistic. As computer processing has become faster and computer graphics capabilities have increased dramatically, this problem should no longer be a limiting factor. The graphics cards on today's computers can render very complex particle systems that can simulate even the intravascular turbulent flow of contrast medium.

Another approach is to use stored real X-ray images and overlay the interventional medical devices and contrast medium over them. To produce such an overlay, real X-ray images taken from different angles are needed, so that the computer can interpolate images from angles other than those stored. Such an approach gives very detailed and realistic X-ray images. The drawback is that it is very time-consuming to create new cases, since the X-ray images need to be specifically recorded from a certain number of angles.

The virtual patient consists not only of a representation of anatomical structures but also of some form of physiological representation. The physiologic parameters (e.g., pulse, blood pressure, electroencephalogram, etc.) are presented to the trainee on a monitor. The model also allows for drug interaction, so that the virtual patient reacts to a drug infusion (or similarly reacts when a drug infusion is needed). The physiological model of the patient can also react to medical device manipulations.

The User Interface: Interacting with the Virtual Patient

The simulator is not "the real thing." Certain steps in a simulated procedure will differ from the actual clinical patient procedure, and learning frameworks need to be administered that are not present in real life. Therefore, a simulator has some kind of user interface (UI) through which the trainer and trainee can communicate with the simulation software on topics that vary from choosing which type of catheter to use as the virtual representation of what is inserted into the interface device to manipulating individual images and image series that have been captured from the simulator screen.

The most direct interaction with the virtual patient is through the manipulation of interventional devices. The trainee pushes, pulls, and rotates guidewires and catheters, and expects to see and even feel the result. Several approaches to evaluating this interaction exist. The simplest is to measure the inserted length of the medical device and the degree of rotation, then map these measurements exactly in the virtual anatomy. Of course, parts of the virtual anatomy can still be associated with resistance (e.g., resistance will always be the same at a particular anatomical location), and this information is transmitted to the trainee as a haptic feedback. In this one-to-one model of direct mapping, only one path through the anatomy is possible, and all side branches of the main vessel cannot be entered. This approach is very straightforward for the computer, since the inserted length of the interventional device corresponds directly to a position within the virtual anatomy. Only one possible way to navigate the anatomy, however, will exist.

A more complex approach to mapping the wire/catheter positioning within the virtual anatomy is to calculate reactive forces acting on the medical devices. These forces depend on the material properties of the virtual device, the properties of the virtual anatomy, and the calculated position of the virtual medical device. In these instances, the inserted length of the interventional device will not have a one-to-one correspondence to the position of the virtual device. Thus, if the trainee pushes a wire through a virtual vascular structure and encounters a lot of resistance, the result could be that the tip of the wire is fixed in position while the rest of the wire is buckled up inside the vessel. In the first simple model noted above, this situation would not happen. Either the guidewire tip would continue to move forward or resistance would make it stop, and it would be impossible for the trainee to insert more wire.

Many types of interventional devices exist that interact with the virtual patient in other than just a push/pull or rotation motion. For example, balloon catheters and balloon expandable stents are first put in place and then inflated. This inflation is a point of interaction, and it changes the parameters of the virtual patient. Some simulators allow inflation of the balloon, and the computer reads the pressure reached. This value is then used to calculate the resulting geometric change in the vessel, which will result in a change in blood flow. The result can also be predetermined, and the trainee is then only allowed to "fully" inflate the balloon. If a stent is present on the balloon, it is then visualized within the virtual patient.

Contrast media injection provides another form of interaction with the simulator through the UI. Contrast media injection can be performed by pushing a button in the UI—with resultant simulation of a power injector—or through a syringe attached to the computer. With such "manual" injections, the computer then detects that contrast has been injected and renders an X-ray image showing the contrast present. The rendering can be based on flow calculations to get the right amount and speed of contrast injection. If narrowing of a virtual vessel is present, the flow of contrast should make it apparent. And, if the vessel stenosis is removed with a balloon and/or stent, then the flow should change and the imaging of the contrast injection in the area of previous virtual stenosis should reveal patency.

Embolization devices also are available to interact with the virtual patient. They can consist of visible coils and particles that are placed or injected to stop the flow of blood into a specific virtual vascular structure, such as an aneurysm, or an abnormal vessel, such as an arteriovenous malformation pedicle.

Embolic protection devices and expanding stents are similar in construction, and interact with the simulation in similar ways—either through a special handle, or by using a guidewire in a catheter together with a covering sheath. The filter or stent is completely virtual, with only the method of deployment visible to the trainee. An embolic protection device typically consists of a wire and a delivery sheath, which are inserted together. The interface device detects both the wire and the sheath. When the devices are in the desired position, the sheath is retracted and virtually uncovers a filter, which opposes the vessel wall. The computer calculates how much friction the filter should have (if any) on the vessel wall, and this calculation provides the haptic feedback felt by the trainee.

Every action (i.e., the movement of a device, the injection of contrast medium, the inflation of a balloon, the deployment of a filter, the administration of a drug, etc.) can be tracked and stored on the computer. These actions then become the metrics that will be associated with a specific trainee and a specific instance of training. Because a simulator is able to keep track of a number of different users, each trainee must log in on the computer before his or her training session commences. The specific training case is then selected, and the computer will store the user identifier together with the specific training case, a time stamp, and the metrics associated with that training instance. Trainees can then compare the metrics of repeated, serial studies to see how they change over time and with the number of performed cases. Trainees can be compared to their peers. Trainers can also set performance criteria for trainees by identifying acceptable metrics. These criteria can also be set up in the computer software, so that the trainee knows the goal metrics and can practice until the required proficiency level is reached.

The metrics can consist of anything that can be measured. If desired, every turn of a catheter can be logged. Typically, a set of trigger points will be recorded. For example, a signal will be sent to the computer when the trainee engages a diagnostic catheter into the ostium of the renal artery, when a balloon is inflated, or when a certain force is exceeded with the guidewire.

These signals can also trigger other actions. Many simulators allow some form of scripting to allow for the occurrence of complications, but not all complications are scripted. Complications can be allowed to occur randomly, thus allowing the trainee to practice handling specific adverse events. For example, an oversized balloon could trigger a dissection, or an endovascular catheter could trigger a vascular spasm. The trainee must react to these critical events in an appropriate way and within a certain amount of time, or other complications could be triggered. As a result, the scenario that each trainee experiences is unique since it depends on his or her reactions and behaviors.

CONCLUSION

Initially, simulators were limited by the computing power of computers. All calculations necessary for an interactive system were required in real-time. In the 1990s, it was impossible to render realistic anatomy in real-time on a personal computer, or even on a graphics supercomputer. It was also impossible to do advanced, real-time, physics-based calculations of the behavior of medical devices that interact with a virtual anatomy. This led to the careful design of learning objectives and simulation tasks. Today, computing power is no longer the limiting factor. The rendered virtual X-ray images are very realistic, and the behaviors of virtual devices are increasingly approaching real life. Therefore, it is the goal of simulation to make the virtual patient into a one-to-one replacement of the real patient, in order to maximize training. Today, many of those who use simulators ask for more specific programmed procedures and expect to do procedures almost as they would be done on real patients. As simulation becomes more accessible to trainers and trainees, it will become increasingly evident that simulators are excellent training tools. In the future, with increasing simulator realism, it will become difficult to distinguish between the simulated and the real procedure. The look and haptics of both will be very similar.

As mentioned previously, a trend is noted toward integrating more complex equipment into simulation training (e.g., robotic systems for invasive procedures). Equipment is becoming more and more complex, and requires training in a realistic environment. It has become possible to integrate different types of equipment into the simulation environment, since today most equipment is computer based and has the ability to communicate with other systems (Figure 3.3).

This equipment integration allows for more complex team training. The movements of team members, as well as their individual interactions

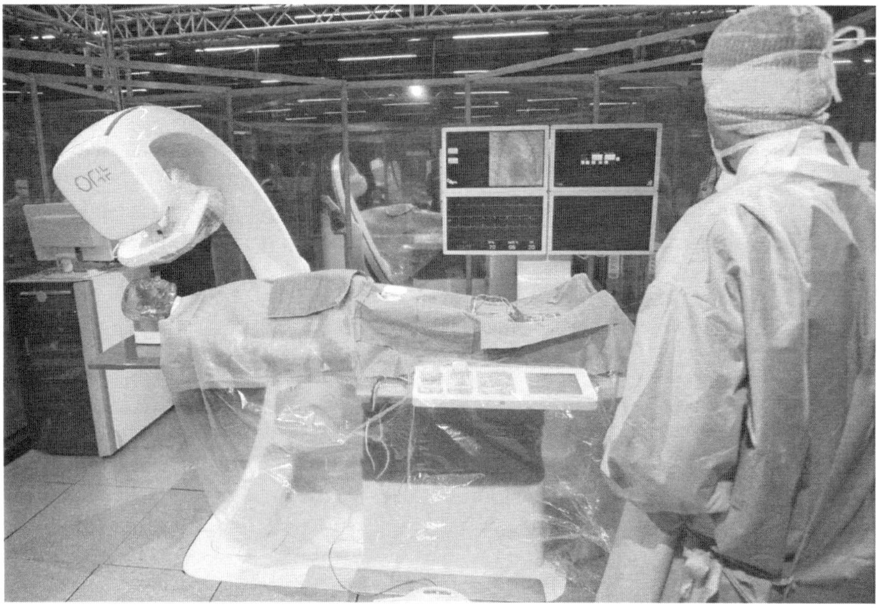

FIGURE 3.3 VIST® system integrated in full catheterization lab mock-up for team training, Orcamp™. Reproduced by courtesy of Orzone AB.

with patients and equipment, can be monitored and recorded in ways not previously possible.

Clinical computerized equipment will be able to exchange information more directly with simulators, so that the boundaries between a simulator as a pure training and assessment tool and as an adjunct to daily clinical practice could diminish. Today, it is possible to use real patient data from scans (e.g., MR and CT) in simulation, but the data does not contain all the necessary information, and the simulation models used are not exact enough to predict outcomes. In the future, with more data of higher quality being acquired, this situation could change. Simulators could become tools not only for highly realistic and qualitative training but also for everyday patient case planning.

RECOMMENDED READING

1. Dawson S. Procedural simulation: a primer. *J Vasc Interv Radiol.* 2006;17:205–213.
2. Gould DA, Kessel DO, Healey AE, et al. Simulators in catheter-based interventional radiology: training or computer games. *Clin Radiol.* 2006;61:556–561.
3. Gould DA. Training on Simulators:Limitations and relevance. Eur J Vasc Endovasc Surg 2007;33: 533–535.
4. Gould DA, Reekers JA, Kessel DO, et al. Simulation devices in interventional radiology: validation pending 2009; 20: S324–S325.
5. Cotin S, Duriez C, Lenoir J, et al. Fried GM, Derossis AM, Bothwell J, et al. New approaches to catheter navigation for interventional radiology simulation. In: Duncan J, Gerig G, eds. *MICCAI 2005.* LNCS 3750. Berlin/Heidelberg: Springer-Verlag; 2005:534–542.
6. Ahmed K, Keeling AN, Fakhry M, et al. Role of virtual reality simulation in teaching and assessing technical skills in endovascular intervention. *J Vasc Interv Radiol.* 2010;21:56–66.
7. Lenoir J, Cotin S, Duriez, et al. Physics-based models for catheter, guidewire and stent simulation. *Studies Health Technol Informatics.* 2006;119: 305–310.
8. Towbin AJ, Paterson BE, Chang PJ. Computer-based simulator for radiology: an educational tool. *Radiographics* 2008;28:309–316.
9. Duncan JR, Glaiberman CB. Analysis of simulated angiographic procedures. Part 1: capture and presentation of audio and video recordings. *J Vasc Interv Radiol.* 2006;17:1979–1989.
10. Duncan JR, Kline B, Glauberman CB. Analysis of simulated angiographic procedures. Part 2: extracting efficiency data from audio and video recordings. *J Vasc Interv Radiol.* 2007;18:535–544.
11. Accessed December 14, 2011 at http://www.hpv.cs.bangor.ac.uk/CRaIVE/projects.php

12. Bucholz EI, Duncan JR. Assessing system performance. *J Vasc Interv Radiol.* 2008;19:987–994.

13. Becker GJ. Simulation and the coming transformation of medical education and training. *Radiology.* 2007;245:7–9.

14. Satava RS. The revolution in medical education—the role of simulation. *J Grad Med Educ.* 2009;1:172–175.

15. Stefanidis D. Optimal acquisition and assessment of proficiency on simulators in surgery. *Surg Clin N Am.* 2010;90:475–489.

16. Derossis AM, Fried GM, Abrahamowicz M, et al. Development of a model fot training and evaluation of laparoscopic skills. Am J Surg.1998;175:482–487.

17. Patel AA, Gould DA. Simulators in interventional radiology training and evaluation: a paradigm shift is on the horizon. *J Vasc Interv Radiol.* 2006;17:S163–S173.

18. Ahmed K, Keeling AN, Fakhry M, et al. Role of virtual reality simulation in teaching and assessing technical skill in endovascular intervention. *J Vasc Interv Radiol.* 2010;21:55–66.

19. Dawson S, Cotin S, Meglan D, et al. Designing a computer-based simulator for interventional cardiology training. *Catheter Cardiovasc Interv.* 2000;51:522–527.

20. Satava R. Emerging trends that herald the future of surgical simulation. *Surg Clin N Am.* 2010;90:623–633.

21. Gould D, Patel A, Becker G, et al. SIR/RSNA/CIRSE Joint Medical Simulation Task Force strategic plan executive summary. *J Vasc Interv Radiol.* 2009;20:7S, S284–S286.

22. Nicholson WJ, Cates CU, Patel AD, et al. Face and content validation of virtual reality simulation for carotid angiography: results for the first 100 physicians attending the Emory NeuroAnatomy Carotid Training (ENACT) Program. *Simulat Healthc.* 2006;1(1 Fall):147–150.

23. Berry M, Lystig T, Reznick R, et al. Assessment of a virtual interventional simulator trainer. *J Endovasc Ther.* 2006;13:237–243.

24. Derossis AM, Antoniuk M, Fried GM. Evaluation of laparoscopic skills: a 2-year follow-up during residency training. *Can J Surg.* 1999;42:293–296.

25. Fried GM, Derossis AM, Bothwell J, et al. Comparison of laparoscopic performance in vivo with performance measured in a laparoscopic simulator. *Surg Endosc.* 1999;13:1077–1081.

4

Simulation Equipment, Commercial and Noncommercial

HUGH J. ROBERTSON, WINTER MELANCON, AND JOAN C. WOJAK

INCREASING INTEREST and research in simulation-based training (SBT) in radiology has stimulated and supported the commercial development of a variety of simulation devices. These devices can be classified in a variety of different ways, as described in chapter 1 (Principles of Simulation). A simple, useful classification of devices for medical SBT divides simulators into four main categories: synthetic/physical models, animal models, human cadaver, and virtual reality (VR) models.[1]

Synthetic physical models include devices simulating vascular anatomy used in SBT for vessel angiography and vascular interventional procedures. Part-task training devices have been developed for SBT of central venous catheter placement, particularly in brachial, cephalic, subclavian, and internal jugular veins. Animal model and human cadaver SBT provide high-fidelity simulations that most closely resemble procedures performed in patients. They are discussed in chapter 2 (Ethics and Regulations of Cadaver Use in Simulation), chapter 17 (Simulation in Spinal Pain Management), and chapter 20 (Simulation in Vascular and Interventional Radiology).

Virtual reality simulation devices have sophisticated computer interfaces that allow realistic simulation of patient interventional procedures. These devices provide computer-derived measurements (metrics) that are useful in partially assessing trainee procedural performance and skill development. Chapter 3 (An Overview of Computer Use in Simulation), chapter 7 (Building and Incorporating Simulation into a Radiology Residency Program Curriculum), chapter 16 (Simulation in Neuroradiology), and chapter 20 (Simulation in Vascular and Interventional Radiology) discuss uses of these devices and highlight the need for progress in further development of these sophisticated simulation tools.

Team-based SBT can utilize both synthetic models and VR (i.e., computer-based) simulation devices effectively. Some aspects of their use are discussed in chapter 12 (Interprofessional Team-Based Training), chapter 13 (Team Training and Crisis

Management: Contrast Reaction Management), chapter 14 (Simulation-Based Training in Intravenous Procedural Moderate Sedation/Analgesia), and chapter 15 (Simulation in Emergency Radiology and Workload Management).

The goal of this chapter is the concise presentation of some commercially available VR and synthetic/physical model simulation devices commonly used in SBT in radiology. Other excellent simulation devices exist and new devices are constantly being developed. Some ideas are presented for simply built, "homemade," low-fidelity part-task training simulation devices. An example of a custom designed specific-use simulation device is described and illustrated.

VIRTUAL REALITY ENDOVASCULAR PROCEDURE DEVICES

Vascular Intervention Simulation Trainer™ (VIST™) System

This high-fidelity, full-size mannequin simulator provides capability for selection and use of specific catheter types for diagnostic and interventional endovascular procedures (Figure 4.1). Modular software allows performance of a large variety of procedures including carotid artery angioplasty and stent placement; intracranial aneurysm coiling and stent placement; coronary artery angioplasty and stent placement; renal, iliac, femoral, popliteal, and below the knee angioplasty; cardiac transseptal catheterization; and foramen ovale closure. Custom-designed procedural scenarios can be provided for specific simulations.

The VIST™-C system is an easily portable system with capability similar to the larger VIST™ system (Figure 4.2).

Mentice, Inc.
1603 Orrington Avenue, Suite 1070,
Evanston, IL 60201, U.S.A.
Telephone: 1-877-636-8423
E-mail: ustechsupport@mentice.com
Corporate headquarters,
Mentice AB,
Rosenlundsgatan 8,
SE-41120 Gothenburg, Sweden
Telephone: 46 31 339 94 00
Website: www.mentice.com.
E-mail: info@mentice.com

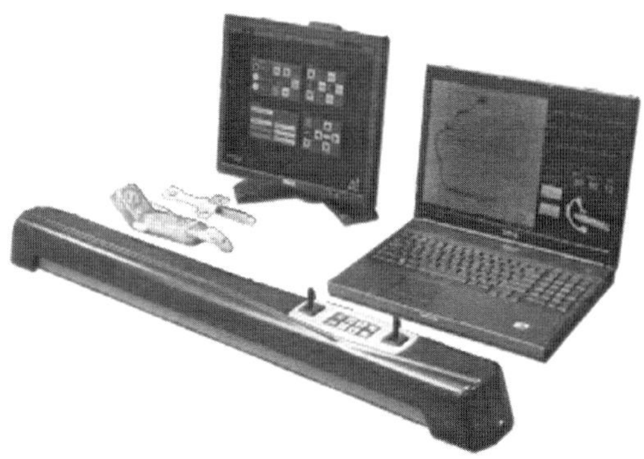

FIGURE 4.2 VIST™-C System, endovascular simulator. Reproduced with permission of Mentice, Inc.

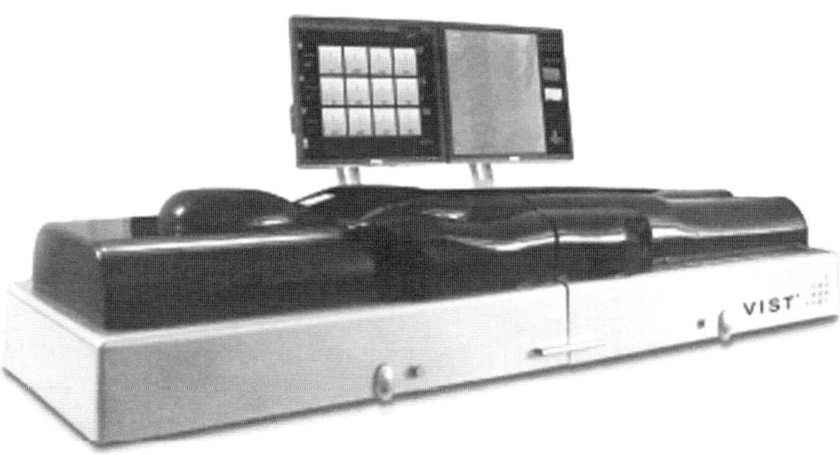

FIGURE 4.1 VIST™, endovascular simulator. Reproduced with permission of Mentice, Inc.

ANGIO Mentor™ Ultimate

This device (Figure 4.3) is a high-fidelity VR stationary system with comprehensive capability for group and individual SBT in endovascular interventional procedures. Training modules are available for carotid artery angioplasty and stent placement, with use of distal embolism protection devices and with monitoring of patient vital signs and vagal reaction. Renal and abdominal aorta, iliac, and femoral artery angiography, and angioplasty and/or stent placement procedures are possible. Intracranial arterial angiography and stent placement simulations can be performed. Coronary artery angiography, angioplasty, and stent placement simulations can be performed while monitoring coronary arterial circulation pathophysiology. More than 100 procedure modules are available for SBT in endovascular procedures using this system. A PROcedure Rehearsal Studio module loads patient-specific computed tomography (CT), magnetic resonance imaging (MRI), and digital subtraction angiography (DSA) studies to permit preprocedural planning and practice.

ANGIO Mentor™ Express is a portable system with capabilities similar to the large stationary ANGIO Mentor™ System (Figure 4.4).

Simbionix USA
Baker Electric Building
7100 Euclid Avenue, Suite 180
Cleveland, OH 44103
Telephone: 216-229-2040
E-mail: support@simbionix.com
Website: http://www.simbionix.com

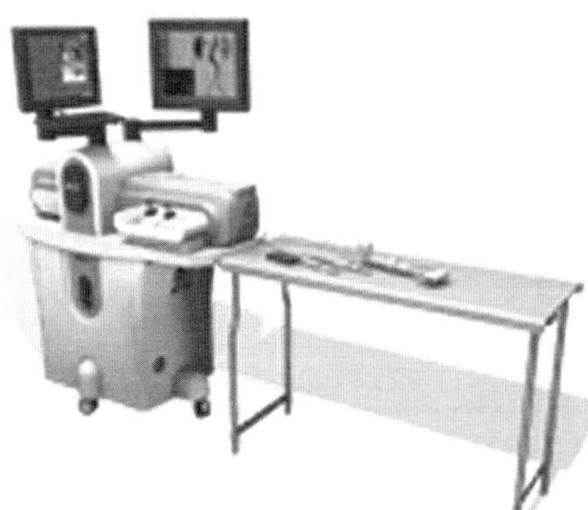

ANGIO Mentor Ultimate

FIGURE 4.3 ANGIO Mentor™ Ultimate, endovascular simulator. Reproduced with permission of Simbionix™ Ltd.

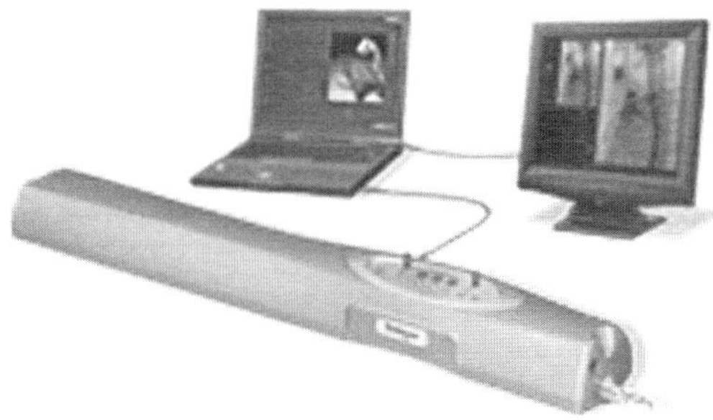

ANGIO Mentor Express

FIGURE 4.4 ANGIO Mentor™ Express, endovascular simulator. Reproduced with permission of Simbionix™ Ltd.

SIMSUITE™

The high fidelity Simantha™ endovascular simulation device (Figure 4.5) incorporates multiple engines and components that provide a realistic VR SBT experience for trainees. Navigation of standard catheters and guidewires in three-dimensional (3-D) vascular anatomy is provided, and the teaching points of the procedure are emphasized by the rules engine. Real-time hemodynamics, oxygen saturations, heart rate, and heart rhythm are provided during procedures. Medications can be given, and effects on blood pressure, heart rate, oxygen saturation, and heart rhythm are documented.

Modular simulation courses are available for cardiac and coronary artery procedures; peripheral vascular, renal, iliac, femoral, and carotid arterial diagnostic and interventional procedures, aortic dissection; intracranial aneurysm coiling, and team training simulation-based procedures.

Medical Simulation Corporation
4643 Ulster Street, Suite 650
Denver, CO 80237
Telephone: 888-889-5882
Website: medsimulation.com

SimMan™ 3G

This very-high-fidelity VR wireless device (Figure 4.6) is the most recent version of the widely used cardiopulmonary resuscitation SBT mannequin. Resuscitation scenarios can be preprogrammed or actively programmed. The wireless device and monitors integrate with existing computer networks. The battery is effective for up to 4 hours before needing recharging. Monitors record two-lead electrocardiograph

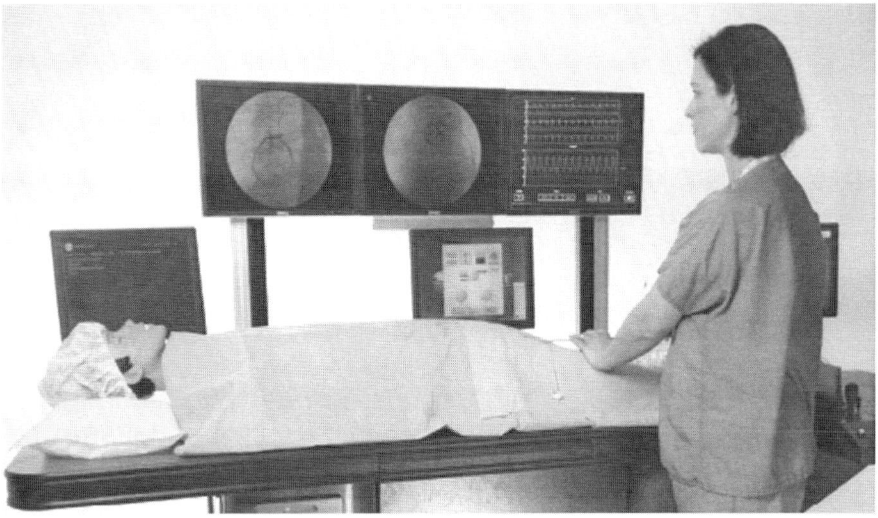

FIGURE 4.5 SIMSUITE™, endovascular simulator. Reproduced with permission of Medical Simulation Corporation.

(ECG), oxygen saturation(SpO_2), carbon dioxide (CO_2), arterial blood pressure (ABP), central venous pressure (CVP), cardiac output, core and peripheral temperatures, and other parameters. Patient voice response is prerecorded or can be simulated by the instructor via wireless microphone.

During cardiopulmonary resuscitation, monitors record chest compression rate, depth of compression, time without compression ("hands-off time"), palpable pulses, respiratory rate, ABP, electrocardiogram (ECG) waveforms, ECG artifacts, critical event recognition (e.g., cardiac arrhythmia), and responses to various drug injections. Modules are available for seizure or trauma SBT.

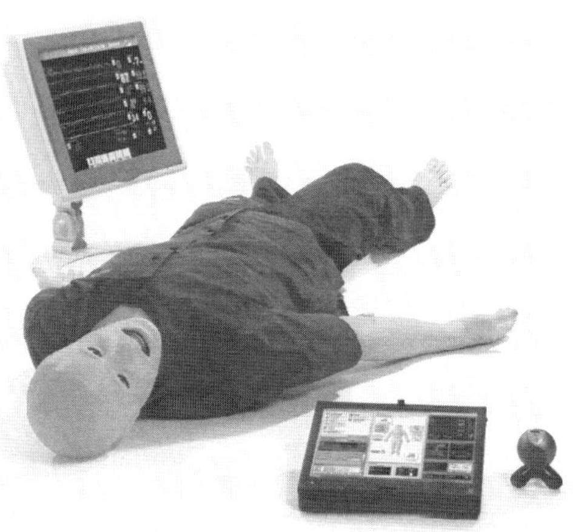

FIGURE 4.6 SimMan™3G, cardiopulmonary resuscitation mannequin. Photo courtesy of Laerdal Medical.

Teamwork SBT with the SimMan™ mannequin (Figure 4.7) provides realistic patient training experiences for deliberate practice of teamwork, leadership, and communication skills in high-risk, low-frequency emergency scenarios. Core skills of airway, breathing, and circulation management are emphasized. Participant debriefing information is generated automatically using event log data synchronized with video images for detailed, immediate feedback on performance.

Laerdal
Customer Service
167 Myers Corners Road
Wappingers Falls, NY 12590
Telephone: 845-295-7770
Web site: www.laerdal.com

ULTRASOUND SIMULATION TRAINING MODELS

Blue Phantom™

BLUE PHANTOM™ FAST MODEL

This life-like upper and lower torso mannequin for SBT in ultrasound for emergency trauma provides excellent ultrasound imaging characteristics for thorax, abdomen, and pelvis (Figure 4.8). Variable amounts of simulated hemorrhage can be added to various areas of the torso. Standard ultrasound equipment is used in the ultrasound SBT. Anatomically

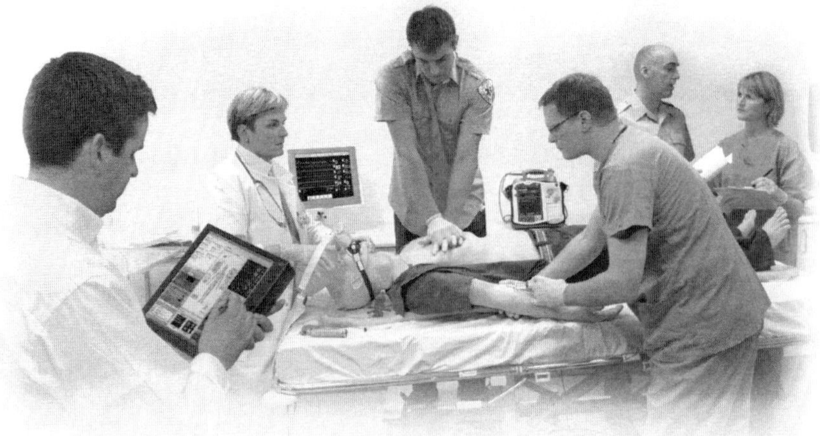

FIGURE 4.7 Teamwork simulation with the SimMan™3G mannequin. Photo courtesy of Laerdal Medical.

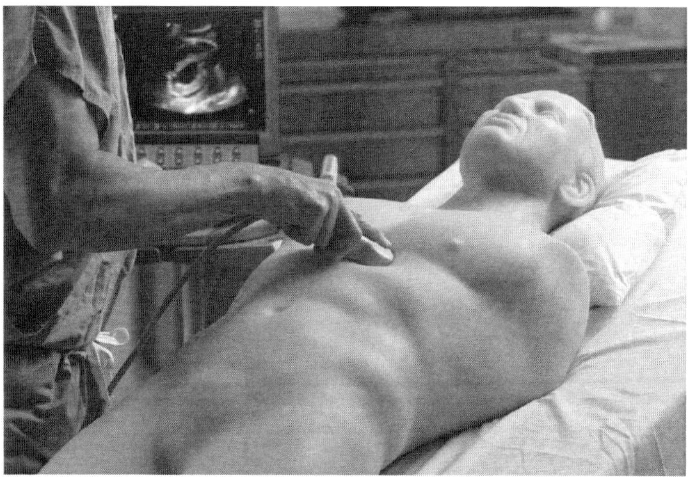

FIGURE 4.8 Blue Phantom™ FAST, ultrasound simulator. Reproduced with permission of Blue Phantom Corporation.

correct images are provided with or without labeling of anatomical structures.

Blue Phantom
8557 154th Avenue Northeast
Redmond, WA 98052
Telephone: 425-881-8830
E-mail: customerservice@bluephantom.com
Website: www.bluephantom.com

ULTRASIM™

This high-fidelity simulation device is a complete ultrasound system simulator with B-mode, color, and spectral Doppler, with an intuitively designed, generic control panel (Figure 4.9). The probes are 3-D position sensors that communicate to the UltraSim™ monitor the position and angle at which the body volume is being scanned. The probes do not emit ultrasound energy. Available modules include abdomen, obstetric, gynecologic, endovaginal, vascular, breast imaging, emergency medicine focused assessment with sonography for trauma (FAST), biliary, pelvic, and abdominal aorta examinations. All necessary clinical data and a detailed analysis are provided for each patient case.

MedSim, Inc.
3215 NW 10th Terrace, Suite 201
Fort Lauderdale, FL 33309
Telephone: 954-563-0855

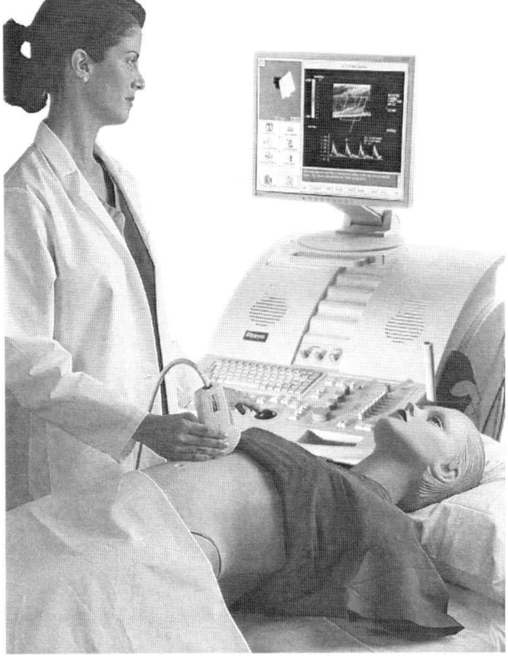

FIGURE 4.9 UltraSim™ ultrasound simulator. Reproduced with permission of MedSim, Inc.

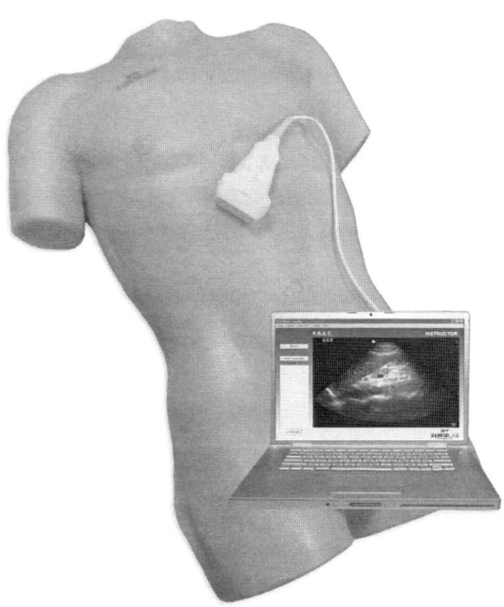

FIGURE 4.10 SonoMan™ System, ultrasound simulator. Reproduced with permission of Simulab Corporation.

E-mail: general@medsim.com
Website: www.medsim.com

SonoMan™ System

This torso mannequin with chest, abdomen, and pelvis components is designed for SBT use with standard ultrasound equipment (Figure 4.10). Separate modules are available for basic instruction in gallbladder and renal disease, abdominal aortic aneurysm, echocardiography, and focused assessment with sonography for trauma (FAST).

Simulab Corporation
1600 West Armory Way
Seattle, WA 98119
Telephone: 866-400-1260
E-mail: info@simulab.com
Website: www.simulab.com

CENTRAL VENOUS ACCESS SIMULATION DEVICES

Blue Phantom™ Central Venous Access Model

This part-task SBT device uses ultrasound guidance for needle puncture and catheter insertion in jugular, subclavian, or axillary vein (Figure 4.11). The device has anatomically correct vascular anatomy and anatomical landmarks. Red and blue colored solutions in plastic tubing simulate vessels and identify venous or arterial puncture. The durable simulated skin over the puncture sites has imaging characteristics of human tissue and can be replaced after extensive use.

Blue Phantom
8557 154th Avenue Northeast
Redmond, WA 98052
Telephone: 425-881-8830
E-mail: customersupport@bluephantom.com
Website: www.bluephantom.com

Life/form Central Venous Cannulation Simulator™

This SBT device includes durable and replaceable simulated skin, and tubing containing colored liquid to simulate internal and external jugular veins, subclavian artery and vein, and common carotid artery (Figure 4.12). Anatomically accurate, palpable landmarks for localization include sternal notch, sternocleidomastoid muscle, and clavicle.

Nasco Healthcare
901 Janesville Avenue,
Post Office Box 901,

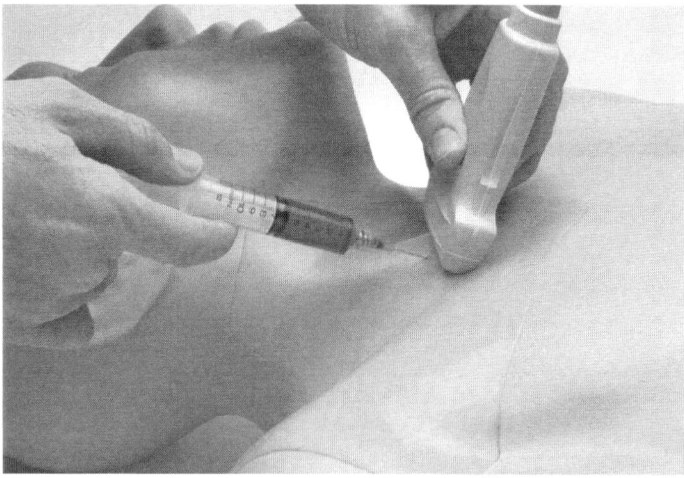

FIGURE 4.11 Blue Phantom™ central venous access model simulator. Reproduced with permission of Blue Phantom Corporation.

Fort Atkinson, WI 53538
Telephone: 1-800-558-9595
E-mail: info@eNasco.com
Website: www.eNasco.com/healthcare

Peter PICC Line™-0600

This simulation device is designed specifically to practice peripherally inserted central catheter (PICC) insertion (Figure 4.13). The replaceable, translucent simulated arm skin allows visualization of cephalic, basilic, and median basilic veins. Tubing to simulate subclavian, axillary, and jugular veins, and the superior vena cava is present. The moveable chin allows simulated practice of the maneuver required to prevent the catheter from entering the jugular vein. Proper PICC line placement can be confirmed by viewing the catheter distal tip in the visible superior vena cava on the side of the model. The ribs and chest wall are palpable, permitting catheter length measurement to the correct intercostal space.

A kit with ribs, vessel tubing, simulated blue venous blood, and covering simulated skin and subcutaneous tissues is provided for device assembly and portability (Figure 4.14).

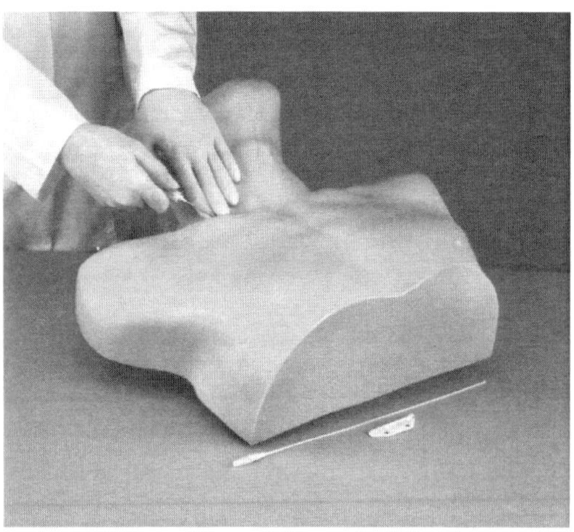

FIGURE 4.12 Life/form™ central venous cannulation simulator. Reproduced with permission of Nasco Healthcare, Inc.

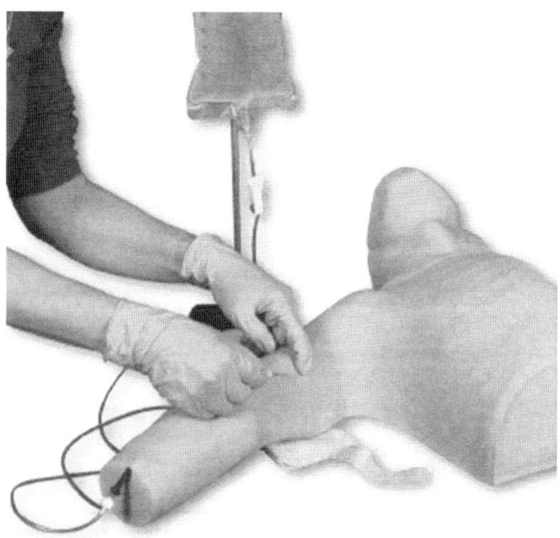

FIGURE 4.13 Peter PICC Line™-0600, peripheral intravenous central catheter placement simulator. Reproduced with permission of VATA, Inc.

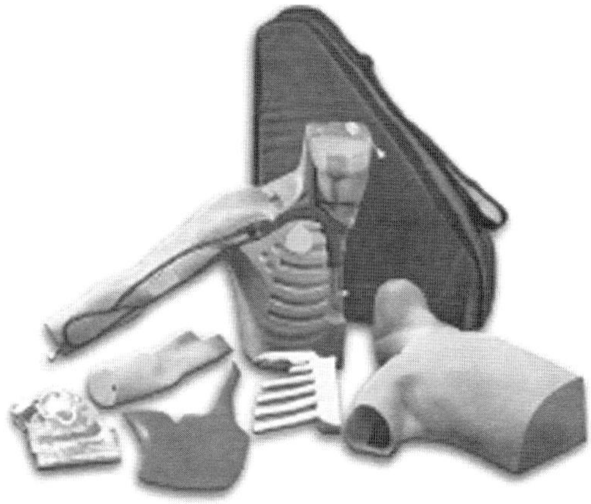

FIGURE 4.14 Peter PICC Line™-0600, components kit. Reproduced with permission of VATA, Inc.

Vata, Inc.
308 South Sequoia Parkway
Canby, OR 97013
Telephone: 503-651-5050
E-mail; info@vatainc.com
Website: www.vatainc.com

LUMBAR PUNCTURE SIMULATION DEVICES

Lumbar Puncture Simulator II

This device simulates the lumbar spine's palpable landmarks (Figure 4.15). Realistic haptic sensation of skin and tissue resistance to needle puncture is provided. Fluid within the simulated thecal sack allows simulated spinal fluid pressure measurement and fluid collection. This device also provides the opportunity for SBT of needle placement into the epidural space. The puncture site simulated skin is replaceable.

Kyoto Kagaku USA Office
3109 Lomita Boulevard,
Torrance, CA 90505
Telephone: 301-325-8860
E-mail: rw-kyoto@kyotokagaku.co.jp
Website: www. kyotokagatu.com

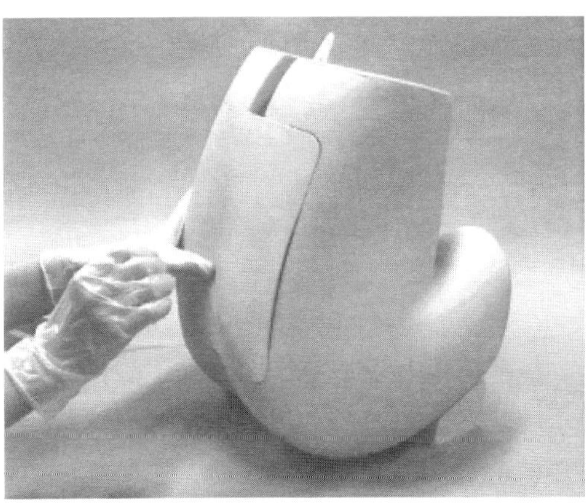

FIGURE 4.15 Lumbar Puncture Simulator. Reproduced with permission of Kyoto Kagaku Company, Ltd.

Life/form™ Spinal Injection Simulator

This SBT device has simulated lumbar spine with vertebrae, central spinal canal with fluid, and palpable vertebral and iliac crest landmarks (Figure 4.16). It can be placed in the lateral decubitus or upright position. Lumbar puncture and lumbar or caudal epidural puncture SBT is possible. The simulated skin at the lumbar puncture site has some haptic characteristics and is replaceable.

Nasco Healthcare
901 Janesville Avenue
P.O. Box 901
Fort Atkinson, WI 53538

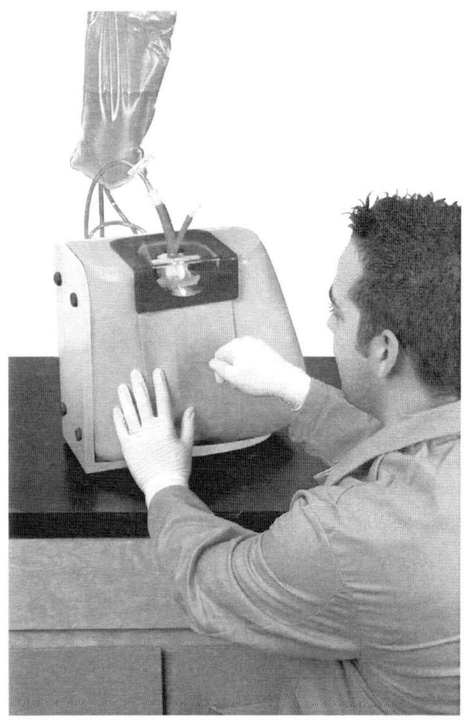

FIGURE 4.16 Life/form™, spinal injection simulator. Reproduced with permission of Nasco Healthcare, Inc.

Telephone: 1-800-558-9595
E-mail: info@eNasco.com
Website: www.eNasco.com/healthcare

CUSTOM-DESIGNED ENDOVASCULAR SIMULATION MODELS

United Biologics Silicone Vasculature

United Biologics, Inc. designs and builds simulation models of a wide variety of arterial and venous anatomical configurations (Figure 4.17). These innovative, custom-designed and manufactured models can be either low- or high-fidelity simulation devices, according to use. The silicone rubber vessel models are rendered seamless, and the vessels can be filled with mildly lubricated fluid for SBT of endovascular procedures. Selective arterial catheter procedures are possible for the aorta, renal, hepatic, mesenteric, iliac, femoral, coronary, brachiocephalic, and intracranial internal carotid, vertebral, basilar, and proximal cerebral arteries. Intracranial vessel models have been designed to practice coiling of aneurysms in typical anatomical locations. A composite model, the Neuro System Model Plus™, was designed to include anomalous origins of brachiocephalic arteries. This device has a bovine carotid artery origin and a type III innominate artery. Simulation-based training with this device teaches proper catheter selection and manipulation through the anomalous arteries to reach the intracranial circulation for required interventional procedures.

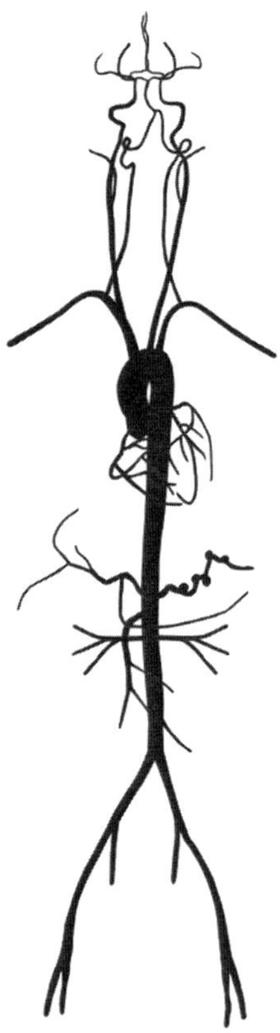

FIGURE 4.17 Endovascular simulator model. Reproduced with permission of United Biologics, Inc.

With United Biologics simulated vasculature, SBT for endovascular clot removal in a simulated stroke model is possible. This high-fidelity simulation model allows realistic practice of microcatheter manipulation and clot extraction device placement without risk to an actual patient.

United Biologics, Inc.
15451 Red Hill Avenue, Suite B
Tustin, CA 92780
Telephone: 877-824-8245
E-mail: info@unitedbiologics.com
Website: www.unitedbiologics.com

DEVELOPMENT OF A VASCULAR FLOW MODEL FOR INTERVENTIONAL STROKE THERAPY

Background

The increasing number of hospitals seeking certification as stroke centers of excellence by the Joint Commission has led to increasing interest in interventional stroke therapy, particularly on the part of hospitals interested in meeting the criteria for Comprehensive Stroke Centers.[2,3] This interest, in turn, has led to an increasing demand for physicians who are trained to provide intra-arterial thrombolysis and mechanical thrombectomy. The traditional pathway for training has been via an interventional neuroradiology (or endovascular surgical neuroradiology) fellowship. The number of fellowship-trained interventional neuroradiologists, however, is not sufficient to meet this increasing demand. As a result, interest has developed in providing specific training in stroke therapy—rather than the full range of interventional neuroradiology—to physicians from other backgrounds, such as interventional radiology and diagnostic neuroradiology.

Current Standards

The Society of Interventional Radiology (SIR) has developed training standards for interventional stroke therapy that outline the cognitive and technical skills necessary and how these skills may be required outside of an interventional neuroradiology fellowship.[4] These standards are primarily intended for physicians who already possess catheter manipulation skills. These physicians do not typically have cognitive training in neurosciences or extensive experience with microcatheters in the cerebral circulation.

The SIR standards mandate specific cognitive qualifications. They also require training in neuro-specific technical skills, as well as documentation of these skills. The skills include selective carotid and vertebral artery catheterization; experience with 3 French or smaller microcatheter/microwire systems; use of Y-connectors, tubing, catheter-flushing techniques; facility with air embolus prevention and guide catheter use.

Comprehensive Stroke Therapy Training

To facilitate acquisition of the necessary cognitive and technical skills, the SIR decided to develop a comprehensive stroke therapy training course. An integral part of the course is a hands-on workshop providing participants experience with the actual types of catheters, wires, flush systems, and techniques commonly used in intra-arterial thrombolysis. As this workshop was being developed, it became apparent that an anatomic flow model simulator that would serve this purpose was not commercially available.

The decision was made to develop a model that would allow selective catheterization of vessels in the setting of Type I–III aortic arches, exchange for a guide catheter, and microcatheter/microwire manipulation to select target vessels in the anterior and posterior intracranial circulation. The model also had to allow demonstration of proper connection, purging, and injection techniques to avoid air embolism. A model that did not require fluoroscopy but could be used with a video camera and monitor was considered essential.

Research into the designers and manufacturers of anatomic flow models utilized for training purposes by vendors of catheters, wires, and other devices designed for intracranial use led to United Biologics, Inc. (Tustin, California) as a potential source for creating the model. This company was willing to help develop a workable model, which they would then be able to market. The first prototype was an anatomically correct representation of the arterial system, extending from the common femoral arteries to the second- and third-order intracranial vessels. The model was made of silicone to simulate the elasticity of vessels and to allow visualization with a video camera system. Continuous, pressurized flow was provided using a proprietary solution designed to decrease friction. The prototype was evaluated using the catheters and wires planned for use in the comprehensive stroke therapy training workshop. All of the technical skills that the participants were expected to learn and demonstrate were test performed.

On the basis of this evaluation, several changes were made. A second camera and monitor were added to simulate biplane imaging. A screen was designed to prevent the user from directly visualizing the intracranial circulation, thereby reproducing the actual patient situation. Modifications were made to the model at the time of the evaluation, and further modifications were recommended to simplify the intracranial portion of the model to allow for better visualization and to provide specific anatomic challenges.

Drawings of the proposed modifications were evaluated, and a revised model was produced. This model was again bench-tested. At this time, all of the skills were demonstrated and recorded for a training video. The final design was approved, and additional models were manufactured for the course. The comprehensive stroke therapy training workshop faculty members were shown the training video and were given the opportunity to practice the skills that they would be teaching. The faculty then worked one-on-one with the workshop participants. The participants were given the list of skills that would be tested and were given time to practice on their own. Each participant was then tested on the required skills, including setting up and purging the flush system, selective vessel catheterization, exchange for a guide catheter, and microcatheter selection of an intracranial target vessel. Feedback from the workshop faculty and participants was positive, and the models will continue to be used; some minor modifications were recommended (see Figures 4.18 and 4.19).

Simulation Equipment, Noncommercial

A fully equipped simulation laboratory requires highly technical, sophisticated, high-fidelity devices

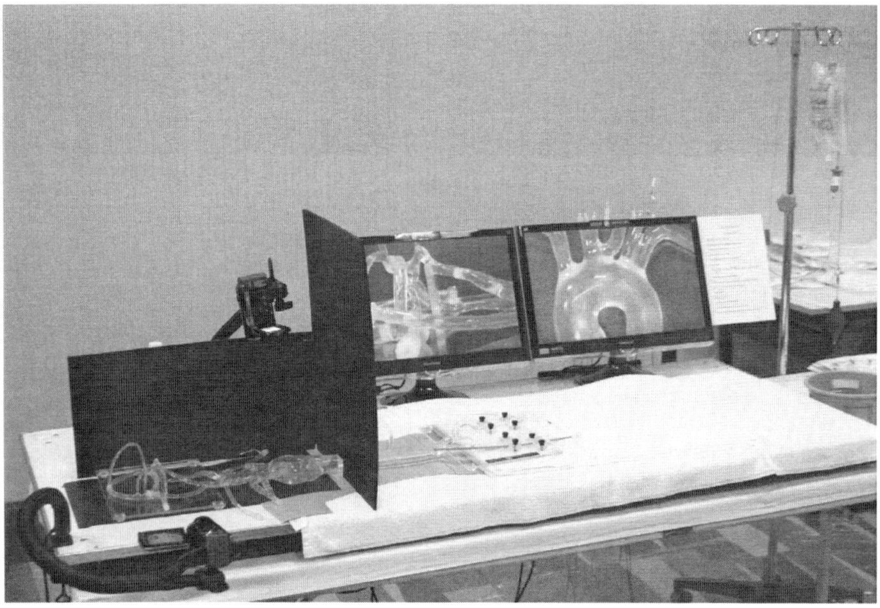

FIGURE 4.18 Endovascular simulator model. Reproduced with permission of United Biologics, Inc.

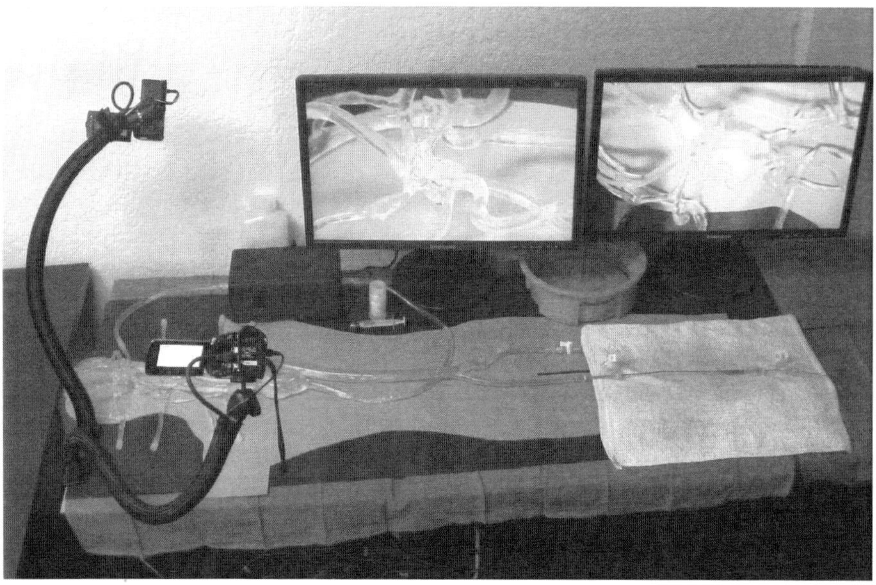

FIGURE 4.19 Endovascular simulator model. Reproduced with permission of United Biologics, Inc.

only available through specialized commercial manufacturers. A definite need also exists for part-task, low-fidelity SBT at the novice trainee level. With the identification of a specific need, a variety of "homemade" inexpensive devices can be made "on site" in the laboratory workshop. Chapter 22 (Simulation in Breast Imaging) describes phantoms for SBT of image-guided breast biopsy using eggplant or layered meat segments with embedded almond "pseudolesions." Turkey or chicken breast with embedded olives has also been used for simulated breast biopsy. The multilayered meat phantom was considered to have tactile sensation (i.e., haptics) similar to human breast tissue on biopsy. The simple phantoms allow SBT for biopsy localization by ultrasound, CT, and MRI.

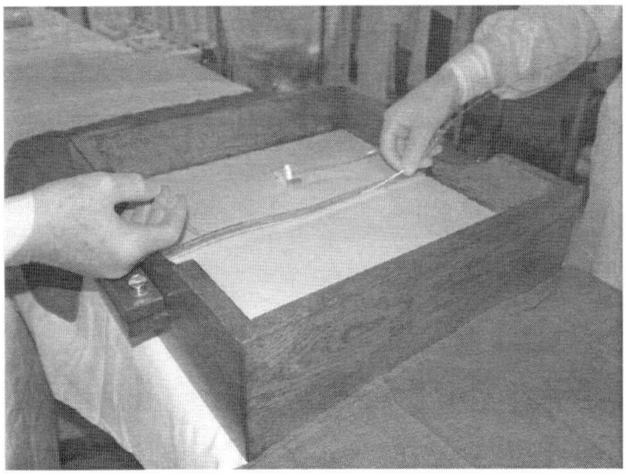

FIGURE 4.20 Seldinger technique vascular entry simulator. Photograph courtesy of Dr. Luis Serrano.

An SBT device for vascular puncture and endovascular catheter insertion (i.e., Seldinger technique) can be simply constructed of wood and plastic tubing, obtained from a hardware store and of a diameter similar to that of an adult common femoral artery. The device shown in Figure 4.20 was constructed of oak side panels, with wooden clamps at both ends to fasten the tubing, and a plywood base. Sheet extruded polypropylene insulation material was placed beneath the tubing. The tubing was resistant to needle puncture, and it was necessary to use a small drill to make an entry site for the needle and the subsequent insertion of guidewire, vascular sheath, and catheter. Micropuncture arterial access can be well demonstrated with this device. The clear plastic tubing allows direct visualization of the procedure. An arterial stenosis can be simulated by application of a plastic or metal clamp, variably narrowing the tubing lumen. A trainee and instructor can work simultaneously on the device. Instruction in this SBT emphasizes the safe vascular insertion of the flexible tip guidewire to avoid potential injury and dissection of the artery wall. Simulation-based training with this simple part-task device is performed with novice trainees before participation in patient arteriography, with the goal of trainee early familiarity with equipment and techniques for safe catheter endovascular placement. This simulation device can also be used for SBT of puncture site closure devices.

CONCLUSION

A basic classification of medical SBT devices includes synthetic/physical models, animal models, human cadaver and virtual reality devices. Some examples of commercially available synthetic/physical and virtual reality devices were presented in this chapter. Other excellent similar devices are available. Examples of simple, low-fidelity part-task training simulation devices are noted that can be built in the workshop from readily available materials. The development and construction of a custom designed specific-use simulation device is noted.

Computer assisted simulation devices used alone have no more practical learning capability than a simple computer game. The development and use of medical simulation devices must be based on absolute, strict criteria. Complex educational, psychological, physiological, physics and engineering principles are used in the simulation device development and construction and in the fabrication of the training algorithm in which it is used.

The specific learning goal necessary from the simulation procedure must be fully verifiable through evidence based performance metrics. The computer based metrics system must reliably report the trainee simulated procedure technical and cognitive errors. Face validity (i.e., the system looks like what it represents), content validity (i.e., the system contains the material for necessary training), construct validity (i.e., critical factors are assessed that relate to the required skill(s) acquisition), and predictive validity (the learning performance on the system correlates with the actual clinical patient procedure performance) are vital factors in the simulation device development and its use in the simulation teaching algorithm.[5–8]

REFERENCES

1. Ahmed K, Keeling A, Fakhry M. The role of virtual reality simulation in teaching and assessing technical skills in endovascular intervention. *JVIR*. 2010;21:55–66.

2. Alberts MJ, Latchaw RE, Selman WR, et al. Recommendations for comprehensive stroke centers: A consensus statement from the Brain Attack Coalition. *Stroke*. 2005;36:1597–1616. [Epub June 16, 2005]

3. Leifer D, Bravata DM, Connors JJ 3rd, et al.; on behalf of the American Heart Association Special Writing Group of the Stroke Council, Atherosclerotic Peripheral Vascular Disease Working Group, Council on Cardiovascular Surgery and Anesthesia, and Council on Cardiovascular Nursing. Metrics for measuring quality of care in Comprehensive Stroke

Centers: Detailed follow-up to Brain Attack Coalition Comprehensive Stroke Center recommendations: a statement for healthcare professionals from the American Heart Association/American Stroke Association. *Stroke.* 2011;42:849–877. [Epub January 13, 2011]

4. Connors JJ 3rd, Sacks D, Black CM, et al.; Society of Interventional Radiology. Training guidelines for intra-arterial catheter-directed treatment of acute ischemic stroke: a statement from a special writing group of the Society of Interventional Radiology. *J Vasc Interv Radiol.* 2009;20:1507–1522.

5. Dawson S. Procedural simulation: a primer. J Vasc Interv Radiol.2006;17:205–213.

6. Gould DA, Kessel DO, Healey AE, et al. Simulators in catheter-based interventional radiology: training or computer games? Clin Radiol. 2006; 61:556–561.

7. Gould DA, Reekers JA, Kessel DO, et al. Simulation devices in interventional radiology: validation pending. J Vasc Interv Radiol. 2009; 20:S324–S325.

8. Gould DA. Training on simulators: limitations and relevance. Eur J Endovasc Surg. 2007; 33:533–535.

SECTION 2

SIMULATION IN EDUCATION

5

Educational Principles in Simulation

SHEILA W. CHAUVIN

RAPID ADVANCES in information and instructional technologies have been observed in recent decades, particularly with regard to simulation. Insights gained from these developments and the research on how people learn best offer opportunities to embrace new ways of thinking about and engaging in teaching and learning.[1] Although simulation technologies offer an increased range of options for teaching and learning, educators and instructional designers still need to be explicit regarding the intended purpose(s), process(es), and outcome(s) of training and education initiatives. This chapter begins with several key definitions and synthesizes relevant educational theories and principles for using simulation in radiology education. The chapter also provides a widely used instructional design framework that can be used for developing simulation-based education—the Assess, Design, Develop, Implement, Evaluate (ADDIE) approach.[2–4] A widely adopted set of criteria pertaining to educational scholarship[5] is described and offers yet another framework for guiding and assuring high-quality training and educational design and implementation. The assessment and evaluation of learner achievement and instructional effectiveness are key ingredients to achieving and sustaining quality education and must be considered at the onset of instructional design, not after implementation has occurred. Although mentioned in this chapter, greater attention is given to assessment in simulation in the chapter that follows. Both chapters have been developed with the intention that readers will use the two together to develop and sustain high-quality simulation-based radiology education.

KEY DEFINITIONS

Drawing on the professional literature, a variety of definitions exists regarding simulation. For example, Fincher and Lewis[6] define simulation simply as a technique that involves a learner (e.g., medical student or resident) and a "patient" (e.g., actor or standardized patient, anatomical model, computer-based application, mannequin). McGaghie[7] offers a more comprehensive conceptualization of simulation that includes the following:

> In broad, simple terms a simulation is a person, device, or set of conditions which attempts to present [education and] evaluation problems authentically. The student or trainee is required to respond to the problems as he or she would under natural circumstances. Frequently the trainee receives performance feedback as if he or she were in the real situation. (p. 9)

McGaghie further notes that simulation-based teaching and evaluation methods share several common features that include the following:

- Learners can be situated in complex scenarios.
- Learners experience cues and consequences that are authentic representations of the real-life setting.
- Learners respond to situations much as they would in real life.
- The extent to which a simulation can replicate real life is never exactly the same (i.e., fidelity) due to limitations such as cost, technological capacity, time, assessment requirements, ethics, and safety.
- Simulations can reflect a wide variety of formats that can focus on either individual or group learning and performance.
- Simulations can involve a variety of simulator technology, such as a simple inanimate anatomical model, a programmable simulation module, or a high-fidelity, physiologically responsive, mannequin-based human patient simulator.
- Simulations for evaluation purposes can reflect decisions and consequences that can range from no to low to high-stakes impact on the learner.

In terms of educational design, *simulation* refers to the design and process of teacher and learner engagement, whereas *simulator* refers to the actual things being used in a specific situation (e.g., materials, equipment, people) to mimic or represent the relevant features of the real-life phenomena being represented in an activity or process (e.g., patient scenario, teaching module, tutorial, assessment procedure). In fact, multiple simulators could be used in a single simulation exercise; this is often referred to as a *hybrid approach* (e.g., standardized patient and virtual reality [VR] trainer, computer-based avatar patient and mannequin simulator). Other simulation-based formats have also been used in radiology (e.g., numerical modeling or clinical/disease-related research applications), but the purposes of these are not primarily focused on teaching and education and are not addressed in this chapter.

Distinguishing simulation and simulator can be particularly helpful when determining the optimal realism necessary for accomplishing desired learning or assessment outcomes. As shown in Table 5.1, Meller[8] published a typology for classifying the level of realism (P1–P4) and the elements of engagement (i.e., passive, active, interactive) that can be represented in simulators for medical education. For example, a paper-based patient case with a set of radiologic images would reflect a realism element of P1; the learner engaged directly or immersed in a simulation-based exercise with teacher-facilitated after-action debriefing reflects a level of realism akin to P4.

SIMULATION-BASED FORMATS AND RELEVANCE TO TEACHING, LEARNING, AND ASSESSMENT

A wide range of simulation-based formats are possible in which different types of simulators (i.e.,

Table 5.1 Meller's typology of simulators for medical education

ELEMENT	LEVEL OF REALISM NECESSARY TO ACHIEVE LEARNING OR EVALUATION OUTCOMES
P1	Patient and/or disease process
P2	Procedure, diagnostic test, or equipment being used
P3	Physician or paraprofessional (e.g., learner engaged in the simulation activity)
P4	Professor or expert practitioner (e.g., teacher involved in the simulation activity)
p	Passive element—static, exists to enhance the authenticity or realism of simulator
a	Active element—change during simulation is programmed, can stimulate learner response(s)
i	Interactive element—dynamic changes that occur in response to features during the simulation activity, such as in response to actions taken by the learner

materials and equipment) are used. For example, traditional formats using simple simulator technologies include face-to-face role plays, case-based discussions, and learners' use of paper-based case scenarios in problem-based learning that reveal increasing amounts of information as learners work through the scenario, a process referred to as "successive disclosure."[9] The complexity of simple simulations (e.g., paper-based cases) can be further enhanced by the inclusion of radiologic images (e.g., X-rays, computed tomography [CT] or magnetic resonance imaging [MRI] scan), a mock patient chart, and/or radiologic diagnostic reports to increase the realism or fidelity of the simulation exercise. Simulation can also be incorporated into discussions of real patient cases (e.g., during rounds). For example, the teacher who uses "what if" type questions skillfully to promote divergent and higher-order thinking is using a form of simulation in that the actual patient being discussed serves as a stimulus or "jumping off point" for creating simulated patients that extend learning. With just a few "what if" questions, learners could find themselves engaged in considering four or five patient scenarios, instead of just that of the person they actually have in their care. Simulation involving other humans in standardized formats reflect a higher level of complexity and can include the use of simulated patients or standardized patients (i.e., trained actors to portray specific patient problems)[9] and patient educators (i.e., patients with actual clinical problems who are educated to work with teachers and learners in a specific instructional format).[10]

Other forms of simulations can use various levels of technological complexity. For example, simulation utilizing low-fidelity simulators can range from simple task trainers for learning and performing specific maneuvers or procedures (e.g., knot-tying boards, transfer tasks related to minimally invasive procedural skills) to anatomical training simulators (e.g., intravenous line placement and central line trainers). Simulators reflecting mid-level fidelity include some computer-based patient cases and problem-based patient case software (e.g., DxR™ clinical cases, available at http://www.dxrclinician.com/) and mannequin-based simulators without computer-driven physiology (e.g., those used in basic and advanced life support trainings).[10–12] With rapid developments in recent years, the availability of technologically complex simulators has increased and includes choices such as high-fidelity, computerized, mannequin-based human patient simulators (e.g., Medical Education Technologies, Inc., METI, http://www.meti.com) and VR simulators (e.g., LapMentor or AngioMentor, http://www.simbionix.com). When designing activities and materials for simulation-based teaching and learning and/or assessment, one needs to think carefully about the level of complexity required to achieve an appropriate level of realism (e.g., psychological, contextual, and technological fidelity) for mastering the intended learning objectives. Achieving good alignment among learning objectives, teacher and learner characteristics, simulator(s), and overall simulation experience is absolutely critical to assuring effective and cost-efficient use of simulation in education. To underestimate the level of fidelity can result in not achieving intended outcomes and wasting scarce resources, such as time and expertise. To overestimate the level of fidelity might result in achievement of learning outcomes, but waste of precious resources when a lower-fidelity scenario would have been sufficient. The potential also exists that learners will not achieve intended learning outcomes when fidelity is overestimated due to cognitive and sensory overload. In such situations, learners are overloaded by unnecessary stimuli and have insufficient cognitive processing capacity to use prior knowledge and experience to make sense of new learning.[13]

Relative to simulation-based radiology education, at least two levels of design could be considered: curriculum and instruction. These two terms often are used synonymously, but important distinctions are worth mentioning. Grant[14] defined *curriculum* as consisting of intended goals and objectives, content, experiences, process, and outcomes at a broad level. *Curriculum design* is a systematic process for specifying elements of the overall learning program, as well as other key elements such as entry requirements, length of enrollment, allowable variation and accommodations for progressing through the courses and experiences, and the assessment system and criteria by which satisfactory completion is determined (i.e., graduation, certification). Particularly in professional education, curricula are often subjected to accreditation standards and review. Definitions of instructional design pertain to a specific teaching, learning, or assessment experience that is intended to achieve specific short-term learning and development outcomes.[13,15–17] Thus, the purposeful threading of multiple experiences to address one or more broad goals contributes to a curriculum. Although the scope of educational design differs at the curriculum and instructional levels, both can be guided by the applications of principles and best practices derived from the literature on the science of learning (i.e., how people learn) and the science of instruction (i.e., how to help people learn).[13] Of note, the results of a recent meta-analysis comparing the effectiveness of web-based versus classroom instruction revealed that, in determining effective learning, the instructional methods used were more important than the type of media used.[18]

EDUCATIONAL THEORIES AND MODELS RELEVANT TO SIMULATION-BASED EDUCATION

Generally, a theory or conceptual model provides a widely applicable explanation of natural phenomenon that has been confirmed through observations, experimentation, and logical reasoning across different settings. These general explanations produce principles or generalized statements that can be used to predict and guide future actions and activities (e.g., teaching and learning). A large collection of theories of learning and education exist in the literature, and these reflect a range of perspectives. A small number of relevant theoretical perspectives are presented in this chapter as a basis for educational principles that educators can use specifically in designing and implementing simulation-based radiology education and training.

Custers and Boshuizen[19] contrast psychological and educational theories of learning. Psychological theories of learning are limited to the processes that occur within a learner's mind, whereas educational theories of learning are more expansive and also include deliberate teacher and instructional design features, and ecological or contextual features that can affect individual and group learning. For this chapter, emphasis is given to educational theories because of the explicit attention paid to contextual features and purposeful intent to influence learning (e.g., teacher and learner qualities, actions, and interactions; teaching methods; and physical and psychosocial features of the learning environment). For readers who desire additional information about psychological theories of learning, Custers and Boshuizenis[19] provide an excellent summary.

TAXONOMIES OF LEARNING AND THINKING

A number of taxonomies and conceptual models describe various levels of thinking and learning that can be used to guide decision-making about the level at which to initiate learning and how to progress systematically to a higher level. An age-old taxonomy developed by Benjamin Bloom and colleagues[20] has been widely used over many decades to communicate and plan for various domains and levels of thinking and learning. Although developed originally to guide assessment and evaluation of learning, this framework (typically referred to as *Bloom's taxonomy*) is useful for defining educational goals and learning objectives/outcomes, creating corresponding activities and materials, and conducting appropriate assessments. Bloom's taxonomy includes three domains: cognitive (i.e., knowledge), psychomotor (i.e., skills and behaviors), and affective (i.e., attitudes, values). Table 5.2 shows the various levels of Bloom's taxonomy for each of the three learning domains, reflecting the interpretation that

Table 5.2 Bloom's taxonomy in the cognitive, affective, and psychomotor domains

LEVEL	COGNITIVE (KNOWLEDGE)	AFFECTIVE (ATTITUDE)	PSYCHOMOTOR (SKILLS)
1	Recall (information)	Receive (awareness)	Imitate
2	Understand	Respond (react)	Manipulate (follow directions)
3	Apply (Use)	Value (understand and act)	Develop precision
4	Analyze	Organize (in terms of personal value system)	Articulate (combine, integrate skills)
5	Synthesize	Internalize value system (adopt behaviors associated with value(s))	Naturalize (automate, become expert)
6	Evaluate (Judge)		

seems most applicable to simulation-based education and training. Noteworthy, Bloom's cognitive domain has been used by educators and trainers considerably more than the other two.

Since the introduction of Bloom's taxonomy, others have contributed varying interpretations of the levels within each of the domains. For example, an updated taxonomy for the cognitive domain by Anderson and Krathwohl[21] retained the levels, but simply reversed the last two levels and refined the synthesis level to include explicitly the aspect of creating/building as more challenging than evaluation. Others have argued differently. Although there is no true consensus on one interpretation, Bloom's original taxonomy and order of levels continues to prevail, and this taxonomy is a widely used framework, especially in education, workplace performance, and training.

Miller's pyramid,[22] shown in Figure 5.1, is another taxonomy or framework that has been used frequently to conceptualize the various levels or stages of learning and performance, particularly in medical education. Starting at the bottom of the pyramid, "knows" reflects initial acquisition of factual, declarative knowledge, akin to Bloom's knowledge level (recognition and recall of information), and is typically targeted with introductory level learning (e.g., lectures, demonstrations, reading). Miller's "knows how" level is similar to Bloom's comprehension level of thinking and learning. At this level, learners can demonstrate fundamental understanding through explanations and descriptions. Applying knowledge and skills to real-life situations is not achieved until Miller's "shows how" level of learning (akin to Bloom's "application"). Although perspectives vary somewhat at the higher levels of Bloom's and Miller's conceptual frameworks, Bloom's higher-order thinking abilities (i.e., analysis, synthesis, evaluation, and the more contemporary concept of creating) coincides with Miller's "does" level. Learning, thinking, and performing at this level reflect the integration of new knowledge, skills, and attitudes into everyday practice and the full use of abilities for dealing with the ill-structured and ever-evolving situations encountered in the professional work environment (e.g., diagnosing a patient problem). Although simulation-based teaching, learning, and assessment can be used effectively for the lower-order knowledge and abilities, simulation is usually most effective for addressing learning outcomes that involve higher-order abilities in the cognitive, affective, and psychomotor domains.

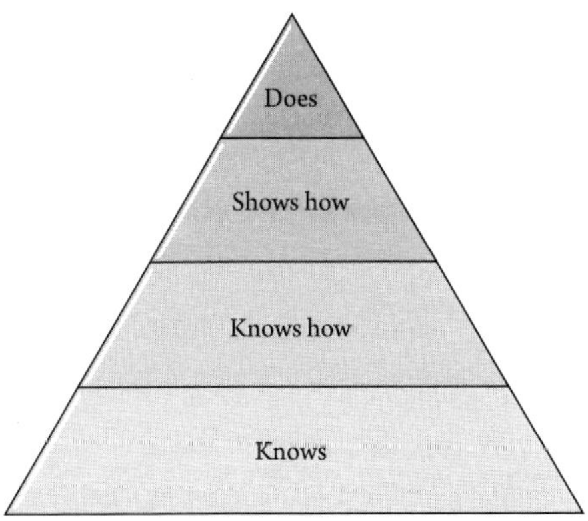

FIGURE 5.1 Miller's pyramid for assessing clinical competence.

Like Bloom and Miller, Kirkpatrick[23] developed a taxonomy that has been widely used for both designing and evaluating instruction. The four levels of Kirkpatrick's training effectiveness taxonomy focus on the overall training/educational program and reflect the following: reaction to the education/training experience (e.g., satisfaction, perception of program quality); learning (e.g., acquisition of new or increased knowledge, skills, and/or attitudes); behavior (e.g., actual change in targeted behavior in the workplace or real-life application setting resulting from the education/training); and result or outcome (e.g., long-term impact on one or more aspects of a learner or targeted client group, or the organization as a whole, in terms of the initial purposes of the education/training, including return on investment in training).

CONCEPTUAL MODELS AND THEORIES OF LEARNING

Adult Learning Theory

Pedagogy is typically used to reflect teacher- and content-centered instruction that has been traditionally associated with teaching children. Malcolm Knowles and colleagues[24] conceptualized the term *andragogy* to distinguish methods used to facilitate adult learning. This theory was based on the assumptions that adults are independent, self-directed learners who are driven more by intrinsic motivators than external ones. Further, Knowles and colleagues emphasized the importance of the adult's prior experiences in learning and believed that adults wanted to integrate and apply learning to relevant situations and real-life problems. More contemporary interpretations of Knowles' theoretical framework have emphasized the relevant role of independent, self-directed learner characteristics, rather than chronological age. The seven principles of adult learning theory are summarized in Table 5.3. Regarding self-directed learning, Candy[25] identified more than 100 characteristics from the literature, of which he indicated that the most important characteristics of learners included confident and competent learning behavior; curious, open, creative, self-motivated; disciplined and methodical; analytic, logical, and reflective; collaborative and interdependent with others; responsible and persistent; and self-aware.

From an educational standpoint, self-directed learning can be facilitated by designing explicit opportunities and supportive structures that engage learners in assessing and identifying their gaps in knowledge and skills; critically appraising new information and comparing it to what they already know, can do, and perceive; asking questions to clarify, expand, and enhance knowledge and to correct misunderstandings; reflecting critically on their learning progress and achievement of expected outcomes; and using insights to continue learning. These skills are recognizably as important as the clinical knowledge, and technical and nontechnical skills required for achieving competence and expertise in radiology practice, and they must be practiced. Simulation-based education is particularly well-suited for facilitating self-directed learning skills, but teachers must be explicit in communicating to learners their expectations for learning outcomes (i.e., discipline-based content and skills) and learning behaviors.

Experiential Learning Theory

Kolb[26] conceptualized learning as a four-stage process grounded in an individual's experiences; these include concrete experience; observation during and reflection on experience to form concepts; formulation of concepts, generalizations, principles, and rules; and testing concepts, generalizations, principles, and rules in new situations/experiences. Kolb described learning as an ongoing process that could begin with any of the four stages. Traditional formats of medical education (e.g., apprenticeship approaches, internships, residency rotations) reflect opportunities for Kolb's four-stage process of doing, watching, thinking, and feeling, and incorporate both active involvement in testing and reflecting on experiences as a basis for learning and developing. The extent to which such processes are explicitly addressed and realized varies. However, when designing and using simulation-based education and training, opportunities exist to optimize learning by incorporating explicit, concrete, realistic experiences, and sufficient opportunities to test, reflect, and practice applying principles and rules during and after experiences.

Table 5.3 Education principles for designing and implementing effective teaching and learning derived from selected learning and educational theories

1. Establish and maintain an effective learning environment that is safe, respectful, and where learners can feel comfortable expressing themselves, experimenting with new experiences, learning with and from each other, and from their mistakes and misunderstandings.
2. Actively engage learners in planning content, curriculum, and appropriate teaching, learning, and assessment methods.
3. Provide ways for learners to diagnose their own learning needs to facilitate self-reflection and to engage intrinsic motivation.
4. Allow for learners to have reasonable control over their learning (e.g., formulating, selecting, or prioritizing their own learning objectives) (this fits directly with #3).
5. Involve learners in identifying or selecting resources and strategies they believe will work best for learning and achieving their objectives.
6. Engage learners to carry out their personal learning plans while providing continuous support.
7. Facilitate and engage learners in self-assessment of their learning as a means to develop their skills in critical analysis, reflective practice, and self-responsibility for continuous learning and improvement.

Constructivist Theory

Constructivist theory is another conceptual framework that can be used to optimize the effectiveness of simulation-based training (SBT) and education. This theory conceptualizes learners as active participants who use their prior knowledge and experiences to make sense of situations and create or *construct* new meanings. In the process of making new meanings, learners make decisions about when and how to modify their knowledge. Identifying and resolving inconsistencies between prior knowledge and new experiences facilitate learning through construction and reconstruction of information, skills, and perspectives. Four principles of constructivism are promoted as critical for effective teaching and learning processes: teachers are guides who facilitate learning, not transmitters of information; teachers must structure learning to help learners access appropriate and accurate prior knowledge and create opportunities for learners to identify inconsistencies between their current understandings and new experiences to facilitate construction of new meaning; learning activities must facilitate learners' active engagement in using relevant problems and situations; and sufficient time must be allocated for in-depth exploration, resolution of inconsistencies, and reflection on new experiences to construct new knowledge and understandings.[13,27–29] For some educators, adoption of this theory would require important changes in self-perceived roles and behaviors in teaching.

Within the constructivist theoretical framework, two distinct perspectives can be considered: cognitive and social. *Cognitive constructivism* emphasizes how the individual learner understands things (e.g., in terms of developmental stages and learning preferences or styles), with an emphasis placed on the mind and cognitive processes of making new meanings (e.g., Bruner).[30,31] On the other hand, *social constructivism* emphasizes the primary importance of social interactions among individuals for constructing new meaning and understanding—new knowledge. Relative to simulation-based education and training, particular attention is given to the theoretical perspectives of social constructivism, most prominently emphasized in the literature by Vygotsky.

Vygotsky[32] emphasized the critical role of interaction between the social nature of learning and what the learner brings to the situation (i.e., what one already knows and how this is shared and compared with that of others). Vygotsky argued that learning was enhanced beyond what an individual could do alone through guidance from experts and collaboration with peers and near-peers (learners who are one step ahead), particularly when the focus of teaching and learning was just beyond a learners' current level of achievement. With this in mind, he introduced a concept regarded as the *zone of proximal development* (ZPD) to represent the next step beyond current achievement, one that is challenging, but achievable with help. Another way to think about this ZPD is to define the scope of challenge or press that "stretches" the abilities of learners to progress toward independent performance. In exceeding this ZPD, the learner is stretched beyond a reasonable expectation to succeed, to a point at which the learner is wary of likely failure.

In a social constructivist learning environment, effective learning is facilitated through systematic use of modeling (e.g., expert demonstrating) and coaching (e.g., the learner practices component skills first with teacher/coach monitoring, encouragement, and assistance, and—once mastered—integrates component skills to achieve the total constellation of skills associated with a complete task or performance). As the learner develops knowledge, skills, and independent abilities, the teacher gradually reduces support and instruction until the learner can perform the task independently. These types of actions contribute to regulating difficulty level (e.g., staying within the optimal ZPD), supporting learner involvement and performance, and promoting reflection to enhance understanding and guide improvement. The systematic and purposeful use of these actions to promote learning and performance is commonly referred to as *scaffolding*.[28,33–35] By scaffolding learning, the teacher can optimize the learner's ZPD, thus providing sufficient challenge to promote growth while maintaining self-perceptions of achieving success.

Related to the important role of self-perceptions, Bandura,[36] in his own work regarding social learning theory, recognized the self-judgments that people make about their own abilities and how these influence their actions. These judgments, called *self-efficacy* may or may not be objectively accurate, but they represent the learners' self-judgments and beliefs about their abilities to deal effectively with different situations. Such beliefs are real to learners and influence how they seek, engage, and succeed in tasks. Self-efficacy is a key consideration in both design and implementation of simulation-based education and can serve a specific bridge function to actual learning and behavior change. The use of simulation-based education and training that targets the enhancement of learners' self-efficacy can contribute to enhancing learners' engagement in the real-life setting, particularly in terms of learners' seeking out new learning opportunities and persisting in their learning, even when tasks are difficult or challenging.

Bandura[36] identified four sources of information from which individuals form self-efficacy, including, in decreasing order of strength, actual achieved performance, observations of others, verbal persuasion, and physiological state. Simply said, successful experiences raise self-efficacy and failures lower it. Thus, having had prior success; observing others perform successfully with an unfamiliar task; receiving encouragement, mentoring, and coaching from teachers, near-peers, and experts (i.e., verbal persuasion); and feeling safe in the learning environment (i.e., physiological state) all influence self-efficacy and the extent to which a learner will pursue and persist with learning, even when faced with a challenging task or situation. Enhancing learners' self-efficacy (e.g., confidence or belief that one can perform successfully), targeting one's ZPD,[32] facilitating positive and productive interactions among teachers and learners (i.e., learning climate), and adopting principles of adult learning promotes engagement and persistence in learning. This is particularly important for effective simulation-based education and especially for complex, immersive, and high-fidelity simulation experiences.

Reflective Practice in Learning

The role of reflection during and after experiences is important to promoting deep learning and higher-order thinking skills and for reinforcing successful performance and improving areas in need of improvement and further development. Advances in understanding how people learn have revealed the importance of learners taking control of their own learning (i.e., self-responsibility), of which reflection is one important aspect. In learning theories that reflect adult and active learning, experiential and constructivist perspectives emphasize the aspect of thinking about, predicting, and monitoring one's thinking and learning, as has been previously noted in this chapter. Flavell[37] and Bransford et al[33] note the importance of helping learners to develop and use these metacognitive abilities. The use of reflective practice and metacognition also promotes the development of expertise and transfer of learning to everyday practice and new situations. Schon[38,39] differentiated reflective practice occurring during experiences as *reflection-in-action* and use of reflection after experiences as *reflection-on-action*. In simulation-based education and training, reflection-in-action is often facilitated by requiring learners to "think aloud" during learning activities, to make explicit their thinking and reflective processes or to provide explanations and rationales for answers, actions, and decisions. Reflection-on-action is often accomplished through individualized and team-based after-action debriefing discussions that follow SBT tasks and scenario experiences. Even preparatory briefings (e.g., at the beginning of a patient scenario) can be used to promote reflection on prior knowledge and experiences and how these apply to the new encounter. Raising awareness about the use of reflection can also encourage the use of reflection-in-action during simulation-based learning activities.

Situated Learning Theory and Communities of Practice

Lave and Wenger's[40] conception of *legitimate peripheral participation* reflects a situated learning or situated cognition theory in which learners' development is facilitated by their involvement in a *community of practice* (CoP). These theorists and others (e.g., Barab et al[41]) have described a community of practice as a sustained social network of individuals who develop and share knowledge and understandings within a set of shared norms, values, and practices (e.g., members of a profession). Lave and Wenger further conceptualized that learning is facilitated by a CoP as individuals are drawn into the interactions of its members through increasing levels of participation. For example, an individual might first engage with a professional community as an observer and from the periphery of the group. As the learner develops knowledge and skills, and becomes socialized into the CoP, he is drawn into the center of the group's activities. Thus, the CoP becomes a strong motivator for the learner to become increasingly engaged in its activities. The learner constructs new understanding and meaning through observing, doing, reflecting, and participating with others.

Learning occurs within the context of everyday practice and is not removed from the messiness of real-life; learning includes solving everyday problems, making sense through interactions with others, and benefitting from the shared knowledge, practices, and norms of the CoP. Creating simulation-based experiences that reflect such situated learning features enhances both learning and transfer of learning to practice, particularly for high-stakes and rare situations, and encourages team development and responsibility for self and others' learning and performance. Given the ever-increasing capability of communication and information technologies (e.g., discussion boards, blogs, synchronous and asynchronous group and team-based learning modules), a CoP need not be limited to geographic proximity. Thus, new possibilities exist for fostering learning from and with each other within a social network of individuals. For example, VR simulation and Internet-based simulation modules might be used with teams of radiology residents and faculty facilitators drawn from several programs.

Two other theoretical perspectives that fit well with situated and constructivist learning are *cognitive apprenticeship* and *cognitive flexibility*. Cognitive apprenticeship views learning as an interactive process between teacher and learner, in which thinking is made explicit and the learner constructs understanding from observing, reflecting, and approximating the teacher or expert cognitive processes (e.g., thinking, reasoning, rationale-building, problem-solving) (e.g., Brown et al[42]). Cognitive flexibility theory[43,44] views use of knowledge as very context dependent and is concerned with how initial learning is transferred to everyday practice through the use of many complex and ill-structured domains (e.g., medicine and solving patient problems).

Thinking and learning using many different cases require learners to restructure and adapt use of knowledge as they respond to problems and situations. For example, learning might start with one case and progress to multiple other patient cases that can be derived by changing one or more features of the initial case (e.g., "what if" variations of the case). As an illustrative example, Jonassen, Ambruso, and Olesen[45] described their use of cognitive flexibility theory to design a hypertext program on transfusion medicine, in which many different clinical cases were included for learners to diagnose and treat, using various sources of information within the program. Educational principles derived from cognitive flexibility and that can be applied to simulation-based education and training include that learning must provide multiple variations of the content; that teaching and learning must occur with learners actively engaged in using cases to construct knowledge; that learning materials should reflect rich, context-dependent stimuli for learning and avoid simplistic representation(s) of the content domain(s); and that sources from which learners can draw information should be integrative, not compartmentalized. In terms of developing simulation-based cases (e.g., for high-fidelity simulation scenarios), educators should develop rich, realistic patient presentations for the highest-level learners and then scaffold the learning to the level of the learner (i.e., one can scale back more easily than ramp up the complexity of cases for appropriate learning). The use of structured debriefings and think-aloud strategies could also be incorporated to combine principles of cognitive apprenticeship and cognitive flexibility.

The Complementarity of Mastery Learning, Mastery Teaching, and Deliberate Practice

Various theoretical perspectives described thus far coalesce around the key principles of active engagement with others, building upon prior knowledge, and constructing knowledge and new meaning that can be applied to multiple contexts and ill-structured problem situations. Flexibility and facility of thinking and multiple opportunities to practice, reflect, use feedback, and refine learning and performance emphasize teaching and learning processes to achieve mastery. Benjamin Bloom[46] introduced the *Learning for Mastery* model that was later expanded by Block and Burns[47] and termed *Mastery Learning*. Both models were based on the fundamental premise that all people can learn and master targeted outcomes; the differentiating factor was time—some people learn faster or slower than others. In the Mastery Learning model, the following fundamental features must be aligned consistently:

- Baseline, diagnostic assessment
- Clear and sequenced learning objectives reflecting increasing difficulty
- Involvement in specific objectives-based learning activities
- Established minimum "mastery" criteria for each instructional unit that must be achieved before advancing to the next unit
- Formative assessment at the end of each unit
- Corrective feedback and continued practice and learning in an instructional unit until the mastery criteria are met.

Complementary to Block and Burn's model of Mastery Learning was Madeleine Hunter's *Mastery Teaching model* of lesson design[48,49] that focused primarily on the initial teaching and learning of targeted content and skills. Included in the model were anticipatory set (i.e., motivation, readiness assessment, introduction) and statement of learning objectives; objectives-based instruction and modeling; checking for understanding (monitor and adjust teaching to support learning); guided practice (e.g., support, assistance, coaching, scaffolding); and independent practice. Incorporated into both the Mastery Learning and Mastery Teaching models were the notion of practice, focused and with specific and timely corrective feedback, and encouragement. In more recent years, this concept of practice has been further examined, particularly in regard to mastery and the development of expertise.[50,51] *Deliberate practice*, now a widely accepted term, is characterized as engagement of highly motivated learners in concentrated, intensely focused practice, guided by a clearly articulated learning objective or task that reinforces current level of abilities and stretches the learners' range of performance to advance development (similar to Vygotsky's ZPD). Focused, repetitive practice is assessed by rigorous and explicit assessment. Practice is interspersed by specific and timely feedback (from simulators or teachers)

Table 5.4 Seven evidence-based principles of effective teaching[33,53]

1. Learners' need to access sufficient and appropriate prior knowledge enhances their learning.
2. How learners organize knowledge influences how they learn and apply what they know. (e.g., strive to weave *tapestry* instead of *cheesecloth*-type neural associations among concepts, principles, generalizations).
3. Learners' motivation generates, directs, and sustains what they do to learn. (i.e., goals play a key role; both value and expectancies are critical features of motivation). Value relates to learners' interest, and perceived importance and expectancy relates to the learners' perception of the extent to which the goal is attainable (i.e., reasonable expectation).
4. To develop mastery, learners must first learn fundamental skills within a targeted domain, then practice integrating them to the point of fluency and reasonable automaticity, and finally, learn when to apply what they have learned appropriately in various contexts. (i.e., Sprague and Stuart's three elements of mastery.)[54] Sprague and Stuart also describe a novice-to-expert trajectory based on two dimensions: competence and consciousness. The two-dimensional model yields four levels of expertise: *unconscious incompetence* (i.e., unaware of errors and what one needs to know); *conscious incompetence* (i.e., aware of knowledge and skill deficiencies); *conscious competence* (i.e., aware of and attentive to necessary knowledge and skills); *unconscious competence* (i.e., knowledge and skills are integrated and automatic, doesn't require explicit attention to perform).
5. Deliberate practice (i.e., goal-directed, focused practice with specific feedback) is critical to learning. Goals direct practice, help us evaluate the observed performance, and give appropriate and specific feedback that in turn guides additional practice and achievement of goal-related performance (i.e., mastery).
6. Learners' current level of development interacts with the learning environment (e.g., social, emotional, and intellectual climate), and these features influence learning (e.g., teacher-learner, learner-learner interactions, safe climate, focused on learning with and from each other—cooperation and collaboration vs. competition). It is important to have clear communication of expectations and performance standards, and to reduce anonymity (i.e., recognition of learners and enhancing accountability, professional learning environment, reveal inconsistencies, and embrace conflict as opportunity for growth and learning).
7. To become self-directed learners, individuals must learn to assess the demands of a given task, accurately self-assess their knowledge and skills, plan how to proceed with the task, self-monitor progress, and adjust strategies as needed. (i.e., role of meta-cognition—National Research Council 2001—"process of reflecting on and directing one's own thinking" [page 78])[55]

resulting from careful monitoring to correct errors and promote continued, focused (i.e., deliberate) practice. Advancement to another task or learning objective does not occur until the preestablished mastery standard has been achieved. The continuing cycle of focused practice and focused feedback with the press for continuous improvement is most characteristic of the use of deliberate practice. The use of simulation to promote deliberate practice for achieving mastery has been shown to be among its most promising applications.[52]

In summary, what educational principles can be derived from these theories and models of learning and instruction? Table 5.4[33,53,54,55] summarizes seven key principles of effective teaching that build upon those pertaining to adult or active learning and that were summarized in Table 5.3. Together, these provide an evidence-based framework on which simulation-based educational experiences and materials can be developed and implemented.

Specific to simulation-based learning environments, Issenberg et al[56] provide results of a systematic review of the literature to answer the question, *What are the features and uses of high-fidelity medical simulations that lead to most effective learning?* This Best Evidence in Medical Education (BEME) review revealed ten key findings regarding the features and aspects of simulation teaching and learning experiences that were shown to positively influence learning. These findings provide a set of educational principles identified previously and offer specific guidance for designing and using simulation-based teaching and learning. In reviewing these findings, it was apparent that most reflected elements of instructional design, while others also reflected either organizational or individual features of simulation-based teaching and learning. Table 5.5[56,57] presents ten guiding educational principles, the percentage of articles in the study (n = 109) for which empirical evidence supported each principle, and a brief annotation. For the purposes of this chapter, the principles have been further organized according to individual/learner, instructional design, and/or organizational features that influence training effectiveness. Issenberg and colleagues developed these principles based specifically on the evidence from studies of high-fidelity simulation experiences. However, in light of the more general educational principles summarized in Tables 5.3 and 5.4, these principles are also applicable to a wide range of possible simulator types and experiences.

ADDIE: A PRACTICAL, SYSTEMATIC APPROACH TO INSTRUCTIONAL DESIGN AND IMPLEMENTATION

The ADDIE model is one approach to curriculum development that represents widely adopted principles of educational and instructional design, as summarized in Figure 5.2.[2,3,15,58] Organized into five key stages (i.e., *A*ssess, *D*esign, *D*evelop, *I*mplement, *E*valuate), the ADDIE model provides a general and systematic approach that can be used effectively for developing and refining SBT and education programs, regardless of the selected simulation technology(ies) or the extent to which they are used with more traditional instruction methods (e.g., lecture, small group discussion). Further, the ADDIE model supports curriculum development as a collaborative venture among faculty, learners, content experts, and consultants for educational design, assessment, evaluation, and other relevant aspects (e.g., technology). Particularly for education and training utilizing simulation technology, collaboration is essential to ensure that all appropriate design experts (i.e., content, technical, instructional, evaluation) and implementation stakeholders (e.g., department heads, clerkship/course/program directors, learners, practitioners, and industry partners) are engaged to facilitate positive adoption (i.e., buy-in), successful implementation, and long-term sustainability of high-quality educational programs and activities. The importance of this cannot be overstated, given the high costs (e.g., people, time, technology, and money) associated with simulation-based teaching, learning, and assessment. Applying

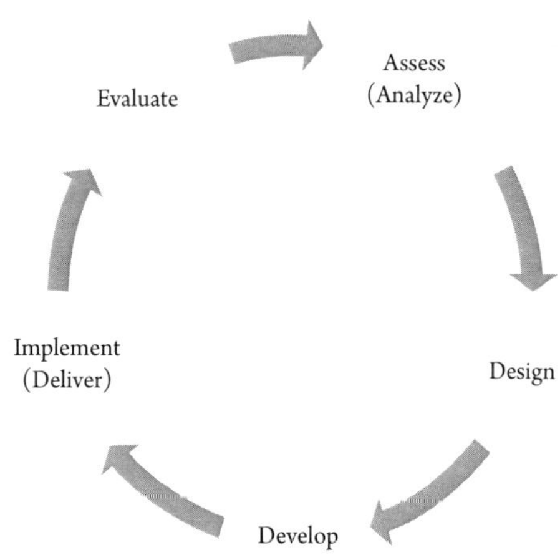

FIGURE 5.2 The ADDIE approach to curriculum and instructional design.

Table 5.5 Educational principles for designing and implementing simulation-based teaching and learning experiences using high-fidelity simulators[56,57]

EDUCATIONAL PRINCIPLE	FEATURES				ANNOTATION
	%[A]	D[B]	I	O	
1. Define specific, observable learner outcomes and benchmarks.	6	✓	✓		Learners are more likely to master expected outcomes if they are clear and appropriate for their level of learning.
2. Establish evidence of the selected simulator as a valid teaching/learning tool.	3	✓			Learning and transfer of learning to real-life practice is enhanced when the choice of simulator(s) and the simulation-based learning environment reflect an authentic approximation of the real-life complexity of situations, principles, and tasks (i.e., face validity). Doing so promotes "suspended disbelief" and learners' opportunities for meaningful hands-on experience.
3. Integrate simulation-based experiences into the overall curriculum/program (i.e., avoid stand-alone simulation-based exercises).	25	✓		✓	Simulation-based learning experiences should not be adjunctive or optional. Learners' (and faculty) are more likely to take such experiences seriously if they are integrated into the overall curriculum, performance evaluation, and the everyday educational schedules and routines. Further, simulation-based experiences should be incorporated as opportunities for deliberate practice, in addition to their engagement in actual patient care where transfer can be facilitated and reinforced.
4. Simulation-based experiences should accommodate multiple learning methods.	10	✓		✓	Identify and develop simulation-based education opportunities that fit the range of appropriate learning methods used in the curriculum (e.g., lectures, small group tutorials, independent learning/practice stations, faculty-facilitated simulation-based scenarios for individual and team learning).
5. Develop simulation-based experiences that reflect controlled learning environments.	9	✓			Simulation-based exercises should reflect "safe" learner- and learning-focused environments that take advantage of "teachable moments," learning from mistakes, and opportunities for deliberate practice.
6. Strive to use simulators that can support a wide range of patient problems and situations.	10	✓			Using simulators and simulation-based designs that can sample from a broad range of patient situations, characteristics, and problems will contribute to strengthening and standardizing curriculum and learning experiences. This can be particularly true for situations reflecting a limited range of patient exposure or rare, but important clinical situations.
7. Design and use simulations to provide standardized, reproducible experiences that can accommodate learners' individualized needs.	9	✓	✓		Effective feedback, either from teachers or via some aspect of the simulation-based design, are critical to accurate learning and avoiding faulty or erroneous learning of knowledge and skills.

(*continued*)

Table 5.5 (continued)

EDUCATIONAL PRINCIPLE	FEATURES			ANNOTATION
8. Maximize use of simulation for opportunities to engage in deliberate practice.	39	✓	✓	Creating simulation-based education and training to reflect standardized, reproducible experiences also supports opportunities for repetitive practice. However, practice needs to be focused, deliberate, and coupled with timely and specific feedback. The deliberative and repetitive cycles of practice and feedback is referred to as "deliberate practice" and are a necessary component to facilitating development of expertise.
9. As learners achieve at one level of learning, they should be progressively challenged to performance at higher levels of difficulty.	14	✓	✓	Learning is enhanced when learners can progress to higher levels of ability at their own pace. Scaffolding the level of challenge motivates and sustains learner engagement and persistence when the press for achievement is reasonable and perceived to be attainable. Simulations should be designed to accommodate systematically and consistently increasing levels of difficulty or complexity, so that learners can build upon their progress and achieve at higher levels of mastery. Although the shape of individuals' "learning curves" will vary and be influenced by their different rates and pace of learning, the long-term learning goals and the standards by which success or competency is determined remain the same for all (i.e., mastery).
10. Purposeful and effective feedback is the single most important element of simulation-based teaching and learning.	47	✓		Although feedback may be provided in a variety of ways (e.g., automatically provided via the simulator technology or provided in real time by a teacher), effective feedback should reflect several fundamental features. In many forms of simulation-based education and training, effective use of debriefing techniques can be instrumental in promoting reflective practice and effective use of feedback. Several key features of feedback are critical to assure effectiveness. Effective feedback should be specific to the individual and the task/performance, timely, and provided in a way that encourages continued effort. Effective feedback should also be given in a way that maintains learner dignity and helps the individual learn to monitor and self-assess progress toward mastery and maintenance of quality performance.

[a]Percentage of articles ($n = 109$) reviewed in Issenberg, et al. (2004, 2005)[56,57] that offered supporting evidence of important features and aspects of high-fidelity simulation that lead to effective learning.

[b]Features: D, Design; I, Individual; O, Organization

the ADDIE model as a systematic and ongoing cyclical process of development, implementation, evaluation, reflection, and refinement/expansion incorporates these processes into everyday practices of training and education and facilitates long-term use and continuous improvement. To use the expanded and cyclical ADDIE model, educators and other stakeholders engage with each other in completing the five steps or stages of curriculum and instructional design that are shown in Figure 5.2

The following paragraphs provide additional explanation.

Assess

- *Needs assessment*: Using appropriate methods, gather relevant information about specific needs, including those of learners, course/program, and school. Methods might include any combination of the following that are appropriate to the curriculum or course of interest: direct observation, survey, interviews, focus groups, review of results from learners' past performances, program accreditation standards, criteria for licensure and certification, reviews of relevant research and contributions to the professional literature, and input from stakeholders (e.g., practitioners, recipients of our learners/graduates). Needs assessment processes also target issues of resource availability, feasibility, receptivity to innovation and change, and organizational support.

Design

- *Context*: Define the educational context in which the curriculum or course will be implemented, including the learner group(s) and the context or target to which we expect the learning to transfer (e.g., specific knowledge application, competency, or desired behavior in everyday practice).
- *Goals*: Identify the major goals to be addressed by the curriculum or course. These should be clear statements of learner outcomes that require multiple steps of development or learning to achieve.
- *Learning objectives*: Develop specific, learner-centered and observable objectives (or expected learning outcomes) that fit with the major curriculum goals and will be achieved by learners completing the curriculum or course. That is, achieving a sequence of specific learning objectives leads to the achievement of a learning goal. Educators should consider what will be the primary, secondary, and tertiary learning objectives to be addressed by the simulation-based experience(s). The process of developing goals and objectives will help to identify the learning context that will be best for achieving the intended education and training outcomes. Further, basing simulation scenarios on real-life experiences, rather than on hypothetical ones, will facilitate decisions about the type(s) of simulator, simulation-based format, and specific case distracters that are necessary to achieve an optimal level of realism that facilitates learners' suspended disbelief and assures an effective learning experience. For further discussion of the various types of learning objectives and how these can enhance the effectiveness of simulation-based education experiences, please see Kozmenko et al.[59]
- *Assessment*: Early in the instructional design process, envision how learning goals and intended objectives/outcomes can be assessed. Develop the assessment framework and define assessment methods for evaluating both processes and outcomes appropriate to the goal(s) and learning objectives. For example, acquisition of factual knowledge might be assessed best through a multiple-choice test. However, assessing basic competency for angioplasty with vascular stenting or ultrasound-guided central line might be best accomplished through direct observation by trained assessors during mannequin-based or VR simulation, and/or, at the appropriate time, during real-life patient cases. Observation-based performance criteria, valid and reliable tools (including observer training and calibration), and endorsed standard setting for successful performance are also essential elements of assessment development. As the education and training experience, materials, and activities are developed, it will be necessary to revisit the assessment aspects of instructional design to finalize details and instrumentation, establish appropriate evidence of validity and reliability, and prepare assessors adequately. Doing so will ensure a good fit between teaching, learning, and evaluating. (For additional information pertaining to assessment, please refer to chapter 6 (Assessment in Simulation).
- *Facilitators*: Identify individual and organizational features that can facilitate or support the curriculum or course.
- *Obstacles*: Identify potential challenges and obstacles, and realistic coping strategies to address and overcome them. Like facilitators, these can occur at the individual and organizational levels.
- *Content*: Define the core content to be addressed (e.g., competencies, best practices, breadth and depth) and design the content structure (e.g., scope and sequence) appropriate to the learner group and the goals, objectives, and educational setting. Specify any prerequisite experiences, knowledge, or skills that are required for success in the curriculum/course, and assure that there is sufficient opportunity for learners to achieve these prior to the planned simulation-based experience.

Develop

- *Methods*: Identify and develop methods and associated activities for the teaching and learning process and for conducting formative and summative assessments, including the sequence and timing of these activities. Carefully plan scenarios and how these progress systematically to achieve standardized implementation from one occasion to the next. For example, for immersive, scenario-based, high-fidelity simulations, writing a thumbnail sketch of the real patient scenario (e.g., a one-page story) and then using this with the objectives to create a storyboard of the various scenes are important first steps to developing the educational experience or training session. (For expanded and practical discussion of these design features, please see chapters in Section XIV of Kyle and Murray).[60]

- *Resources and materials*: Develop teaching, learning, and assessment materials. Acquire necessary resources for implementation (e.g., equipment, supplies, space, personnel, technology, finances, administrative and implementation support). For example, when developing and refining the storyboard for a scenario-based simulation session, educators can simultaneously create a materials list of the various audio, video, digital files (e.g., heart and lung sounds, X-rays, CT and MRI scans, etc.), equipment, clinical and nonclinical props, actors, and so on that will be needed for each scene and the progressive disclosure of patient information and events within the scenario. Using real-life patient cases can facilitate acquisition of the images, sounds, and props needed to support appropriate levels of realism for learning and assessment. Just as the scenario needs to be carefully planned, so does the after-action reflection, which is often facilitated through a structured or semi-structured debriefing discussion. This component is where considerable learning, insight, and commitment to expanded learning and practice occurs, and it must not be left to chance. For a discussion about the debriefing environment and a tool to assess the quality of debriefing discussions, Gururaja Paragi et al[61] is a useful reference.

Implement

- *Pilot study*: Conduct a pilot or field test of the simulation-based curriculum or module, including assessment procedures (typically, a small-scale implementation).
- *Refine and finalize*: Use results of the pilot study to make necessary adjustments or refinements to the curriculum, scenarios, context features, and supporting materials (e.g., cases, scenarios, curriculum materials, assessment instruments). Pilot study results can also be particularly helpful in refining prompts and trigger questions for the introductory briefing at the beginning of a session (e.g., setting ground rules) and for debriefing discussions that occur after a simulation experience. Finalizing a facilitator guide and any written or onscreen directions for learners is an important component of assuring that full implementation will proceed in a standardized way.
- *Implement*: Implement the full-scale curriculum, course, or training session or series.

Evaluate

- Conduct assessments of learner performance (individual and cohort) and program effectiveness.
- Examine formative and summative results in terms of intended processes and outcomes of the educational program (i.e., program evaluation).
- More attention and detail are given to evaluation in chapter 6 (Assessment in Simulation).
- Provide feedback to faculty, learners, and other stakeholders.
- Use results and feedback process to identify areas in need of redesign, refinement, and/or expansion. It is important to include all relevant stakeholders in the use of evaluation results for both formative (i.e., improvement) and summative (i.e., decision-making) purposes.
- Repeat the ADDIE cycle to achieve desired enhancement and/or expansion.

Quality as Scholarship of Teaching and Learning

Six attributes of scholarship have been widely adopted by the medical education community, and these provide an additional set of criteria by which educators can assess and assure high quality in curriculum and instruction. Now commonly referred to as the *Glassick criteria*, the criteria provide a basis of quality in the design, assessment, and ongoing refinement of both educational materials and processes in simulation-based education and training.[5,62–64] The six attributes and associated guiding questions are as follows:

- *Clear goals*: Have you clearly defined the purpose(s)? Have you taken into account important questions regarding teaching and learning processes? Are the objectives realistic and achievable for the targeted learner group and allotted time frame?

- *Adequate preparation*: How does the training/education demonstrate an understanding of relevant literature and best practices (both in terms of disciplinary content and teaching, learning, and/or assessment methods)? How has the work been influenced from prior experiences, knowledge, and skills (e.g., previous implementation of the same or similar training or curriculum, educator knowledge and skills related to both content and educational practices)? How have you assured sufficient and appropriate resources (e.g., expertise, personnel, equipment, technological support, time, learner preparation)?
- *Appropriate methods*: Do the selected methods fit the purpose, goals and objectives, and teaching/learning context? Are the methods used effectively? How have methods been modified to accommodate situational changes (e.g., setting, timing, coordination with other prior and subsequent educational experiences)? Is/are the appropriate simulator(s) being used? To what extent does an optimal fit exist between intended learning outcomes, the *fidelity* of simulators, and the overall simulation-based experience?
- *Significant results*: To what extent has the training/education achieved or exceeded goals and objectives? How does the work contribute substantially to others (e.g., learners and colleagues) and to the field? What are the specific forms of evidence (quantitative and qualitative)? How are the results used to promote exploration, expansion, and enhancement at the individual/learner, group, and total cohort levels (e.g., by self, by others, collaboratively with others)?
- *Effective presentation*: How is the education/training presented to others (e.g., learners and faculty) for orientation and preparation for expected roles and to assure quality implementation? How are the results of the education/training presented to others (e.g., learners and faculty) for assessing and facilitating continuous improvements at the learner, group, and program levels? Are the presentations clear, unambiguous, and appropriate for the intended audience(s)? Is the work presented in a way that others can use or build upon it?
- *Reflective critique*: Individually and with colleagues and/or learners, what processes are used to examine the extent to which education/training and/or assessment processes and intended outcomes are realized? How are evaluation results used to refine and expand teaching and learning? Has there been reflection and reflective collaboration with others to examine why or why not? How does the education training and/or assessment fit within the larger relevant context? How might this work contribute to the program, school, and/or professional field? How can you, the faculty, or colleagues build upon this work?

CONCLUSION

In summary, a wide range of simulators and simulation methods is available for enhancing radiology education. Among the most prominent principles of best educational practices is that instructional design matters beyond the choice of technology. A recent report by Issenberg[65] revealed that best outcomes of simulation-based education will be achieved when multiple simulation-based components and different types of simulator technology are integrated with the overall educational program or curriculum (i.e., not as stand-alone, adjunct, or supplemental options for learning). In fact, Issenberg observed two major flaws in contemporary practices in simulation-based education: the lack of faculty development efforts to assure that faculty members are well-prepared as teachers to use and maximize the educational potential of chosen simulators and simulation-based methods, and the separateness or isolation of simulation-based educational components from the rest of the curriculum and educational program. Simulation should be used to complement learners' professional education and success in actual patient care. In the case of radiology education, the complementarity of simulation might be achieved at various levels of learning and within multiple contexts (e.g., introduction, preparation, verification of minimum competency for actual patient care, practice of rare or crisis situations). Adopting Bloom's taxonomy and constructivist views of learning and instruction, applying a systematic process to designing education (e.g., ADDIE model), selecting teaching methods that reflect mastery learning and deliberate practice, and using the Glassick criteria to assure overall educational quality are among the key components necessary for achieving success in simulation-based radiology education.

FOR FURTHER READING

In addition to the models and educational principles presented, this selective list of recommended readings can further facilitate the design and implementation of SBT for radiologic applications.

1. Chauvin SW. Disseminating research and implementing change. In: Norman GR, van der

Vleuten CPM, Newble DI, eds. *International Handbook of Research in Medical Education, Vol. II,* Chapter 32. Dordrecht, The Netherlands: Kluwer Academic Publishers; 2002:997–1038.

This chapter provides a comprehensive review of theoretical frameworks and practical strategies for using the results of research and evaluation in facilitating successful innovation and change. It includes an extensive list of relevant reference citations.

2. Cooke M, Irby DM, O'Brien BC. *Educating Physicians. A Call for Reform of Medical School and Residency.* The Carnegie Foundation for the Advancement of Teaching, Preparation for the Professions. San Francisco: Jossey-Bass; 2010.

This book summarizes an extensive study of physician education by the Carnegie Foundation for the Advancement of Teaching. The book addresses the major issues faced in physician education today. In addition to its findings and recommendations, the book provides multiple, context-specific examples of many of the theoretical frameworks and educational principles reflected in this chapter and is a useful resource for further reading and thinking about the role, design, and use of simulation-based education and training in radiology education for the future.

3. Custers EJFM, Boshuizen HPA. The Psychology of Learning. In: Norman GR, Van der Vleuten CPM, Newble DI, eds. *International Handbook of Research in Medical Education,* Chapter 5. Dordrecht, The Netherlands: Kluwer Academic Publishers; 2002:163–203.

This is an excellent summary of the research and resulting theoretical perspectives on the psychology of learning. The authors discuss these perspectives particularly in terms of their application to and relevance for medical education.

4. Issenberg SB, McGaghie WC, Petrusa ER, et al. *BEME Guide no. 4: Features and Uses of High-Fidelity Medical Simulations That Lead to Effective Learning.* Dundee, UK: Association for Medical Education in Europe; 2004.

Commissioned by the Best Evidence in Medical Education (BEME) collaborative, this systematic review of the literature pertaining to simulation provides a comprehensive review and discussion of evidence-based features and uses of high-fidelity simulation for teaching and learning. At the time of this literature review, most published reports identified did not reflect empirical studies. In fact, only 109 of the 670 articles met the inclusion criteria for this review. Specific guidelines based on the findings of the 109 articles included in the review are provided and discussed in terms of future use of simulators in teaching and learning processes and the implications for future research. A summary of the complete report was also published in *Medical Teacher* 2005;27:10–28.

5. Kyle RR Jr., Murray WB. *Clinical Simulation: Operations, Engineering, and Management.* Burlington, MA: Academic Press; 2008.

This book includes an extensive array of chapters targeting theoretical perspectives, educational design principles, teaching strategies specific to simulation-based learning environments, and the practical matters related to designing, implementing, and sustaining clinical simulation (e.g., use of props, technology for simulating various clinical scenarios, use of audio and video technology), and assessment and research considerations. This is an excellent resource for exploring in greater depths many of the educational principles highlighted in this chapter, for which page limits constrained the level of detail and discussion.

REFERENCES

1. Patel AA, Gould DA. Simulators in interventional radiology training and evaluation: a paradigm shift is on the horizon. *J Vasc Intervent Radiol.* 2006;17:S163–S173.

2. Goldstein IL. *Training in Organizations,* 3rd edition. Pacific Grove, CA: Brooks/Cole; 1993.

3. Kraiger K. *Creating, Implementing, and Managing Effective Training and Development: State-of-the-Art Lessons for Practice.* San Francisco: Jossey Bass; 2002.

4. Rothwell WJ, Butler MN, Hunt DL, et al. *The Handbook of Training Technologies: An Introductory Guide to Facilitating Learning with Technology—From Planning to Evaluation, Instructional Technology and Training Series.* San Francisco: John Wiley and Sons; 2006.

5. Glassick CE, Huber MT, Maeroff GI. *Scholarship Assessed: Evaluation of the professoriate,* An Ernest L. Boyer Project of the Carnegie Foundation for the Advancement of Teaching. San Francisco: Jossey-Bass Publishers; 1997.

6. Fincher RM, Lewis LL. Simulations Used to Teach Clinical Skills. In: Norman GR, Van der Vleuten CPM, Newble DI, eds. *International Handbook of Research in Medical Education,* Chapter 16. Dordrecht, The Netherlands: Kluwer Academic Publishers; 2002:499–535.

7. McGaghie WC. Simulation in professional competence assessment: Basic considerations. In: Tekian A, McGuire CH, McGaghie WC, eds. *Innovative Simulations for Assessing Professional Competence.* Department of Medical Education, University of Illinois at Chicago; 1999:7–22.

8. Meller G. A typology of simulators for medical education. *J Digital Imag.* 1997;10(3Suppl1): 194–196.

9. Barrows H. A taxonomy of problem based learning methods. *Med Educ.*1986;20:481–486.

10. Ker J, Bradley P. Simulation in Medical Education. In: T. Swanwick, *Understanding Medical Education Series.* Edinburgh, UK: Association for the Study of Medical Education; 2007.

11. Kneebone R. Simulation in surgical training: Educational issues and practical implications. *Med Educ.* 2003;37:267–277.

12. Maran NJ, Glavin RJ. Low- to high-fidelity simulation—a continuum of medical education? *Med Educ.* 2003;37(Suppl 1):22–28.

13. Mayer RE. Applying the science of learning to medical education. *Med Educ.* 2010;44:543–549.

14. Grant J. Principles of Curriculum Design. In: T. Swanwick, ed. *Understanding Medical Education Series.* Edinburgh, UK: Association for the Study of Medical Education; 2006.

15. Diamond RM *Designing and Improving Courses and Curricula in Higher Education.* San Francisco: Jossey-Bass; 1989.

16. Reigeluth CM, ed. *Instructional-Design Theories and Models: A New Paradigm of Instructional Theory, Vol. II.* Mahwah, NJ: Lawrence Erlbaum Associates; 1999.

17. Reigeluth CM, Carr-Chellman AA, eds. *Instructional-Design Theories and Models: Building a Common Knowledge Base, Vol. III.* New York: Routledge; 2009.

18. Sitzmann T, Kraiger K, Stewart D, et al. The comparative effectiveness of web-based and classroom instruction: a meta-analysis. *Personnel Psychol.* 2006;59:623–664.

19. Custers EJFM, Boshuizen HPA. The Psychology of Learning. In: Norman GR, Van der Vleuten CPM, Newble DI, eds. *International Handbook of Research in Medical Education,* Chapter 5. Dordrecht, The Netherlands: Kluwer Academic Publishers; 2002:163–203.

20. Bloom B, Engelhart MD, Furst EJ, et al. *Taxonomy of Educational Objectives: Handbook 1, The Cognitive Domain.* New York: Longman; 1956.

21. Anderson LW, Krathwohl DR, eds. *A Taxonomy for Learning, Teaching, and Assessing: A Revision of Bloom's Taxonomy of Educational Objectives.* New York: Longman; 2001.

22. Miller GE. The assessment of clinical skills/competence/performance. *Acad Med.* 1990;65: S63–S67.

23. Kirkpatrick DL. *Evaluating Training Effectiveness: The Four Levels.* San Francisco: Bennett-Koehler; 1994.

24. Knowles M, Nadler L, Nadler Z. *Andragogy in Action: Applying Modern Principles of Adult Learning.* San Francisco: Jossey-Bass; 1984.

25. Candy PC. *Self-direction for Lifelong Learning: A Comprehensive Guide to Theory and Practice.* San Francisco: Jossey-Bass; 1991.

26. Kolb DA. *Experiential Learning: Experience as the Source of Learning and Development.* Englewood Cliffs, NJ: Prentice-Hall; 1984.

27. Kaufmann DM, Mann KV, Jennett P. Teaching and Learning in Medical Education: How Theory Can Inform Practice. In: Swanwick T, ed. *Understanding Medical Education Series.* London, UK: Association for the Study of Medical Education; 2000.

28. Jonassen D. Designing Constructivist Learning Environments. In: Reigeluth CM, ed. *Instructional-Design Theories and Principles, Vol. II,* Chapter 10. Mahwah, NJ: Lawrence Erlbaum Associates; 1999:215–239.

29. Kaufmann DM. Applying Educational Theory in Practice. In: Cantillon P, Hutchinson L, Wood D, eds. *ABC of Learning and Teaching in Medicine,* 2nd edition, Chapter 1. London, England: BMJ Books; 2010:1–4.

30. Bruner J. *The Process of Education.* Cambridge, MA: Harvard University Press; 1960.

31. Bruner J. *Toward a Theory of Education.* Cambridge, MA: Harvard University Press; 1966.

32. Vygotsky LS. *Mind in Society: The Development of Higher Psychological Processes.* Cambridge, MA: The Harvard University Press; 1978. (Originally published New York: Oxford University Press; 1930).

33. Bransford JD, Brown AL, Cocking RR. How *People Learn: Brain, Mind, Experience, and School.* Washington, DC: National Academy Press; 2000.

34. Wood DJ, Middleton R. A study of assisted problem-solving. *Br J Psychol.* 1975;66:181–191.

35. Wood DJ. *How Children Think and Learn,* 2nd edition. Oxford: Blackwell Publishers, Ltd.; 1998.

36. Bandura A. *Social Foundations of Thought and Action: A Social Cognitive Theory.* Englewood Cliffs, NJ: Prentice Hall; 1986.

37. Flavell JH. Metacognitive aspects of problem-solving. In: Resnick L, ed. *The Nature of Intelligence.* Hillsdale, NJ: Erlbaum; 1976:231–236.

38. Schon DA. *The Reflective Practitioner: How Professionals Think.* New York: Basic Books; 1983.

39. Schon DA. *Educating the Reflective Practitioner: Toward a New Design for Teaching and Learning in the Professions.* San Francisco: Jossey-Bass; 1987.

40. Lave J, Wenger E. *Situated Learning: Legitimate Peripheral Participation.* Cambridge, UK: Cambridge University Press; 1991.

41. Barab SA, Barnett M G, Squire K. Building a community of teachers: navigating the essential tensions in practice. *J Learn Sci.* 2002;11:489–547.

42. Brown JS, Collins A, Duguid P. Situated cognition and the culture of learning. *Educ Res.* 1989;18:32–41.

43. Spiro RJ, Coulson RL, Feltovich PJ, et al. *Cognitive Flexibility Theory: Advanced Knowledge Acquisition in Ill-Structured Domains.* Technical Report No. 441. University of Illinois at Urbana-Champaign, Champaign, IL: Center for the Study of Reading; 1988.

44. Spiro RJ, Jehng J. Cognitive Flexibility and Hypertext: Theory and Technology for the Non-linear and Multidimensional Traversal of Complex Subject Matter. In: Nix D, Spiro R, eds. *Cognition, Education, and Multimedia.* Hillsdale, NJ: Erlbaum; 1990: 163–205.

45. Jonassen DH, Ambruso DR, Olesen J. Designing a hypertext on transfusion medicine using cognitive flexibility theory. *J Educ Hypermedia Multimedia.* 1992;1:309–322.

46. Bloom B. Mastery Learning. In: Block JH, ed. *Mastery Learning: Theory and Practice.* New York: Holt, Rinehart & Winston; 1971:47–63.

47. Block JH, Burns RH. Mastery Learning. In: Shulman LS, ed. *Review of Research in Education,* Vol. 4. Itasca, IL: Peacock; 1971:3–49.

48. Hunter MC. Teaching is decision-making. *Educ Leadership.* 1979;37:62–67.

49. Hunter MC. *Mastery Teaching.* El Segundo, CA: TIP Press; 1982.

50. Ericcson KA, Krampe RT, Tesch-Römer C. The role of deliberate practice in the acquisition of expert performance. *Psychol Rev.* 1993;100:363–406.

51. Ericcson KA. Deliberate practice and the acquisition and maintenance of expert performance in medicine and related domains. *Acad Med.* 2004;79:S70–S81.

52. Ericcson KA. An expert-performance perspective of research on medical expertise: the study of clinical performance. *Med Educ.* 2007;41:1124–1130.

53. Ambrose SA, Bridges MW, DiPietro M, et al. *How Learning Works: Seven Research-Based Principles for Smart Teaching.* San Francisco: Jossey-Bass; 2010.

54. Sprague J, Stuart D. *The Speaker's Handbook.* Fort Worth: Harcourt Publishers; 2000.

55. Zimmerman BJ, Schunk DH (eds). Self-regulated Learning and Academic Achievement: Theoretical Perspectives. Second Edition. Mahwah, NJ: Erlbaum; 2001.

56. Issenberg SB, McGaghie WC, Petrusa ER, et al. Features and uses of high-fidelity medical simulations that lead to effective learning. *Med Teacher.* 2005;27:10–28.

57. Issenberg SB, McGaghie WC, Petrusa ER, et al. *BEME Guide no. 4: Features and Uses of High-Fidelity Medical Simulations that Lead to Effective Learning.* Dundee, UK: Association for Medical Education in Europe; 2004.

58. Rothwell WJ, Kazanas HC. *Mastering the Instructional Design Process: A Systematic Approach,* 2nd edition. San Francisco: Jossey-Bass; 1998.

59. Kozmenko VV, Kaye AD, Morgan B, Hilton, CW. Theory and Practice of Developing an Effective Simulation-Based Clinical Curriculum. In: Kyle RR Jr., Murray WB, eds. *Clinical Simulation: Operations, Engineering, and Management.* Burlington, MA: Academic Press; 2008:135–152.

60. Kyle RR Jr, Murray WB. *Clinical Simulation: Operations, Engineering, and Management.* Burlington, MA: Academic Press; 2008.

61. Paragi R, Yang T, Paige J, Chauvin SW. Examining the effectiveness of debriefing at the point of care in simulation-based operating room team/ training. *Advances in Patient Safety: New Directions and Alternative Approaches, Vol. 3. Performance and Tools.* AHRQ, 2008. Publication No. 08-0034-3. Retrieved from http://www.ahrq.gov/downloads/pub/advances2/vol3/Advances-Gururaja_7.pdf

62. Boyer EL. *Scholarship Reconsidered: Priorities of the Professoriate.* Princeton, NJ: The Carnegie Foundation for the Advancement of Teaching; 1990.

63. Glassick CE. Boyer's expanded definitions of scholarship, the standards for assessing scholarship, and the elusiveness of the scholarship of teaching. *Acad Med.* 2000;75:877–880.

64. Association of American Medical Colleges. *Advancing Educators and Education: Defining the Components and Evidence of Educational Scholarship.* Summary Report and Findings of the Group on Educational Affairs Consensus Conference on Educational Scholarship, 2007. Retrieved from https://services.aamc.org/publications/index.cfm?fuseaction=Product.displayForm&prd_id=196&cfid=1&cftoken=2EEBC846-0397–03E9-BB08F5094BE60D9D

65. Issenberg SB. The scope of simulation-based healthcare education. *Simul Healthc.* 2006;1: 203–208.

6

Assessment in Simulation

SHEILA W. CHAUVIN

TEACHING, LEARNING, and assessment are interactive and dynamic components of quality education. Educators are often drawn to the use of simulation—given the level of realism that is possible—but the evidence of what *works* in simulation is still limited. The quality of assessment instruments and procedures directly impact the usability of results for determining learners' abilities, providing feedback, examining the effectiveness of training and education (including simulation-based methods), and making decisions about ongoing improvements and resource allocations. Designing and using assessment in simulation-based education (SBE) is tedious, time-consuming, and expensive, given the necessary areas of expertise in domain-specific content, instrument development, measurement, statistical analysis, educational development and change, and knowledge in simulation-based theatrical perspectives that are also important.

Given the broad scope of assessment and evaluation, this chapter focuses on a set of fundamental concepts and principles in assessment and evaluation. Specific references are made to information presented in chapter 5 (Educational Principles in Simulation) on educational principles that is also relevant to assessment (e.g., simulators, simulation formats, and conceptual frameworks). Its intention is to serve as a reference for addressing and designing assessment and evaluation components for SBE in the field of radiology. The chapter concludes with several recommended sources for further reading.

ASSESSMENT AND SIMULATION

Assessment has an important role in SBE, and, likewise, simulation technologies can contribute to enhancing the effectiveness of assessment in certain situations. In SBE, assessments can be accomplished with and without the use of simulators and simulation formats. For example, assessments of factual and applied knowledge taught and learned using SBE and training can be accomplished with written knowledge tests (e.g., multiple-choice or constructed response items), oral case discussions, computer-based simulation options (e.g., video patient cases, part-task trainer exercises), or high-fidelity simulation-based scenarios. Assessments of technical and nontechnical (i.e., combined cognitive and interpersonal) skills can be assessed by trained observers during actual patient care or by using a set of standardized simulation-based scenarios or stations in either a simulation center or in the clinical environment as an in situ simulation-based assessment.

Simulation can be used to enhance the measurement qualities of assessments, particularly those targeting higher-order abilities and the verification of readiness and competency for providing actual patient care. For example, assessments can be designed to use specific simulators and simulation formats to examine the extent to which learners have achieved particular knowledge, skills, and attitudes (KSAs) targeted by non-SBE components. For example, after a series of lectures and/or small-group case discussions, an assessment of learners' abilities to synthesize clinical content and skills might include a set of computer-based simulation stations in which they diagnose "patients" and make clinical decisions based on their medical records and/or specific radiologic and laboratory tests. Such simulation-based assessment tasks are sometimes referred to as physician "in-basket" assessments or objective structured clinical examinations (OSCEs). Simulation-based assessments might also be used to verify individuals' minimum competency in a particular domain or for a particular skill before allowing them to advance in the educational program or to assume particular responsibilities (e.g., taking night call in the reading room, performing image-guided biopsies on patients). Similarly, assessing knowledge and skills for high-stakes or rare situations may not be feasible in the real-life setting, but simulation-based assessments could offer a reasonable alternative for verifying competence. Regardless of whether simulation is used in a learner assessment, key questions involving who, what, when, how, and why should be considered. When assessments involve simulation, it is important to remember that a simulation can never completely mimic real life, but can only approximate it. Therefore, the level of both physical (i.e., engineering) and functional (i.e., psychological) fidelity needs to be considered in terms of what is necessary and sufficient for achieving the goal of a particular assessment.[1–3] Fortunately, a set of fundamental concepts and strategies can be used to guide effectively the design and implementation of assessment instruments, as well as the use of results for making decisions about learners and programs.

ASSESSMENT CONCEPTS, STRATEGIES, AND TOOLS

Even though the terms "assessment" and "evaluation" are often used synonymously, they are, in fact, distinct yet closely related concepts. Understanding the similarities and differences between these terms facilitates making good decisions about the who, what, how, when, and why of selecting, designing, and using assessment. Other concepts that are fundamental to designing and implementing quality assessment and evaluation instruments include formative versus summative assessment, normative versus criterion-related assessment, and performance assessment versus program evaluation. Each pair of terms is discussed briefly in the following paragraphs to highlight essential assessment principles, strategies, and tools.

Assessment Versus Evaluation

At the simplest level, assessment refers to the specific measurements, tools, and procedures used to gather systematically information about a learner, team, program, or other object of interest.[4–6] Within an SBE program, a comprehensive learner assessment might include each of the following: direct observation of a learner's performance using a detailed checklist, a written test targeting factual and applied knowledge, a set of assessment stations using simulators and/or standardized patients in a simulation center that includes observation checklists and some performance data collected automatically by a simulator, and an unannounced standardized simulation scenario conducted in the actual clinical environment (i.e., in situ) using similar observation checklists and simulator-captured performance data.

The concept of evaluation reflects judgments at specific points in time when all relevant assessment results are gathered and compared to preestablished criteria or standards for the purposes of making decisions about the merit, worthiness, or outcomes achievement of a learner, team, program, or other object of interest.[5,7] Evaluation is commonly used to reflect curriculum- or program-level examination and decisions. In education, however, particularly in North America, the term evaluation is frequently used interchangeably with assessment and to reflect the decision-making points in both student assessment and program evaluation.[8] For the purpose of clarity in this chapter, the term *assessment* reflects the processes and decisions about learner-specific performance. The term *evaluation* reflects program-specific processes and decisions that sometimes involve the use of aggregated learner assessment results (e.g., a class or cohort) to answer one or more questions about a course curriculum or degree program. Consequently, in this context, assessment fits within the larger category of evaluation.[9]

Clarifying the relationship between learner assessments and program evaluation contributes to determining how assessments and resulting decisions should be incorporated into training and educational program designs. Situating the consequences of assessment and evaluation for individuals and groups within the larger context of educational program and professional practice is also important. For example, performance on the United States Medical Licensing Examinations (USMLE) Step 3 has multiple consequences for learners (e.g., enrollment and advancement in residency, graduation, credentialing). Performance on this examination at the cohort level also reflects consequences for a given educational program (e.g., recruitment, curriculum, accreditation status).

Therefore, to achieve effective learner assessment and educational program evaluation, educators must agree upon the purpose(s), expected learning outcomes, achievement standards, and tools and processes for assessing sufficient samples of the targeted knowledge, behaviors/skills (technical and nontechnical), and affective abilities. Educators must also determine what needs to be done to assure that accurate and dependable assessment results are obtained (e.g., well-designed and verified assessments, trained assessors) and analyzed at appropriate times to determine progress and achievement of established criteria. In defining expectations and using criteria, educators must consider carefully why assessment is being done and determine whether assessment results are of equal importance or if some type of weighting protocol is needed to accurately represent the expected competencies and educational outcomes.[5,6,10]

Formative Versus Summative Assessment

Freeman and Lewis[5] address the question, *Why are you doing assessment?* in terms of *formative* and *summative* purposes. The primary purpose of formative assessment is to produce specific, data-based *feedback* regarding how learning and performance are progressing toward expected levels of achievement. For example, a detailed assessment checklist of required behaviors or technical skills that are directly observed would provide the necessary descriptive and diagnostic information for giving specific, focused feedback to learners as they engage in deliberate and focused practice toward mastery.[11–14] Formative assessments typically use informal, ungraded methods that are embedded within teaching and learning activities and that reflect low-inference measurement (e.g., assessment of directly observed, specific behavior) and low-stakes consequences (e.g., decisions impact current, specific performance and not global or long-term academic status). In contrast, summative assessment is used to make data-based decisions about whether a learner is ready to perform or advance to the next level of education or professional practice. Typically, summative assessments represent formal, graded activities that are separate from teaching/learning activities, and they reflect high-inference measurement (i.e., combined abilities, multiple steps or performances) and high-stakes consequences for individuals (e.g., pass/fail, licensure, certification). Typically, summative assessments can also contribute to overall program evaluation (e.g., promotion rates, graduation rates, internal review, accreditation).[15]

Selecting and designing quality assessment starts with being clear about the purposes and intentions for which you will use assessment results. For example, a mid-year assessment might compare a learner's performance on a knowledge test, clinical performance assessment, and a set of simulation-based procedural assessments to a set of preestablished benchmarks or criteria for determining satisfactory progress and providing feedback to the learner (i.e., formative assessment). The same or a highly similar set of assessment activities could be used at both mid-year and year-end to support educational effectiveness and learner success. At the cohort and program level, such a semi-annual assessment process would reflect program evaluation for formative and summative purposes, respectively.

Other features can be designed within formative and summative assessments to address important aspects of achievement criteria. For example, formative and summative assessments can be designed as *announced* or *unannounced* activities, depending on the purposes and targeted abilities. Announced assessments are designed to produce evidence of the extent to which individuals or groups/teams can demonstrate goal-based knowledge, skills, and affective abilities (i.e., *can do* or demonstrate best abilities). Unannounced assessment activities target the extent to which individuals regularly demonstrate knowledge, skills and affective abilities (i.e., *do/choose to do* or demonstrate normative or everyday abilities). Unannounced assessments are more typical of summative than formative purposes, including assessment of the extent to which objectives-based learning has transferred from training to everyday practice. These types of assessments can contribute to decisions about individual achievement and program effectiveness.

Norm-Referenced Versus Criterion-Referenced Assessment

The terms *norm-referenced* and *criterion-referenced* assessment might be familiar. In general, norm-referenced assessments are based on comparing an individual's performance to that of others who also completed the assessment (e.g., percentile rank or a standard score). For example, assessments using standardized knowledge tests for medical licensure and specialty board certifications are based on norm-referenced criteria. In contrast, criterion-referenced assessments compare an individual's performance to a preestablished set of mastery criteria, instead of to the performance of other test takers. Although norm-referenced assessments could be developed and used in SBE, criterion-referenced assessments are more typical. Regardless of approach, standards need to be set. A discussion of standard setting methods is not possible with the space limitations of this chapter, but Yudkowsky, Downing, and Tekian[16] provide an excellent introduction and overview of several common methods.

Performance Assessment Versus Program Evaluation

When designing assessment, consider both the learners and the program as a whole. Performance assessment is related to the individual learner (e.g., for procedural competency) or the group/team (e.g., for teamwork effectiveness), as determined appropriate for the targeted educational learning objectives and goals. Performance assessments are typically differentiated from knowledge assessments (e.g., multiple-choice tests) and include systematic assessments of observed performance (e.g., skills/behaviors) or products of specific performance (e.g., projects, papers, portfolios). A wide variety of methods are available and can include direct observations of performance in real or simulated situations, acquisition of outcome data automatically captured by simulators or derived from chart review for real-life practice, and examination of products generated by the learner (e.g., learning portfolio, project, model, case write-up, or interpretive report).[10,17,18] The use of simulators and simulation-based formats can be particularly effective for assessing learners' applied knowledge and the simultaneous demonstration of technical/procedural proficiencies, thinking skills, and decision-making effectiveness across different situations (see chapter 5 [Educational Principles in Simulation] for additional explanation). Although knowledge tests (e.g., faculty-developed or standardized examinations) are not typically considered performance-based assessments,[6] when they are structured to solicit individuals' applied knowledge (e.g., patient scenarios, interpretation of a computed tomography [CT] scan, use of patient information, and results of diagnostic tests to make clinical decisions), they do indeed represent a form of low-fidelity simulation-based assessment. In such instances, these types of knowledge tests can be used for preparatory/readiness to learn, formative, and summative purposes.[10,19] Table 6.1 summarizes a set of common guidelines for developing and using performance-based assessments.

Program evaluation, as mentioned previously, involves the use of aggregated learner assessments within or across program periods. Depending on the selected assessment data, evaluation of program quality can be examined in terms of implementation processes (i.e., formative component) and the achievement of program-related goals or outcomes (i.e., summative component). A wide variety of conceptual frameworks and approaches are available for conducting program evaluation.[20–22] Although a discussion of program evaluation models and methods is beyond the scope of this chapter, considering how learner assessments might also support program evaluation needs (e.g., cohort mean scores on a knowledge test, a set of simulation-based skills stations) should be included when designing specific assessments to maximize use of precious time, resources, and expertise. Consultation with education evaluation experts is highly recommended to maximize the use of learner assessment in educational program evaluation.

Table 6.1 Guidelines for developing and using performance-based assessments

STAGE	ACTIVITIES
Predevelopment	Analyze and establish purposes and goals. Design an assessment plan or blueprint: • Fit assessment types to objectives (e.g., formats, low- vs. high-inference). • Describe assessment types and implementation/administration procedures. • Identify resources needed up front and to maintain. • Finalize assessment plan with stakeholders.
Development	Develop assessment: • Best practices, literature review, expert panel • How should assessment questions or instructions be presented to learners/assessees (e.g., announced or unannounced assessments)? • What stimuli are needed to prompt learners? • What will be the learner's response mode? • What are the criteria for judging responses/performances? • What scale structure is appropriate for assessing performances (e.g., rating scale, anchors, number of levels/scale points)? • What are examples of performances for each level of response? • Refine assessment instrument and administration as indicated. Develop assessment administration directions: • Standardized assessment situation that can be replicated • Complete and accurate (pilots and field testing are essential) • Modify and finalize directions based on field test results. • Collect example behaviors. • Use example behaviors to score responses according to criteria. • Develop preliminary scoring guide. • Develop an appeals guide. Pilot assessment and use results to refine instrument. Retest and submit to expert panel for final review. Finalize instrument.
Preassessment Administration	Identify or select assessors, administration support staff. Train and certify assessors, staff: • Retrain/Recalibrate assessors who do not meet assessor certification standards. Pilot assessment administration and use results to refine assessment administration (including assessors). Inform learners of assessment expectations and orient them to the assessment process.
Assessment administration	Implement assessment: • Finalize assessment schedule and logistics planning (who, when, where, etc.). • Use an objective coordinator (not an assessor) to examine implementation processes. • Monitor and recalibrate, as needed, to ensure validity and reliability.

(continued)

Table 6.1 (continued)

STAGE	ACTIVITIES
Post-assessment administration	Implement scoring protocol. Maintain and store confidential assessment data. Management system of results (e.g., database). Summarize and prepare score reports (e.g., individual, cohort, assessor). Use assessment results to inform future programming and teaching/learning methods. Evaluate effectiveness of assessment implementation: • Debrief regarding processes and value of assessment activities. • Examine measurement qualities of assessment (e.g., validity and reliability issues). • Revisit and revise assessment components, as indicated.

Validity and Reliability

Establishing evidence of validity and reliability are fundamental components of assessment and the appropriate, justifiable use of results for decision-making. Simply stated, validity is the extent to which assessment data are accurate and representative for a particular purpose/decision. On the other hand, reliability refers to the consistency or dependability of the assessment data. That is, reliability estimates reflect the extent to which data could be replicated if assessments were repeated. Assessment data may be reliable (i.e., consistent, replicable), but not valid (i.e., accurate, representative). Assessment data cannot be valid, however, if they are not reliable. For example, assessing an individual's visual acuity with a standard eye examination may be highly reliable, but not valid as an assessment for reading a magnetic resonance imaging (MRI) scan correctly.

Establishing evidence of validity and reliability is never finished work. Educators must be diligent in examining how assessment methods and measures interact with assessment situations across time, individuals, settings, and purposes to produce data. When selecting established assessment instruments and procedures, it is important to review the primary evidence reported for validity and reliability. You must also consider and evaluate the extent to which the prior uses of the assessment(s) are similar to your intended assessment activities (e.g., purpose, learners, content and skills, task demand, setting, consequences). Additional research may be necessary to establish validity, particularly if your intended use of an assessment instrument or procedure differs in important ways (e.g., learner or setting characteristics) from its prior application(s). Even when similar, you will still want to establish sufficient evidence of validity and reliability of the data you gather for your own application to assure quality, rigor, and appropriate use of assessments. Obviously, the higher the stakes or consequences of assessment (e.g., for learners, the educational program, society), the stronger the evidence of validity and reliability needs to be to support decision-making and its consequences.[15] Correspondingly, assessments reflecting low-stakes, strictly formative purposes (e.g., those that might occur during a simulation session for providing feedback and coaching during practice) can be used appropriately with less evidence of validity and reliability.

ESTABLISHING VALIDITY

Particular attention must be given to establishing evidence that supports the accuracy of interpretation(s) of the results (e.g., scale or subscale scores) and corresponding decisions (e.g., pass/fail, competent/not competent). Said another way, validity is based on the extent to which an assessment instrument or method produces data representing what it was designed or purported to measure. Thus, instead of asking the question, *Is this valid?* one should really be asking the question, *Are these data/results valid for this intended purpose or decision?* For example, data gathered using a direct observation checklist may be valid for assessing residents' abilities in a specific assessment of a simulation-based exercise for providing feedback, but not valid for assessing medical students' abilities during an elective radiology rotation for the purpose of determining a grade.

Kane[23] explained validity as systematic, multifaceted investigative processes through which data are gathered and evidence is provided to define the constructs of assessment and to argue for or against a particular interpretation of assessment results. Messick[24] argued that all forms of validity represent collectively a single, unified framework of construct validity. Early approaches to establish the validity of data obtained with a particular assessment included various activities to establish types of validity, such as face, content, criterion (i.e., predictive and concurrent), and discriminant. In 1999, a new conception of a unified validity framework was introduced, consisting of six aspects of validity: content, substantive, structural, generalizability, external, and consequential. Table 6.2 summarizes the six aspects of validity in terms of requisite evidence and associated methods.

When designing and using assessments in SBE, each aspect of validity becomes important, not only for methods, tools, and processes of assessment (e.g., checklist items, observer training and calibration), but also for the selection, design, and use of simulators and the specific simulation context.[17,25] Elements of the structure and fidelity of simulation formats are as important to effective assessment as they are to teaching/learning processes, as was addressed in chapter 5 (Educational Principles in Simulation). Standards of best practice and additional guidance regarding assessment and the various aspects of validity are provided in the *Standards for Educational and Psychological Testing.*[4] The general guidelines shown in Table 6.1 reflect these standards of best practices in assessment design and use. Other references that serve as useful resources include Holmeboe and Hawkins,[7] Downing and Yudkowskey,[6] and Johnson et al.[10]

ESTABLISHING RELIABILITY

All assessments contain some degree of measurement error, resulting from a variety of sources (e.g., variation across assessors, assessees, occasions, settings, or use of assessment items/measurement). Simply stated, *true score* represents the person's actual ability, whereas *observed score* is the result obtained using the selected assessment tool that includes both true score and error. The goal of establishing reliability in assessment is to design, select, and use measurements and processes that produce scores that maximize the true score and minimize error, so that results can be dependable and trusted for making decisions.

The reliability of assessments can be strengthened through good practices of instrument development and establishing sufficient evidence of its validity.[6,7,10] In simulation-based environments, the reliability of assessments is also influenced by the features of the actual simulator and simulation format in terms of its replicability across repeated implementations.[25–27] Thus, reliability can be enhanced by paying careful attention to the details of the simulation context that were addressed in chapter 5 (Educational Principles in Simulation). Such details include the simulation setting, its preparation, the fidelity of the simulators and the simulation format. In addition, pilot and field testing cannot be overemphasized for developing both assessments and simulation-based tasks and scenarios. Issues related to the standardization and consistency of simulation-based experiences for instruction that were discussed in the previous chapter are equally relevant to assessment.

Selecting assessors and establishing rigorous training, calibration, and recalibration of assessors is another important means to achieving consistency in assessments and minimizing variation within and among assessors. A particular threat to reliability is the phenomenon referred to as *assessor drift*. Over time, without adequate assessor training and routine calibration, assessors tend to drift or deviate from the intended interpretation from established criteria. For example, an assessor's personal preferences for doing a particular procedure can drift into the assessment context and influence how he or she observes, interprets, and scores observed performance. Also, assessors may become harder or easier in their assessments as they complete multiple assessments (e.g., due to fatigue or the influence of performances of previous assessees). Personal qualities of an individual being assessed, recent observations or encounters with assessees (i.e., positive or negative), or physical features of a product (e.g., attractiveness of portfolio layout not related to content) can also influence assessor behavior and cause them to drift from the established criteria. Such deviation can reflect either "halo" (i.e., positive bias)

Table 6.2 Six aspects of a unified framework of validity as conceptualized by Kane[24]

VALIDITY	EXAMPLE EVIDENCE	EXAMPLE METHODS
Content	• Assessment items, instrumentation, simulation tasks and scenarios reflect relevant and representative content; technical quality.	• Best practice(s) in targeted domain • Literature review • Content expert review
Substantive	• Assessment includes sufficient representation of relevant knowledge, skills, abilities in the domain(s) of interest. • Simulated scenario includes sufficient prompts/triggers to elicit representative, relevant responses, maneuvers, behaviors.	• Best practice(s) in targeted domain • Use of established standards or algorithms (e.g., breast imaging protocol) • Task analysis • Content expert review • Direct observation of real-life practice and/or experts
Structural	• Assessment process and scoring criteria fit the cognitive, psychomotor, and effective domains and underlying constructs of the domain(s) of interest.	• Assessment structure representative of real-life abilities • Instrument development and refinement (e.g., content, structure, wording, order, response scales, labels, scoring protocols) • Implementation issues (e.g., assessor training and calibration, administration procedures, timing, setting, preparation of learners/assessees)
Generalizability	• Assessment scores represent targeted abilities across settings, tasks, and groups; not limited to the particular assessment task or context in which it is administered.	• Statistical analysis (e.g., factor analysis, generalizability analysis)
External	• Relationships between assessment scores and other measures of the targeted domain reflect expected values.	• Criterion-related validity studies (predictive and concurrent) • Discriminant validity studies (e.g., assessment discriminates between novice and expert performances)
Consequential	• Intended and unintended effects; assessment scores are accurate and appropriate. • Issues of bias, fairness, justice, aspects of correct and incorrect decisions (i.e., false-positive and false-negative decisions) are included. • Reasonableness of assessment, sufficient sampling, opportunity for assessee to perform is present.	• Compliance with the Standards for Educational and Psychological Testing (AERA, APA, NCME, 1999) • Standard setting methods (e.g., Angoff[42]; Yudkowsky, Downing, and Tekian[16])

or "pitchfork" (i.e., negative bias) effects. Assessors who exhibit general preferences or tendencies to be particularly harsh are often called "hawks," and those who are significantly less harsh are called "doves." These examples are all potential sources of assessor bias and error that affect the reliability of assessments and require specific attention in instrument development and assessor training and calibration/recalibration activities.[10,25] For some types of assessments, the use of trained assessors who are not content experts may be possible and indicated to enhance reliability without sacrificing validity.

Still other sources of error can affect the reliability (and validity) of assessments. For example, each rating in an observation-based assessment involves the following chain of events: the assessor first observes a behavior/response, interprets it, compares the interpretation to the item (another level of interpretation), records a rating, and then the overall data are at some point judged in terms of the overall purpose of the assessment. At each step, the potential for error exists. Logistical features of an assessment can also contribute to errors. For example, an assessor may miss seeing a key maneuver or behavior because of poor eyesight, arriving late, and/or being in a poor position to adequately see and hear individuals and other phenomena in the assessment setting. Also, assessments based on the observation of live performances are generally easier to witness accurately than are those typically based on video recordings. Design features of assessment tools and scoring procedures, and setting rules for optimal assessor position and performance in the assessment environment can minimize or alleviate such sources of assessor error. Rigorous training and routine calibration exercises for assessors can enhance the accuracy and consistency of assessments and minimize these types of threats to reliability. Simply said, the assessment instrument is only as valid and reliable as the person using it. Johnson et al[10] provide a useful overview and a set of steps for designing and implementing effective assessor training for observation-based assessments (e.g., simulated and real-life assessment contexts) and for assessing products of performance-based assessments (e.g., using scoring rubrics with portfolios, patient write-up, written/constructed responses).

Despite the importance of assessor training, overcoming the logistical challenges of accomplishing training with busy clinical faculty is often difficult. Thus, the quality of instrument development and refinement and assessor guidelines becomes particularly important for facilitating reliable assessments. For example, clear descriptions of performance criteria and scoring options on observation checklists, rating scales, and scoring rubrics used enhance the accuracy and consistency of assessments from one occasion to the next within assessors and across assessors. Again, Johnson et al[10] provide useful step-by-step guidance and examples, as do Gable and Wolf,[28] and Colton and Covert.[29] Excellent resources for developing checklists are also available from Stufflebeam[30] at www.wmich.edu/evalctr/checklist, as well as from Bichelmeyer[31] and Adler, et al[32]

Another strategy to enhance the reliability (and validity) of assessment data involves making decisions for instrument design regarding the appropriate use of "low-inference" or "high-inference" assessment items. Low-inference items reflect clear descriptions of discreet behaviors or processes (e.g., inserted catheter correctly without hesitation) or specific outcomes (e.g., specific cardiac rhythm or status of a patient simulator) that can be easily and directly observed and assessed. With low-inference items, there is less opportunity for variation in interpretation. In contrast, high-inference items reflect global assessments for which multiple behaviors, steps in a process, or characteristics of an outcome must be synthesized and interpreted by the assessor to judge the performance. For example, an assessor might observe an individual's execution of a procedure and then render an overall assessment using a scale of expertise (e.g., Dreyfus,[33] that reflects the following levels of expertise: novice, advanced beginner, competent, proficient, and expert).

Scalese and Issenberg[26] present a scoring framework using two dimensions of scoring: the target of scoring—process or outcome, and the type of assessment—explicit and implicit. Their categorization of explicit scoring of process (e.g., behaviors or steps on a checklist) and outcome (e.g., observable or recorded status features or specific outputs of a patient simulator) is similar to the description of low-inference assessments. Their use of implicit process and outcome scoring reflects assessment decisions that are characteristic of high-inference items. That is, multiple behaviors or features (e.g., fluidity and efficiency of movement, technical ability in using instruments, and overall efficiency of task performance) must be synthesized to make a judgment about an overall ability or task completion to render an assessment rating.

Depending on the purpose and format of an assessment, more than one aspect of reliability may need to be addressed; these can include test–retest (stability), internal consistency (e.g., KR20,

Cronbach's α), parallel-forms reliability (involving two parallel or equivalent forms of a measure), and interrater reliability or agreement. A variety of statistical methods are available, and calculating such reliability estimates is straightforward. Consultation with an educational researcher and/or statistician (e.g., in offices of medical education research and development), can be instrumental in learning more about establishing various types of reliability and which method(s) are best for particular assessment and evaluation purposes. Also, a wide variety of excellent measurement books are readily available that include sections on reliability.

QUALITATIVE METHODS

Validity and reliability are concepts that relate to quantitative assessment methods. In most forms of performance assessment, results are quantitative. Even assessment methods that employ qualitative or subjective judgments are often transformed to a quantitative result (i.e., score/rating) through some type of rubric or systematic method of conversion (e.g., global rating using a three-point scale, observation checklist using behavior descriptions and a numerical rating scale, assessment rubric that uses multiple levels for each of several domains). For particularly complex, high-level, performance-based assessments, a purposeful combination of quantitative and qualitative methods may be needed (e.g., a mixed methods approach[34,35]).

When qualitative assessment methods are necessary, specific standards of rigor and associated methods for establishing evidence are available and should be used.[36,37] For example, the qualitative research methods referred to as *triangulation* (i.e., confirming interpretations based on multiple sources of evidence), *peer review* and *audit trail* (e.g., reviews of data and interpretation by knowledgeable peers, other experts), and *saturation* (i.e., continuing to collect data until no new information is being produced) reflect aspects of validity in a qualitative context and may be applicable to assessment development and use. Such methods are used to minimize error and demonstrate the trustworthiness of data for drawing interpretations and conclusions. A *juried assessment* involving multiple assessors and a consensus decision at the end of an oral examination is one example of a qualitative assessment method. Within the context of program evaluation, observations, document reviews, interviews, and focus groups are among the various methods that can be used. When qualitative methods are warranted for learner assessment and/or program evaluation, educators should consult qualitative researchers and the professional literature as needed.[36,37]

TARGETS OF ASSESSMENT

Identifying the specific target or focus of assessment will facilitate the best use of assessment and simulation methods and optimize precious resources. Assessment targets should align closely with the purposes, goals, and intended learning outcomes to achieve an optimal "goal–tool" match. For example, assessing declarative/factual knowledge does not require the use of expensive, complex simulation technology when a well-constructed multiple-choice test might be adequate. If the assessment target reflects the combined abilities of knowledge, procedural competence, and effective clinical reasoning and problem-solving, however, a simulation-based assessment involving authentic patient scenarios provides a better goal–tool match for verifying such competence for practice in the real-life setting.

In terms of program evaluation, the targets of assessment may include aggregated results of individual and/or team assessments (e.g., group summary results) and additional measures (e.g., survey responses from learners and/or faculty members about specific simulation-based experiences). Such targets will likely be important for demonstrating training effectiveness, educational quality, and the achievement of accreditation requirements. Results of various cohorts can also be used for long-range and strategic planning and continuous improvement in areas such as resident recruitment, faculty development planning and support, and program-level resource planning and acquisition. Finally, program evaluation planning should take into account the individual and organizational features that can influence or be influenced by the simulation-based training and education program (e.g., receptivity to various simulation and assessment methods). Consequently, program evaluation may require additional activities (e.g., learner and faculty perceptions questionnaires, interview or focus groups with educational leaders and stakeholder groups within and outside the program/organization). For example, individuals who receive or work with radiology residents in the clinical settings during training and after graduation could provide important input for enhancing future education, training, and assessment initiatives and improvements. A comprehensive summary of the literature on using evaluation results to facilitate innovation and change can be found in Chauvin.[38]

DOMAINS AND LEVELS OF ASSESSMENT AND EVALUATION

The previous chapter on educational principles included information on various domains of learning (e.g., knowledge, skills, attitudes) that included both technical (e.g., clinical procedures) and nontechnical (e.g., interpersonal and communication skills, teamwork) abilities. Bloom's taxonomy[39] identified various levels of learning in each of the cognitive, performance, and affective domains. Millar's[40] pyramid of learning, and Kirkpatrick's[20] four levels of evaluation for training effectiveness were also described as assessment frameworks that have had significant influence on instructional and educational design practices. A return to these frameworks is recommended here to provide useful guides for identifying the relevant range of levels at which learners are intended to perform when designing domain-specific assessments. Keep in mind that the level at which learners are assessed should match the teaching and learning level that was targeted (i.e., goal–tool match). Also, consider what learners must ultimately know and be able to do in the real-life context of professional practice. For example, are the targeted domains for knowledge, skills, and/or attitudes performed in the real world of practice as an individual competency or as a team? For a given level of learners, what should they be able to do in the real-life setting at a particular point in time? Choices for assessment in the simulation-based educational program should reflect as best as possible the real-life context and performance requirements to facilitate relating assessment results to job-related competency. Further, paying particular attention to the verbs used in goals and objectives can help confirm the highest level of expected performance that should be targeted in assessment activities (e.g., knows, knows how, shows how, or does).

Keep in mind that it is not necessary for every assessment to address every level of achievement. Assessments should target the relevant level or range of levels within a targeted domain that is most critical to verifying achievement of the expected competence or proficiency at a particular point in time, before proceeding to the next level of learning or performance. These specific assessment targets or criteria can be thought of as the *critical performance indicators* (CPIs) within a selected assessment method. Identifying the CPIs will facilitate effective decision-making about the tools, context, format, and timing of assessment activities. For example, declarative or factual knowledge can be assessed with a multiple-choice test, basic technical competence for a procedure might require only a part-task trainer or a computer-based skills trainer, but applied knowledge, clinical reasoning, team-based problem-solving and decision-making during the execution of a complex clinical procedure will require a sophisticated simulation or real-life assessment context.

When designing high-fidelity simulation scenarios, one should strive to achieve the highest level of realism possible to maximize the use of such resource-intensive materials. Thus, it is typically much easier to "scale-back" the complexity or difficulty of such scenarios for use with novice learners (e.g., medical students) than to attempt to "ramp up" a simple scenario for use with advanced learners (e.g., residents or practitioners). In addition, selected components of a rich scenario might also be repurposed to use in a focused, technical skills assessment or in combination with a non–simulation-based assessment (e.g., create a video trigger for an oral examination).

TOOLS, PRINCIPLES, AND STRATEGIES TO ACHIEVE ASSESSMENT AIMS

Although not exhaustive, the Accreditation Council for Graduate Medical Education—American Board of Medical Specialties (ACGME-ABMS) Toolbox of Assessment Methods[41] (http://www2.aap.org/sections/uniformedservices/competencytooltable.pdf) lists 13 categories of assessment tools and provides a starting point for planning and developing an effective assessment system for simulation-based education and training. Other types of assessment tools may also include learner and faculty questionnaires that are more useful for answering questions about program outcomes and effectiveness than for individual or team acquired learning or competence. Figure 6.1[6,7,20,40] provides an overview of the common types of assessment tools and the most typical levels of assessment for which each is used for learner assessment and program evaluation. Within each of these categories are variations that can be used to accommodate specific purposes, decisions, and consequences. More detailed explanations for these various types of assessment tools and their uses can be found in the AGME Outcomes Project documents and other previously cited publications.[6,7]

Assessment Tool	Learner Outcomes (Miller's Pyramid)				Program Outcomes (Kirkpatrick's Taxonomy)			
	Knows	Knows How	Shows	Does	Reaction (L1)	Learning (L2)	Behavior (L3)	Outcomes (L4)
Written Examinations (e.g. Multiple-Choice Questions)	✓	✓				✓		
Standardized Oral Examinations	✓	✓				✓		
Chart Stimulated Recall Oral Examinations	✓	✓				✓		
Procedure, Operative, or Case Logs			✓			✓	✓	
Record Reviews			✓	✓			✓	✓
Patient Surveys				✓			✓	✓
Learner Surveys (e.g., satisfaction, self-reported behaviors, or self-efficacy)					✓			
Faculty Surveys (e.g., perceptions)					✓			
Portfolios	✓	✓	✓	✓	✓	✓	✓	✓
Checklist Evaluations of Live or Recorded Performance (observation-based)			✓	✓		✓	✓	✓
Global Ratings of Live or Recorded Performance (observation-based)			✓	✓		✓	✓	✓
Multi-sourced Feedback (i.e., 360-degree) Evaluation Instruments			✓	✓		✓	✓	
Standardized Patient Examinations			✓	✓		✓	✓	
Objective-Structured Clinical Examinations			✓			✓	✓	
Simulations and Models		✓	✓	✓		✓	✓	✓
Projects and Products	✓	✓	✓	✓	✓	✓	✓	✓

FIGURE 6.1 Categories of assessment tools typically used for addressing learning and program outcomes of an educational program

A variety of other types of assessment tools that use simulation technology of various forms and levels of complexity are available (e.g., paper-based case discussions for oral examinations, table-top exercises, simulation-based "in-box" exercises, and virtual reality environments). These variations of scenario-based assessment provide options for achieving the optimal goal–tool match discussed previously in this chapter. With each comes the weighing of time, resources, cost, and feasibility. Descriptions and discussion of these various options are beyond the limits of this chapter. Sufficient information is available in the literature, but not necessarily within medical education. For example, table-top exercises represent a low-fidelity simulation format that can be used effectively for team-based assessments, but they have not been used as much in medical education as in public health—particularly in recent years, pertaining to the training and evaluation of competencies associated with emergency and bioterrorism. Similarly, paper-based cases and in-basket simulation exercises have been used for decades in business and leadership training, but substantially less so in medicine. The use of virtual reality environments for assessment has been pursued extensively within the military and computer sciences fields.

CONCLUSION

Assessment and simulation activities can be complex, tedious, and resource-intense enterprises. However, using the fundamental principles and best practices of assessment discussed in this chapter, accessing the published literature in relevant fields within and outside of medicine, and collaborating with other educators engaged in SBE and colleagues who have expertise in assessment and evaluation can help one design and use quality and value-added assessments in simulation-based radiology education programs that are feasible, valid, reliable, and sustainable.

FOR FURTHER READING

In addition to the information on assessment presented here, this selective list of recommended readings can further facilitate the design and implementation of assessment tools for radiologic applications.

1. Case SM, Swanson DB. *Constructing Written Test Questions for the Basic and Clinical Sciences*. Philadelphia: National Board of Medical Examiners; 1996.

2. Childs JM, Bell HH. Training Systems Evaluation. In: Charlton SG, O'Brien TG, eds. *Handbook of Human Factors Testing and Evaluation*, 2nd edition, Chapter 21. Mahweh, NJ: Lawrence Erlbaum Associates; 2002:473–510.

3. Downing SM, Yudkowsky R, eds. *Assessment in Health Professions Education*. New York: Routledge; 2009.

4. Holmboe ES, Hawkins RE, eds. *Practical Guide to the Evaluation of Clinical Competence*. Philadelphia: Mosby-Elsevier; 2009.

5. Johnson RL, Penny JA, Gordon B. *Assessing Performance: Designing, Scoring, and Validating Performance Tasks*. New York: Guilford; 2009.

REFERENCES

1. Meller G. A typology of simulators for medical education. *J Digital Imag.* 1997;10(3Suppl 1):194–196.

2. Maran NJ, Glavin RJ. Low- to high-fidelity simulation—a continuum of medical education? *Med Educ.* 2003;37(Suppl 1):22–28.

3. Mayer RE. Applying the science of learning to medical education. *Med Educ.* 2010;44:543–549.

4. American Educational Research Association, American Psychological Association, National Council on Measurement in Education. *Standards for Educational and Psychological Testing*. Washington, DC: American Educational Research Association; 1999.

5. Freeman R, Lewis R. *Planning and Implementing Assessment*. London: Routledge-Falmer; 1998.

6. Downing SM, Yudkowsky R. Introduction to assessment in the health professions. In: Downing SM, Yudkowsky R, eds. *Assessment in Health Professions Education*. New York: Routledge; 2009:1–20.

7. Hawkins RE, Holmboe ES. Constructing an evaluation system for an educational program. In: Holmboe ES, Hawkins RE, eds. *Practical Guide to the Evaluation of Clinical Competence*. Philadelphia: Mosby; 2008:216–237.

8. Goldie J. AMEE education guide no. 29: evaluating educational programs. *Med Teacher.* 2006;28:210–224.

9. Mehrens WA. *Measurement and Evaluation in Education and Psychology*, 4th edition. New York: Holt, Rinehart & Winston; 1991.

10. Johnson RL, Penny JA, Gordon B. *Assessing Performance: Designing, Scoring, and Validating Performance Tasks*. New York: Guilford Press; 2009.

11. Block JH, Burns RH. Mastery Learning. In: Shulman LS, ed. *Review of Research in Education*, Vol. 4. Itasca, IL: Peacock; 1971:3–49.

12. Bloom B. Mastery Learning. In: Block JH, ed. *Mastery Learning: Theory and Practice*. New York: Holt, Rinehart & Winston; 1971:47–63.

13. Ericcson KA, Krampe RT, Tesch-Römer C. The role of deliberate practice in the acquisition of expert performance. *Psychol Rev.* 1993;100:363–406.

14. Ericcson KA. Deliberate practice and the acquisition and maintenance of expert performance in medicine and related domains. *Acad Med.* 2004;79:S70–S81.

15. Pugh C. Simulation and High-Stakes Testing. In: Kyle RR Jr, Murray WB, eds. *Clinical Simulation: Operations, Engineering, and Management.* San Diego, CA: Elsevier; 2008:655–666.

16. Yudkowsky R, Downing SM, Tekian A. Standard Setting. In: Downing SM, Yudkowsky R, eds. *Assessment in Health Professions Education.* New York: Routledge; 2009:119–148.

17. Norcini JJ, McKinley DW. Assessment methods in medical education. *Teaching Teacher Educ.* 2007;23:239–250.

18. Shumway JM, Harden RM. The assessment of learning outcomes for the competent and reflective physician. *Med Teacher.* 2003;25:569–584.

19. Hawkins RE, Swanson DB. Using written examinations to assess medical knowledge and its application. In: Holmboe ES, Hawkins RE, eds. *Practical Guide to the Evaluation of Clinical Competence.* Philadelphia: Mosby; 2008:42–59.

20. Kirkpatrick DL. *Evaluating Training Effectiveness: The Four Levels.* San Francisco: Bennett-Koehler; 1994.

21. Stufflebeam DL, Shinkfield AJ. *Evaluation Theory, Models, and Applications.* San Francisco: Jossey-Bass; 2007.

22. Worthen BR, Sanders JR, Fitzpatrick JL. *Program Evaluation: Alternative Approaches and Practical Guidelines,* 2nd edition. White Plains, NY: Longman; 1997.

23. Kane M. Validation. In: Brennan RL, ed. *Educational Measurement,* 4th edition. New York: American Council on Education/Greenwood; 2006:1764.

24. Messick S. Validity. In: Linn RL, ed. *Educational Measurement,* 3rd edition. New York: American Council on Education/Macmillan; 1989:13–104.

25. Patel AA, Gould DA. Simulators in interventional radiology training and evaluation: a paradigm shift is on the horizon. *J Vasc Intervent Radiol.* 2006;17:S163–S173.

26. Scalese RJ, Issenberg SB. Simulation-Based Assessment. In: Holmboe ES, Hawkins RE, eds. *Practical Guide to the Evaluation of Clinical Competence.* Philadelphia: Mosby-Elsevier; 2006:179–200.

27. McGaghie WC, Issenberg SB. Simulations in Assessment. In: Downing SM, Yudkowsky R, eds. *Assessment in Health Professions Education.* New York: Routledge; 2009:245–268.

28. Gable RK, Wolf MB. *Instrument Development in the Affective Domain: Measuring Attitudes and Values in Corporate and School Settings,* 2nd edition. Boston: Kluwer Academic Publishers; 1993.

29. Colton D, Covert RW. *Designing and Constructing Instruments for Social Research and Evaluation.* San Francisco: Jossey-Bass; 2007.

30. Stufflebeam DL. Guidelines for Developing Evaluation Checklists: The Checklists Development Checklist (CDC). *The Evaluation Checklists Project,* 2000. Accessed August 1, 2010, at http://www.wmich.edu/evalctr/checklists

31. Bichelmeyer B. *Checklist for Formatting Checklists,* The Evaluation Checklists Project, 2003. Accessed August 1, 2010, at http://www.wmich.edu/evalctr/checklists

32. Adler MD, Trainor JL, Siddall VJ, et al. Development and evaluation of high-fidelity simulation case scenarios in pediatric resident education. *Ambul Pediatr.* 2007;7:182–186.

33. Dreyfus H, Dreyfus S. *Mind Over Machine: The Power of Human Intuitive Expertise in the Era of the Computer.* New York Free Press; 1986.

34. Tashakkori A, Teddlie C, eds. *Handbook of Mixed Methods in Social and Behavioral Research.* Thousand Oaks, CA: Sage; 2003.

35. Linn RL, Baker EL. Complex performance-based assessment: expectations and validation criteria. *Educ Res.* 1991;20:15–21.

36. Patton MQ. *Qualitative Evaluation Methods.* Beverly Hills: Sage; 1980.

37. Huberman AM, Miles MB. *The Qualitative Researcher's Companion.* Thousand Oaks, CA: Sage; 2002.

38. Chauvin SW. Disseminating Research and Implementing Change. In: Norman GR, van der Vleuten CPM, Newble DI, eds. *International Handbook of Research in Medical Education, Vol. II,* Chapter 32. Dordrecht, The Netherlands: Kluwer Academic Publishers; 2002:997–1038.

39. Bloom B, Engelhart MD, Furst EJ, et al. *Taxonomy of Educational Objectives: Handbook 1, The Cognitive Domain.* New York: Longman; 1956.

40. Millar GE. The assessment of clinical skills/competence/performance. *Acad Med.* 1990;65(Suppl 9):S63–S67.

41. Accreditation Council for Graduate Medical Education (ACGME) and the American Board of Medical Specialities (ABMS). *Toolbox of Assessment Methods.* Version 1.1. A product of the joint initiative of the ACGME Outcome Project of the ACGME and the ABMS, 2000. Accessed May 1, 2010, at http://www.acgme.org/outcome/assess/assHome.asp

42. Angoff WH. *Scales, Norms and Equivalent Scores.* Princeton, NJ: Educational Testing Service; 1984.

7

Building and Incorporating Simulation into a Radiology Residency Program Curriculum

LEONARD R. BOK AND JOHN T. PAIGE

SIMULATION IS merely a tool, not a curriculum. As such, it must reside within an effective curriculum, otherwise it is simply a game.[1–5] But, why do we need a curriculum? What is a curriculum? What curriculum does this radiology program require? These questions must be addressed by the radiology program director and the curriculum committee before we can answer the question of how one builds a simulation program and incorporates that simulation program into the radiology residency curriculum.

When building simulation into a radiology residency educational program, it should supplement the current curriculum not supplant it.[4] Simulation is not a complete replacement for the current didactic and clinical curriculum.[4] The potential roles for simulation in health care are manifold and include aptitude testing, early skills acquisition, advanced skills training, career-long training, board examination, credentialing, preprocedural rehearsal, procedural prototyping, and replacement of animal laboratories.[4,5] Armed with the knowledge of what simulators can do, radiology program directors and curriculum committees must ask the question, "Would a simulation experience facilitate this particular curricular goal effectively and efficiently?" If it can, then they must ask "How should it be integrated into this curriculum? Is it appropriate for testing trainee's aptitude? Can it be used in training early or advanced skills? Does it have a role in preprocedural rehearsal? Will its use help improve patient safety?" After determining that simulation would enhance a curricular objective, the program director must then consider the quality of the simulation as an educational and assessment tool by considering its feasibility, its validity (i.e., face, content, construct, predictive validity), its reliability, and its fidelity.[6]

Simulation has been successfully adopted and employed in training and education in several other medical specialties, with perhaps the best example being in general surgery. Early on, Reznick et al[7,8] demonstrated that simulation could be used to assess surgical technical skills and in developing and validating the Objective Structured Assessment of

Technical Skills (OSATS). This simulation-based technical skill evaluative tool complemented the previously developed Objective Structured Clinical Examination (OSCE), a clinical skill–oriented instrument. Seymour et al then demonstrated that virtual reality (VR) training could improve actual operative performance in the clinical environment.[8,9] On the strength of such research, the Accreditation Council on Graduate Medical Education (ACGME) Surgery Residency Review Committee (RRC) mandated, in 2008, that all surgical programs have access to (i.e., would use) a simulation and skills lab.[2] Working with the Association of Program Directors in Surgery (APDS), the American College of Surgeons (ACS) has developed a national surgical skills curriculum for residents. This curriculum has core competencies in 20 basic skills, full procedures, and team training.[2]

In radiology, the way forward using simulation—particularly in endovascular procedures—remains controversial. Some studies demonstrate the validation of simulation-based training (SBT) interventions, whereas others fail to do so.[10–13] Increased clarity may be achieved as more studies provide more data. A Joint Task Force of the Society of Interventional Radiologists (SIR), the Radiology Society of North American (RSNA), and the Cardiovascular and Interventional Radiological Society of Europe (CIRSE) has made recommendations and comments regarding the validation and implementation of SBT curricula,[11,14] with the long-term goal of generating standards for simulation use. In this context, as each radiology residency program chooses to move forward with a simulation program, it is important to recognize the metrics that define the quality of any assessment tool (see chapter 6, Assessment in Simulation). These metrics include feasibility, validity (i.e., face, content, construct, predictive validity), reliability, and fidelity.[6] As was the case in general surgery, over time, the radiology community will need to develop, implement, and validate simulation-based curricula, as well as define core skills.

MODELS OF TRAINING AND KNOWLEDGE ACQUISITION

It is helpful to review where medical education institutions have been in order to determine where they are currently and to set a course for where they should be going. One of the greatest challenges physician educators face today is the transition from the century-old master–apprenticeship model (MAM) of graduate medical education (GME) to an objectives-driven, theoretically based educational model (i.e. the Dreyfus model of knowledge development, tied to the curricular goal of teaching six general competencies in conjunction with the subject matter of the specialty).[15] Radiology is no exception to this challenge. Of even greater importance, this teaching must take place within the context of patient safety and the pursuit of system-wide quality. This change is a great challenge for physician educators because, although physicians are experts in their particular field of practice (i.e., their subject matter), they are not experts in educational theory and design. Historically, using the MAM, subject matter expertise was all that was required of physicians to train neophytes in their particular field. Today, such content expertise alone is insufficient for educating trainees. Fortunately, radiologists who are educators do not have to obtain a Ph.D. in education in order to teach. They do, however, need to learn the basic principles of education and develop skill using the tools of education and evaluation. At times, these physician educators might benefit from seeking expert help from education specialists, psychologists, and psychometricians. Regardless, the professional development of physician educators in principles of education and learning theory is necessary.

Using the MAM, physician educators merely had to go about their business as subject matter experts, and the expectation was that their trainees would learn through the "see one, do one, teach one" approach.[15] In essence, an elaborate formal curriculum was lacking: the physician educator needed only to be a subject matter expert and had no need for educational expertise or the help of those with educational expertise. Learning simply occurred as a by-product of being at work in the clinical environment and performing clinical duties. The focus was on "teaching" medical knowledge and technical skill, with teaching occurring on rounds, at the workstation, or in the operating room. The concept of training was to teach the learner everything he or she needed to know in that field "just in case" that individual ever needed to know it. Knowledge was viewed primarily as static, and the accepted theory of learning held that the apprentice would learn by working with a master clinician in his or her field of expertise.

In contrast, we now teach not "just in case," but also teach how to learn "just in time" because the rate of change has accelerated so dramatically, and practice-based learning is critical. The "just in case" method of MAM teaching has morphed into a "just in time" model associated with the dramatically accelerated rate of new information, technologies, and techniques that make practice-based learning and improvement a critical competency. In 1997, the ACGME, in collaboration with other interested organizations, committed to a new accreditation model based on outcomes rather than on structure and time spent in a residency program. The ACGME reviewed 2,500 articles on physician competency and selected 84 competencies clustered in 13 categories.[15] Ultimately, six competencies were determined to be key: Patient Care, Medical Knowledge, Practice-Based Learning and Improvement, Interpersonal and Communication Skills, Professionalism, and Systems-Based Practice.[15,16] The ACGME also adopted and modified a model of human skill acquisition known as the *Dreyfus Taxonomy* or *Dreyfus Knowledge Acquisition Model*, named after the brothers who first described it in 1980.[15,16] They originally described five levels in the development of a skill; later, Paul Batalden added a sixth.[15,17]

The six developmental levels of skill acquisition in the modified taxonomy represent a hierarchy of increasing ability related to the particular skill in question: novice, advanced beginner, competent, proficient, expert, and master.[15,17] When applied to medicine, the modified Dreyfus Taxonomy can assist in categorizing developmental stages in skill acquisition with the educational level of the learner. For example, a medical student (i.e., someone involved in undergraduate medical education [UME]) would be considered a novice. A first-year resident (i.e., someone involved in early GME would qualify as an early beginner. A senior-level resident (i.e., someone near completion of GME) would have theoretically attained competency or proficiency. Optimally, this individual would have developed the skills sets necessary to allow him or her to evolve to the level of expert or master over the coming years, as part of his or her continuing medical education (CME).[15,16] Based on the stage of development in skill acquisition, individual learners react and respond differently to skilled performance. For example, the novice and early beginner need lists and facts,[17] but the competent physician recognizes contextual or situational aspects, rather than relying on the abstract lists required by the novice or beginner.[17] The proficient physician recognizes whole situations as aspects, but adjusts his viewpoint if things do not seem to fit.[17] The expert relies on intuition and experiences the situation.[17,18] Finally, the master is embedded in the situation, and she loves surprises and enigmas.[16,17,18] This schema of mental stages creates challenges when teaching or learning using the MAM. A novice may not be able to learn effectively from an expert or a master because the novice needs lists and rules, whereas the master intuits from the entire contextual situation without using a formal decision rule.[16,17] Hence, a master in a particular skill may not be able to teach the novice or early beginner the lists and rules these learners require because these things are no longer readily apparent to the master. Fortunately, the use of simulation has the potential to alleviate such problems.

Simulation-based training makes it possible to replace certain aspects of clinical work and didactic teaching with deliberate practice on systems tailored to provide efficient, effective practice embedded in a level-appropriate curriculum. Ericsson and colleagues describe such "deliberate practice" as a distinct process that unfolds over many hours, days, and years, and one through which expert- and master-level performance is developed.[19–22] Their work suggests that up to 10,000 hours are required to attain expertise.[19,21] *Deliberate practice* connotes a very specific style of practice with defined characteristics. It requires time and motivation, and can only be engaged in for discrete periods of time.[2,19] Key components of deliberate practice include initial instruction, structured repeated practice, immediate feedback, and periodic supervision by a master instructor.[19] Hence, within any given domain, deliberate practice occupies a realm outside of work and play.[19,21] It holds great promise for improving the perceptual skills needed in radiology.[20,21]

The Institute of Medicine's (IOM) 2000 and 2001 reports, *To Err Is Human: Building a Safer Health System* and *Crossing the Quality Chasm: A New Health System for the 21st Century*, respectively, brought to light what many in health care, government, and the public considered to be glaring deficiencies in the health care system and in the system of GME; deficiencies that ultimately caused between 44,000 and 98,000 largely preventable deaths annually due to medical errors. The IOM reports suggested an agenda to bring about change,[23,24] focusing particular attention on patient safety and setting an aggressive timetable for change and improvement. Along with other studies, these two IOM reports pointed to an epidemic of medical errors and spurred public, governmental, and medical interests in improving patient safety.[25] These concerns have been instrumental in the development of resident duty hours, as well as the Joint Commission's annual National Patient Safety Goals. Satava has pointed out that, in addition to the patient safety movement, a "revolution" is taking place in medical education as well. This change has begun to supplant the century-old model ushered in by Flexner in 1910, which was founded on undergraduate medical education and the MAM of graduate medical education. Satava argues that "simulation is and will be pervasive," and the most important and dramatic impact will be on patient safety. He considered that skill acquisition and practice will occur in the simulation lab, surgical rehearsal will become a reality, and preoperative warm-up/practice will become possible.[2]

The world is dramatically more complex than it was 100 years ago, and it is information and communication driven. Health care is delivered in large complex systems, and the rate of technical and social change is rapid and often disruptive to our existing technical, professional, economic, and political structures.[2,26] Such forces demand that institutions pay attention to the ACGME's six competencies, as well as to changes in educational methods that include the incorporation of simulation into the curriculum. The objective of radiology residency programs experiencing this "revolution" should be to keep the best of the past while adopting and inventing those methods and tools, such as simulation and the six competencies, that optimize the future.[27] To achieve this goal, GME must be based upon curricula designed to achieve level-specific outcomes in the six competencies and to embrace knowledge, skill, and affective objectives (i.e., Bloom's Taxonomy, see below) while recognizing the curricular implications of the modified Dreyfus Taxonomy (i.e., the six developmental stages of knowledge and skill acquisition).

CURRICULUM DEVELOPMENT

In its broadest sense a *Curriculum*" (i.e., the "big C" variant) is the overall rationale for any educational program.[28] When used in this way, the word is often capitalized to reflect its all-encompassing nature. Additionally, the term *total curriculum* is sometimes used to convey such meaning.[28] For a radiology program, such a Curriculum would have the overarching goal to develop, through residency training, radiologists who are competent or proficient in their specialty and/or subspecialty and who are prepared for lifelong learning and maintenance of certification. In its smaller sense, a *curriculum* (i.e., the "small c" variant) is the program's or rotation's course plan. Other key curricula-related terms that radiology educators should become familiar with include the *hidden curriculum*, the *planned curriculum*, the *received curriculum*, and the *formal* and *informal curriculum*.[28] Curricular development involves planning, implementing, teaching, learning, assessing the learner, and evaluating the effectiveness of the process. Chapter 5 (Educational Principles in Simulation) and Chapter 6 (Assessment in Simulation) provide excellent overviews of the key elemental and assessment principles needed to build and incorporate simulation successfully into a radiology program curriculum.

Before designing any curriculum, an understanding of some of the taxonomies related to learning and thinking and curricular development is necessary. Bloom's taxonomy is one of the best known and frequently used. In his *Taxonomy of Educational Objectives Handbook*, Bloom suggested that curriculum planning should divide objectives into three categories or domains: cognitive, psychomotor, and affective.[28] General statements of goals should then guide curriculum planning toward achieving specific behavioral objectives.[28] In the taxonomy, a hierarchy of achievement exists within each domain. For example, the behavioral objective of "can describe" conveys a different level of achievement than does the objective of "can do." For the most part, this model of education argues for prespecified course objectives, and the acquisition of knowledge is conceptualized largely as a linear process. The target outcomes are declared by the goals and objectives, and the outcomes are assessable and testable. The key here is that a curriculum is explicitly planned to achieve defined certain goals and objectives. Therefore, the teaching plan should include the appropriate use of simulations to advance learning, with the incorporation of assessment and evaluation of the effectiveness or ineffectiveness of the instructional methods. The *ADDIE* (Assess, Design, Develop, Implement, Evaluate) Model of curriculum development is a very useful guide to help keep the radiologist educator on track while planning and implementing curriculum incorporating simulation (see chapter 5, Educational Principles in Simulation).

Predetermined objectives also are important. In proficiency-based training, learning objectives can be derived from proficient or expert performance.[5] Factors that affect the effectiveness of a curriculum include learner motivation and the use of deliberate practice, performance feedback, task demonstration, practice distribution, practice difficulty and practice variability, proficiency-based training, performance assessment, observer ratings, automaticity, workload assessment, and performance anxiety and physiologic measures of performance.[5] These factors should be attended to as one develops, implements, and manages a curriculum that incorporates simulation.

All ACGME-accredited radiology residencies are currently structured along similar lines: curricula must use the six competencies within nine subspecialties, plus physics, as well as contain a set of common core requirements. Each program has level-specific yearly and rotation-specific goals and objectives that generally follow Bloom's taxonomy while incorporating the Dreyfus model of skill development. The ACGME has developed an Outcomes Project whose goal is for the curriculum to be proficiency based.[29] Learner evaluations, therefore, must be tied to the goals and objectives of the program, and assessment should be reliable, valid, easy to use, require reasonable resources, easy to interpret, and have educational impact.[30]

The Internal Medicine RRC has developed milestones for internal medicine residents,[31] and the radiology RRC is currently developing milestones for radiology residencies.[32] It is expected that radiology residency programs will structure their curricula to facilitate timely, successful accomplishment of the milestones. It makes sense to embed simulations in such curricular development to help learners attain the milestones efficiently and effectively while safeguarding patient safety. A key question will be the timing (e.g., massed vs. distributed practice) and location (e.g., center-based vs. in situ) of the SBT.

BUILDING A SIMULATION CURRICULUM

Simulation requires resources: space, supplies, and personnel time and resident time away from other activities. At Louisiana State University Health Sciences Center in New Orleans (LSUHSC-NO), the Russell C. Klein, MD, Center for Advanced Practice (CAP) and the Isidore Cohn, Jr., MD, Student Learning Center serve as large shared resources for SBT within the school of medicine. Within them are advanced endovascular simulators, multistation simulation labs, simulated operating rooms, major physiology simulators, and specialty-specific simulation spaces. The department of radiology has utilized the CAP and Learning Center for airway management SBT, and a set of 10 to 15 scenarios for contrast reaction emergency SBT is being programmed into the computer-based mannequin simulators at the centers to augment video-based contrast reaction instruction currently in use. The department of radiology has also developed a small demonstration-simulation area within its own space, so that radiology programs in the future will benefit from the efficient and effective use of simulation. That said, simulation can be expensive. But, when used properly, simulation can advance the goal of patient safety and improve the efficiency and effectiveness of training.

Because of its expense, care must be taken when considering when, where, and how to integrate simulation into existing curricula. First and foremost, radiology program directors must try to incorporate simulation where it makes the most sense and provides the greatest benefit. Educators have begun to employ SBT for endovascular and other invasive image-guided procedures (see chapter 20, Simulation in Vascular and Interventional Radiology, and chapter 25, Simulation-Based Training for Ultrasound and Computed Tomography–Guided Interventional Procedures). In addition, simulation has been used to teach responses to contrast reactions (see chapter 13, Team Training and Crisis Management: Contrast Reaction Management) and to prepare and qualify residents for on-call duties in the emergency room (see chapter 15, Simulation in Emergency Radiology and Workload Management). Many of these applications are for teaching high-risk, low-frequency events—an ideal use for SBT. These should not be, however, the only areas of interest. Ericsson has pointed out three domains in which researchers have identified superior performance in medicine: perceptual diagnosis, medical diagnosis of patients, and surgery.[20,21] Indeed, he has discussed at some length the literature available on how to define expert versus novice interpretation of radiographs, primarily mammograms.[20,21] Combining this knowledge, related to the development of expertise in radiographic interpretation, with computer-based simulation allows for an acceleration of learning because the learner could review more cancers, more efficiently in a system of deliberate practice than he or she could possibly encounter in the typical clinical practice workflow.[20,21,29] With improved feedback, this approach of incorporating deliberate practice within the curriculum might even allow trainees to advance in ability beyond their mentors, who are subject matter expert radiologists.[20,21]

Furthermore, should practitioners in subspecialties of radiology choose to utilize the deliberate practice approach, their skills could potentially advance further than they would through experience gained in clinical practice alone.[20,21]

It will take time for the full implementation of simulation in a curriculum. The program, therefore, should start where it can find faculty, fellows, or residents who will champion development of the simulation-based curriculum. Alternately, it could find champions in the above-listed areas, where simulation has already begun to be incorporated into training. It is not necessary to wait for the validation of a particular SBT intervention before implementation. Flight simulators were in use long before they were fully validated,[4] and the ACGME provides significant guidance on validating assessment tools. Having experts in education, testing, and statistics, however, is helpful in many cases.[30] Formats to consider for curricula include using both high- and low-fidelity simulation. Many options exist: high-fidelity procedural SBT, low-fidelity procedural SBT, workstation picture archiving and communication system (PACS), computer-based SBT, interprofessional team or single disciplinary crew SBT, and the use of OSCE or OSATS are just a few.

In creating an SBT protocol for any procedure, certain guidelines should be followed. Developing an optimal procedural simulation starts with a definition of the task/procedure to be simulated, including supplies, steps, and desired outcome to define competence or proficiency. The formal method for accomplishing this is through physical and cognitive task analysis (CTA).[33,34] A CTA has been done for several procedures by the Collaborators in Radiological Interventional Virtual Environments (CRaIVE) group in the United Kingdom.[33,34] Alternatively, one can engage in a less formal expert discussion with colleagues before agreeing on typical supplies, steps, and desired outcomes. Expert or proficient performance can be utilized to determine the desired objective outcome to be achieved by the learner.[5] Before starting any training, a pre-simulation demonstration must be prepared that includes background, supplies, steps, and, most importantly, the goals and objectives of the training. The demonstration may be presented by the subject matter expert in person or through a computer module. It may include a pre-test, if appropriate.

Once training has begun, the subject matter expert needs to spend time initially giving basic training. The learners should then have time to practice. The curriculum designer will need to decide whether to utilize massed practice or distributed practice, recognizing the risks of massed practice based on cognitive load theory. Such decisions are typically based upon program structure and resource availability. At LSUHSC-NO, the department of radiology has utilized massed practice with unembalmed cadaver and C-arm fluoroscopy for musculoskeletal procedures, certain interventional radiology simulations, and neuroradiology interventional procedures. The department of radiology has utilized distributed practice for SBT of endovascular interventions using a VR simulator, mammography procedural SBT, SBT related to equipment and supplies familiarization, and training of the Seldinger technique via low-fidelity simulation-demonstration. Whenever possible, distributed, deliberate practice should be the method of choice. It promises to improve educational efficiency and effectiveness, and holds the potential to help radiology educators accelerate the learning curve to mastery in the field.

During any SBT encounter, the learner should have opportunities for feedback either from the device itself or from subject matter experts. For example, the Procedicus Vascular Intervention Simulation Trainer Virtual Reality (VIST™ VR) (Mentice, Gothenburg, Sweden) simulator produces metrics for procedures that are both static (e.g., procedure time, fluoroscopic time, contrast volume used, number of cine-loops) and dynamic (e.g., stent or balloon/vessel ratio, coverage percentage, placement accuracy, residual stenosis, and lesion coverage). Subject matter experts could include faculty, senior residents, or simulation specialists. Whether via device computer metrics or in person (simulation proctor), feedback is critical to optimize learning.[2,6] Performance errors in simulated procedures should be detected and corrected because practicing the wrong thing over and over again is not helpful! For current endovascular simulators, it is not yet entirely clear to investigators which metrics confirm proficiency or the transferring of skills acquired on the simulator to actual clinical practice.[6] A systems point of view can be helpful in designing quality improvement programs, assessment programs, and even curricula.[35] Given the importance of assessment, it is important to understand that many, if not most, radiology faculty have not been trained in assessment techniques, although such training is important to improve reliability and reproducibility of ratings. Checklists and global evaluations with objective anchoring descriptors can be helpful.[13]

At the completion of the training protocol, a final assessment is useful to determine whether the learner has met the predetermined target of proficiency for the level of training. If the learning objective has not been achieved, further practice or a new personal learning plan should be developed. This assessment could be based upon a checklist evaluation, global rating scale, selected machine-generated metrics, or some combination of the three. Finally, after a reasonable number of trainees have participated in the simulation, the program director should determine whether the simulation and associated curriculum are achieving their goals through an analysis of results. If the goals are not being met, the strategy should be modified.

Note that interpreting an imaging study such as a digital radiograph, ultrasound, computed tomogram, magnetic resonance image, positron emission tomogram-computed tomogram (PET-CT), or nuclear medicine study can also be conceptualized as a procedure and can be taught and simulated in the same manner as any other procedure. Physical and cognitive task analysis can be applied to the task of working at the hospital information systems (HIS)–radiology information systems (RIS)–PACS workstation. As discussed above, utilizing PACS-based techniques with the principles of deliberate practice, short periods of distributed practice, and a mix of self-study and faculty mentoring offers the promise of improved efficiency and effectiveness for radiology residency training.[20,21,29]

At the global level, postgraduate year 2/radiology year 1 (PGY2/R1) residents come into the radiology residency as novice or early beginners in the domain of radiology; they may be early beginners in the medicine domain and novices in the radiology domain. The goal of the global radiology residency curriculum is to facilitate each resident's progression to competent or proficient in all six competencies by postgraduate year 5/radiology year 4 (PGY5/R4). Thus, PGY2/R1 residents come to the radiology residency as novices or early beginners in radiology, and the program should design curricular elements, including SBT, targeted to this level. Such design would include deconstructing the task environment into context-free features and providing *rules.*[17] As the radiology 2/radiology 3 (R2/R3) resident progresses to the competent stage, the instructor may point out situational component patterns and provide *guidelines.*[17] As the R3/R4 resident reaches the competent or proficient stage, the instructor may begin discussion of whole situations in context and provide *maxims.*[17]

The expectation is that by the time of graduation the radiology residency curriculum, through attention to the six competencies and level-specific deliberate practice and instruction, will have provided the resident with the skills to be a lifelong learner and participate in lifelong maintenance of certification. Ideally, the skill set that this resident has acquired will allow him or her to achieve expert or even master status as he or she progresses in practice.[15] Ericsson suggests that, in most domains, achieving such levels of expertise is unlikely based upon work alone, unless the practitioner is at a university, is a subspecialist, or engages in deliberate practice.[19,20] The physician at the mastery stage confronts the entire experienced situation intuitively and reacts to it as a whole. The step of the analytic decision rule is gone. If the result is not as expected, the master adjusts. It is important to remember that when a master in a field is teaching a novice, early beginner, competent learner, or proficient learner, the experienced task environment is different for each level. The MAM approach to teaching can break down in such a setting, since the novice may have no idea of what is going on in the mind of the master and vice versa.

An outcomes-based residency with a competency-/proficiency-based curriculum using integrated simulation will likely function quite differently than the current time-based residency and curriculum. For example, in an outcomes-based model, the resident entering a radiology program after 4 years of UME and 1 year of clinical GME would then undergo assessment of knowledge, skills, and attitudes related to radiology through some combination of simulation-based assessment, written exams, OSATSs, OSCEs, and other available methods in order to gauge his or her actual level in the expected areas. A personal learning plan, based on these results, could then be developed for each resident to bring him or her to the target level defined in the goals and objectives for that postgraduate year (PGY) status. Currently, all residents entering a radiology program are assumed to be at the novice or early beginner level in radiology, with a basic knowledge and skill base in all six core competencies; this would include things like an understanding of and ability to perform a procedure utilizing sterile technique, the ability to perform a patient history and physical examination, and the ability to start an intravenous line. Proficiency-based training would argue that this assumption may be inappropriate because trainees have been enrolled in time-based programs. Not all trainees may be at the same level of knowledge and skill in all six competencies.

Another model of training, which is an intermediate approach and is in use at some institutions across the country, is the *Simulation Boot Camp Model.*[36–39] This approach has been used more frequently in surgery,[36] pediatrics,[37] emergency medicine,[38] and obstetrics/gynecology[39] programs, but it is equally appropriate to a radiology residency and is in place in a few radiology programs at this time. Using the boot camp concept, the radiology program director, subspecialty directors, and curriculum committee decide what every resident should know from day one. For example, the items selected might be airway management, recognizing and managing a contrast reaction, and/or recognizing 10–20 key life-threatening finding on radiographs, such as tension pneumothorax, free intra-abdominal air, or intracranial hemorrhage. A teaching program is then designed to include specific goals and objectives and a means of assessment, which in some cases is simulation-based. Like basic life support and advanced cardiac life support, this type of program, which involves massed practice, should probably be repeated at some interval (i.e., converting the massed practice into a distributed practice) because learned material does decay over time. Distributed practice can be useful in reinforcing the knowledge and skill base. Furthermore, cognitive load theory suggests that massed practice itself, if not planned wisely can overload the student's ability to comprehend and absorb the knowledge and skills being taught.

Wherever procedures or unsupervised calls are involved, the clinical rotation–specific, level-specific curriculum goals and objectives should include integrated SBT to give the resident an opportunity to learn the skill on the simulator using a proficiency-based protocol. Prior to performing the procedure on a patient under supervision, an objective assessment can be employed to verify that proficiency has been achieved. In the case of emergency radiology call, the resident would be objectively assessed on a call simulation system (see chapter 15, Simulation in Emergency Radiology and Workload Management) prior to being allowed to take call and read patients' films without direct supervision. Additionally, the resident's progress over time could be tracked utilizing periodic simulation-based reassessments.[36,40] Furthermore, in this residency of the future, residents may be internally credentialed in a given procedure using a combination of objective simulation-based assessments and subsequent supervised, formally scored performance of procedures on patients. Such a model would allow the application of the principle of progressive responsibility throughout the course of residency.[41]

Radiology programs are, for the most part, early on the learning curve with regard to integrating simulation into the curriculum. The LSUHSC-NO experience and the experiences of other programs with an interest in simulation are offered in the subspecialty sections of this book. By learning more about how institutions have approached the integration of simulation into existing curricula, individuals will hopefully be stimulated to develop new ideas, thus helping to advance the use of simulation in radiology. Some of the examples are obvious uses of simulation, and some are not so obvious. This chapter has been focused on the use of simulation in GME, but simulation is also very useful in UME and is expected to become integrated into certifying examinations, credentialing, and CME. In *Radiology,* in October 2007, Gary Becker stated: "medical simulation is as relevant to radiology as it is to other clinical disciplines."[42] Increasingly, with the continued adoption of simulation-based techniques in radiology, this statement is becoming more and more self-evident.

CONCLUSION

The construction of a modern radiology residency curriculum involves building a curriculum that fully incorporates efficient and effective simulation and assessment of competence and proficiency. This endeavor takes time and resources. Radiology programs should begin these efforts now, in order to advance the interests of patient safety, quality care, and resident education. The way forward is not without controversy, and it will take time to validate and optimize these programs. Radiology programs can begin the process by taking available steps on a day by day basis. The program director and associated faculty are subject matter experts; radiologist educators will need faculty development to make this transition gracefully and to optimize outcomes. They will sometimes need guidance from experts in education, testing, psychology, statistics, physics, and other fields. Radiology department chairs, program directors, and radiologist educators will all need to champion and actively assist these efforts.

REFERENCES

1. Patel A, Gould D. Simulators in interventional radiology training and evaluation: a paradigm shift is

on the horizon. *J Vasc Interv Radiol.* 2006;17: S163–S173.

2. Satava RM. The revolution in medical education—the role of simulation. *J Grad Med Educ.* 2009;1:172–175.

3. Gould D, Kessel D, Healey, et al. Simulators in catheter-based interventional radiology: training or computer games? *Clin Radiol.* 2006;6:556–561.

4. Dawson S. Procedural simulation: a primer. *Radiology.* 2006;241:17–25.

5. Stefanidis D. Optimal acquisition of proficiency on simulators in surgery. *Surg Clin N Am.* 90;2010:475–489.

6. Ahmed K, Keeling A, Fakhry M, et al. Role of virtual reality simulation in teaching and assessing technical skills in endovascular intervention. *J Vasc Interv Radiol.* 2010;21:55–66.

7. Reznick R, Reghr G, Macrae, et al. Testing technical skill via an innovative "bench station" examination. *Am J Surg.* 1997;173:226–230.

8. Seymour N, Gallagher A, Roman S. Virtual reality training improves operating room performance: results of randomized, double-blinded study. *Ann Surg.* 2002;236:458–464.

9. Satava R. Emerging trends that herald the future of surgical simulation. *Surg Clin N Am.* 2010;90: 623–633.

10. Gould D. Using simulation for interventional radiology training. *Brit Jour Radiol.* 2010;83: 546–553.

11. Gould D, Reekers J, Kessel D. Simulation devices in interventional radiology: validation pending. *J Vasc Interv Radiol.* 2006;17: 215–216 (reprinted 2009).

12. Neequaye S, Aggarwal R, van Herzeele I. Endovascular skills training and assessment. *J Vasc Surg.* 2007;46:1055–1064.

13. Berry M, Reznick R, Lystig, et al. The use of virtual reality for training in carotid artery stenting: a construct validity study. *Acta Radiol.* 2008;7:801–805.

14. Gould D, Patel A, Becker G, et al. SIR/RSNA/ CIRSE Joint Medical Simulation Task Force Strategic Plan Executive Summary. *J Vasc Interv Radiol.* 2007;18: 953-955 (reprinted 2009).

15. Batalden P, Leach D, Swing S, et al. General competencies accreditation in graduate medical education: An antidote to overspecification in the education of medical specialists. *Health Affairs.* 2002;21:103-111. Accessed December 1, 2011, at http://www.acgme.org

16. Leach DC. Changing education to improve patient care, *Qual Health Care.* 2001;10(Suppl II): ii54–ii58.

17. Dreyfus S, Dreyfus H. *A Five-Stage Model of the Mental Activities Involved in Directed Skill Acquisition.* University of California, Berkeley. Operations Research Center ORC 8-2; 1980:1–6.

18. Gladwell M. *Blink: The Power of Thinking Without Thinking.* Boston: Back Bay Book Co/Little, Brown and Company; 2005.

19. Ericsson KA, Drampe R, Tesch-Romer C. The role of deliberate practice in the acquisition of expert performance. *Psychol Rev.* 1993;100:363–406.

20. Ericsson KA. Deliberate practice and the acquisition and maintenance of expert performance in medicine and related domains. *Acad Med.* 2004;79:S70–S75.

21. Ericsson KA. The making of superior doctors through deliberate practice: what can we learn from the training of chess masters, elite athletes and musicians? Mavin Dunn Keynote Address. 2009, ACGME Annual Educational Conference.

22. Gladwell, M. *Outliers: The Story of Success.* Boston: Little, Brown and Company; 2008.

23. Institute of Medicine. *To Err Is Human: Building a Safer Health System.* Washington, DC: Institute of Medicine; 2000.

24. Institute of Medicine. *Crossing the Quality Chasm: A New Health System for the 21st Century.* Washington, DC: Institute of Medicine; 2001.

25. Stevens D. Finding safety in medical education. *Qual Saf Health Care.* 2002:11;109–110.

26. Satava R. Disruptive visions: surgical education. *Surg Endosc.* 2004;18:779–781.

27. Collins J, Porras J. *Built to Last: Successful Habits of Visionary Companies.* New York: Harper Collins; 1994.

28. Kelly A. *The Curriculum: Theory and Practice,* 4th edition. Thousand Oaks, CA: Sage Publications; 1999.

29. Accreditation Council for Graduate Medical Education. Outcome Project. Accessed July 8, 2011, at http://www.acgme.org/Outcome/

30. Swing S, Clyman S, Holmboe ES, et al. Advancing resident assessment in graduate medical education. *J Grad Med Ed.* 2009;1:278–286.

31. Green M, Aagaard E, Caverzagie K, et al. Charting the road to competence: developmental milestones for internal medicine residency training. *J Grad Med Educ.* 2009;1:5–20.

32. Amis S. Radiology RRC Update Presentation at AUR 59th Annual Meeting, 2011. Boston, MA.

33. Johnson S, Healey A, Evans J, et al. Physical and cognitive task analysis in interventional radiology. *Clin Radiol.* 2006;61:97–103.

34. Collaborators in Radiological Interventional Virtual Environments. Accessed December 1, 2011, at http://www.hpv.cs.bangor.ac.uk/CRaIVE/index.php

35. Bucholz E, Duncan J. Assessing system performance. *J Vasc Interv Radiol.* 2008;19: 987–994.

36. Parent RJ, Plerhoples TA, Long EE, et al. Early, intermediate, and late effects of a surgical skills

"boot camp" on an objective structured assessment of technical skills: a randomized controlled study. *J Am Coll Surg*. 2010;210:984–989.

37. Nishisaki A, Hales R, Biagas K, et al. A multi-institutional high-fidelity simulation "boot camp" orientation and training program for first year pediatric critical care fellows. *Pediatr Crit Care Med*. 2009;10:157–162.

38. Laack TA, Newman JS, Goyal DG, et al. A 1-week simulated internship course helps prepare medical students for transition to residency. *Simul Healthc*. 2010;5:127–132.

39. Pliego JC, Wehbe-Janek H, Rajab MH, et al. OB/GYN boot camp using high-fidelity human simulators: enhancing residents' perceived competency, confidence in taking a leadership role, and stress hardiness. *Simul Healthc*. 2008;3:82–89.

40. Glaiberman C, Jacobs B, Street M, et al. Simulation in training: one-year experience using an efficiency index to assess interventional radiology fellow training status. *J Vasc Interv Radiol*. 2008;19:1366–1371.

41. Group Discussion. Supervision Preconference. ACGME, 2010 Annual Meeting. Nashville, TN.

42. Becker, G. Simulation and the coming transformation of medical education and training. *Radiology*. 2007;245:7–9.

8

Development and Operation of a Simulation Laboratory at a Major Medical Center

GLADYS L. FERNANDEZ AND NEAL E. SEYMOUR

THE APPEARANCE and wide expansion of facilities to deliver simulation-based training (SBT) to health care professionals represent a dramatic shift in the way formative education and assessment of skill occurs. Successful precedents have been established for laboratory-based training for physicians, residents, medical students, nurses, first responders, and allied health professionals of all types. The collective experience of development and operation of specialized centers where such training can occur has been highly variable, and, consequently, no truly prescriptive approach for the establishment of a new SBT facility exists. The necessity for such centers, however, has grown as adoption of SBT has progressively grown. Specialty organizations in surgery have recommended that SBT methods be used as an adjunct to more traditional curricula.[1–3] In surgery, the importance of SBT has been underscored with recent requirements for certification in technical skills training in order to achieve board eligibility status.[4] At a programmatic level, the Surgical Residency Review Committee (RRC) of the Accreditation Council for Graduate Medical Education (ACGME) has explicitly stated that trainee access to a skills training center is required for training program accreditation.[5] In radiology, an increasingly extensive body of literature supports the addition of SBT in the graduate medical education (GME) setting.[6–8] Additionally, much speculation exists regarding a greatly expanded use of simulation in radiology in the near future.[9,10] It is not unreasonable, based on current trends to make the broad assumption that, in the future, simulation-based methods will either supersede or complement current practices related to qualification for medical practice.

Although the development and operation of a simulation laboratory might be undertaken in response to regulatory challenges, preferred motivation should include improving access to high-quality education and a clear vision of learning needs that must be addressed, both now and in the future. Keeping these two factors in mind will help inform planning, funding, and curricula development for the new center. This chapter reviews the facility and device requirements, general issues related to curricular development, and operational considerations that are fundamental to the successful development of a modern simulation center.

ORGANIZATIONAL AND PHYSICAL STRUCTURE

General Considerations

Building a new simulation facility requires individuals in leadership roles who are invested in medical education and knowledgeable in local institutional educational needs. Although experiences vary among established centers, the various descriptions of specific centers in the literature can help guide new simulation center developers.[11–13] The most successful efforts have generally been collaborative and multidisciplinary, and they have been preceded by a sometimes challenging process to establish buy-in from institutional administrative and clinical leadership. Identification of financial resources and training site location, planning for startup material resources (e.g., simulator hardware), and creation of personnel infrastructure are all key components of facility development. In recent years, valuable lessons in architectural and infrastructure planning have been learned and can be shared among institutions. Background research, site visits to other centers, and open communication with those who have experienced such a development process can provide new center planners vital information. Although the size and number of simulation spaces in the center ought to be determined by the anticipated number and needs of learners, some minimum basic space requirements should be met for a reasonable level of capability (Figure 8.1).

A laboratory ought to maintain separate spaces for manikin-based high-fidelity simulation (HFS) (i.e., patient simulation) and technical skills training. At least one configurable patient simulation suite is needed to conduct simulated patient care events, and a larger number is needed to accommodate two or more simultaneous training events. Facilitators and simulator operators ought to have one-way mirror viewing of all patient simulation suites from a control area within an adjacent, distraction-free room (Figure 8.2).

Although separate control rooms are desirable, at Baystate Medical Center, three patient simulation suites are successfully managed from a central room with three control stations. Although the technical skills training area can utilize fixed workbench spaces, the use of folding tables with proper lighting allows the skills lab space to be rapidly configured for multiple activities (Figure 8.3).

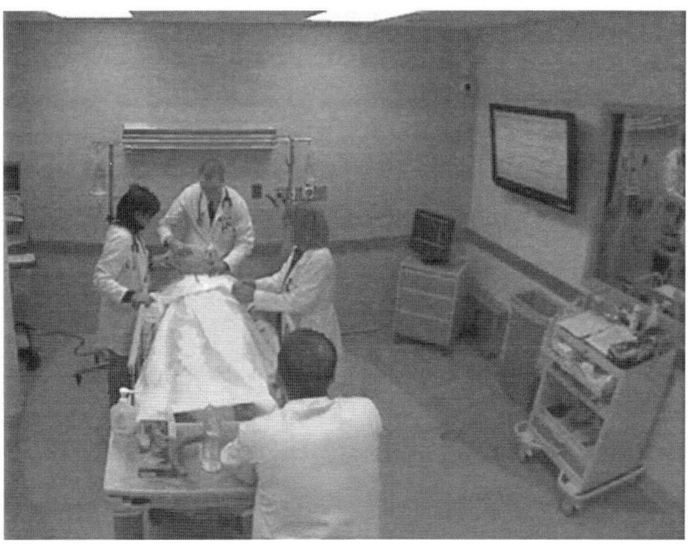

FIGURE 8.1 Patient simulation suite as viewed from a wall-mounted camera used in the framework of the center's audio-video (A-V) management system. The suite can be configured to resemble a variety of clinical spaces, such as an inpatient room, emergency department or intensive care unit room, a postsurgical care unit slot, or an operating room.

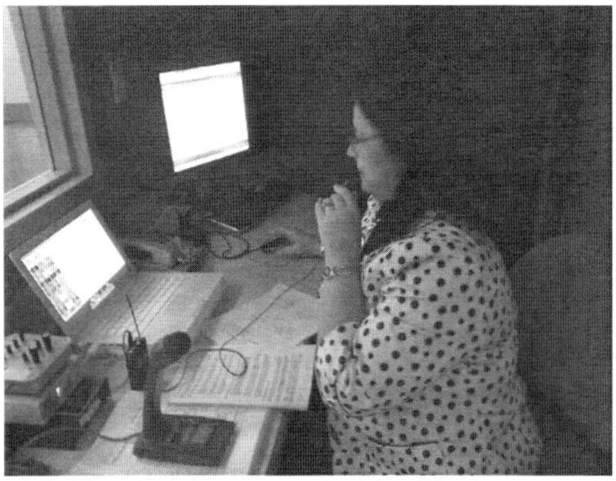

FIGURE 8.2 Control area for simulated patient care in a simulation suite (visible through observation window, with one-way viewing through mirrored glass). Computers at the operator's workstation provide a "heads-up" display for simulator status and control, as well as web browser window with video and audio capture displays that allow bookmarking and annotation of specific events that can be referred to later during debriefing. Information on patient status, including physiologic, laboratory, and diagnostic imaging data, can be delivered into the suite, where participants view it on a wall-mounted display or on an electronic medical record (EMR) workstation.

Basic audio-visual (A-V) recording capabilities are strongly recommended, particularly in the patient simulation area. Other useful space includes a classroom, an office for staff use, and adequate storage areas. Some centers offer workshops that provide information on starting, operating, and maintaining a facility.[11] Sufficient time invested in research prior to finalization of plans may prevent errors in design and misdirected use of budget resources for infrastructure and hardware.

Governance

A clearly understood governance plan for the new simulation center ought to be established, including clearly identified specific leadership roles that leave no uncertainty as to the parties responsible for center supervision and management. Important functions to be addressed include strategic planning, budget stewardship, and operational management. If the simulation center is a medical center resource, its leadership hierarchy might position a center director under a chief academic officer. If, on the other hand, the simulation center is administratively housed within a medical school, the center director might be positioned under the dean for education. At a major medical center, the agency charged with developing the simulation center must generally report to higher-level institutional leadership, for whom the simulation center mission is very likely regarded as secondary to clinical operations. To ensure an authoritative and credible line of communication both back to institutional leadership and down to operational elements, this agency ought to include leaders in continuing medical education (CME), GME, and undergraduate medical education (UME), as well as the simulation center managerial and technical staff. At Baystate Medical Center, a specifically constituted steering committee serves this role. Alternatively, existing infrastructure, such as a GME committee (chaired by the designated institutional officer [DIO]) and/or UME committee, can accomplish this with the proviso that special accommodations be made for services outside the committee's usual scope (e.g., nursing, allied health professions). Operational oversight can be the responsibility of either the full-time center staff or simulation education champions representing the center's active user groups (e.g., clinical departments). At Baystate Medical Center, these individuals meet as a committee to review issues pertaining to educational quality, assignment of resources, and other operational issues. The successful implementation of a simulation program requires high-level support from the leadership of whatever departments or other agencies are engaged in the routine use of the center.

Financial Considerations

A means of securing financial support, both at inception and annually, must be identified in order to maintain the facility and its associated programs. Initial support is generally directed toward funding for the physical plant, hardware, and other materials needed to deliver SBT. Carefully considered purchases of simulator devices, computing resources, equipment warranties, and consumable items constitute the other major early expenditures.

After the center has opened and training has started, a more accurate picture of the operational costs can be put together. The center's managerial staff ought to be responsible for preparation of the budget and financial reports, according to specific institutional requirements. Opportunities for additional support may include revenue for laboratory use associated with CME activities,

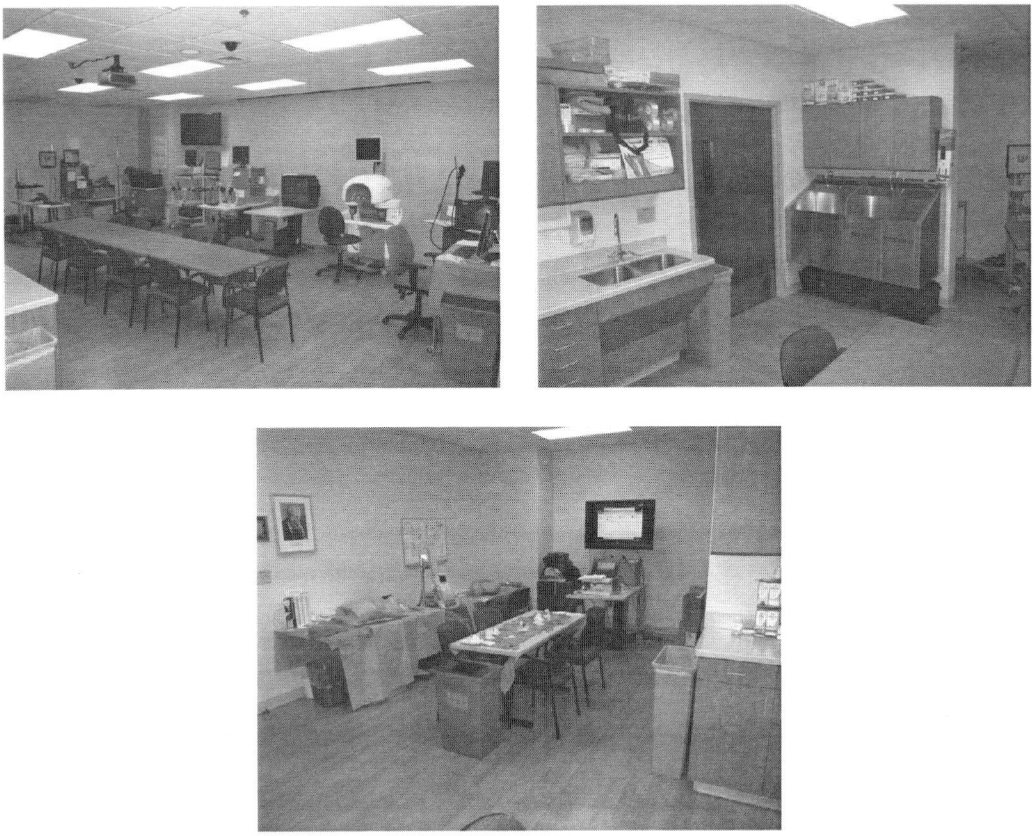

FIGURE 8.3 Although solutions for configuration of a skills training laboratory include fixed benches/task stations with overhead lighting, a configurable technical skills training space offers a degree of flexibility in how the space is used. This design is particularly useful for a small laboratory. Configurations can accommodate group skills training, individual training, and classroom activities. Note the scrub sink, which is at the entrance to the simulated operating room.

external educational programs (e.g., those sponsored by industry), grants, and very importantly, philanthropic support. The simulation center and its needs should be a priority of the institutional development officer charged with facilitating donations.

Physical Plant

A universally applicable basic facility size or design that will meet the needs of all users at all institutions does not exist. Nonetheless, adequate space is essential. The American College of Surgeons (ACS) has suggested that small centers used for basic technical skills training should provide at least 500 square feet of simulation space for accreditation.[1] In general, a minimum threshold size should be determined based on the anticipated scope of use and number of users. As mentioned above, a simulation center ought to have some activity-specific educational areas, briefing and debriefing sites and/or classroom space, and staff work areas, as well as adequate space for storage. The design ought to match the mission, understanding that the need to accommodate activities like standardized patient experiences (e.g., Objective Structured Clinical Examinations [OSCEs]), large CME events (e.g., Advanced Cardiac Life Support [ACLS], Advanced Trauma Life Support [ATLS]), or multiple simultaneous events may require larger facilities with fundamental design features that might not be easy to add later. In many cases, practical limits on size and cost impose the most important restrictions on the scope of the project. In this situation, the argument must be made to maximize the center's size and capabilities within the predefined size and cost restrictions.

The physical location of the center must be considered thoroughly, taking into account accessibility, security, and capacity issues. Locating the facility on the main institutional campus affords access that might otherwise be limited if travel by bus or car were required to a more remote area. This proximity is important for both individual and group activities scheduled during protected educational time. Convenient access is also important for self-directed practice sessions that might occur during periods of opportunity outside normal business hours. Proximity to the clinical environment also facilitates warm-up or rehearsal training sessions. An off-site training facility might have the advantage of imposing a "protected" status on learners, since they are less likely to be drawn away by unexpected clinical events. Such freedom from interruption, however, must be weighed against the disadvantages of travel time, remote access, and lower compliance with training assignments.

Personnel

Irrespective of the model employed, the issue of staffing must be confronted directly and with clear identification of entire or fractional sources of funding for the full-time equivalent(s) (FTE(s)) that will be needed to make the proposed training possible. Simulation center personnel should be able to provide operational support of the skills training, data collection, basic computing, and administrative functions of the center. The extent to which these personnel teach depends entirely on their own qualifications and training. In an ideal situation, one or more FTE simulation center employees are hired, and their efforts are augmented by health care educators from the learners' clinical areas. In addition to teaching, the latter provide subject matter expertise and other content-specific support to the curriculum and to the simulation center full-time staff's curricular efforts. The extent of engagement of these non-center personnel greatly affects the quality of the curricula, as well as the quality of learner participation in training. Encouragement of these individuals is essential and can take the form of recognition (e.g., career advancement, teaching awards), as well as compensation. The inability to compensate faculty members for time spent on this type of activity is a common problem, and it can be a major barrier to more extensive faculty participation in simulation center-based teaching.

Other Resources

The availability of part- or full-time adult education experts and a biostatistician on either a consultative or assigned basis can be a significant help to both the curriculum design process and to any research programs associated with the center. Consultation with institutional health care quality and patient safety personnel can also be of benefit for curriculum development and the alignment of some education programs with institutional goals that might otherwise fall outside formative education activities. Integration Test (IT) or other institutional informatics support for center computing resources is vital, but it may constitute an added expense. These individuals may have to work actively with industry representatives to install and/or maintain some types of simulation devices. Typical issues that might raise security concerns include networking issues with nonstandard equipment and learning management system software in which data storage might occur using servers outside the institution. At Baystate Medical Center, a specific IT technical staff member has been designated to address the simulation center needs.

SIMULATORS AND OTHER TEACHING RESOURCES

Based on each center's specific needs, careful and appropriate planning for the purchase of simulators and other equipment can be made. Key considerations include the types of learner groups to be trained, available space, curriculum considerations, and available financial resources. With needs identified, a prioritization of device purchases should be based on immediacy of learner need, the potential for cross-departmental utilization, potential institutional impact (e.g., alignment with quality assurance ventures), and compatibility with real budget considerations. Due diligence must be given to issues of product usability in the personnel framework in which they will exist and the need for adjunct or supporting equipment and replacement parts, as well as for maintenance contract inclusions/exclusions.

Devices

The procurement of simulators requires a process to justify and assure effective use. Among the factors to be considered are the applicability of the simulator to curricula within the center and its anticipated effectiveness if implemented with local center resources. The latter consideration requires addressing ease of use, capacity to manage anticipated workload, and duty cycle questions prior to purchase. Based on predefined need, a simulation center's device inventory might include bench-top part-task training tools, minimally invasive surgical training devices, flexible endoscopy trainers, and part- or full-patient simulators. Bench-top part-task training devices may include trainers for basic bedside procedures such as phlebotomy, airway management, central venous catheter placement, lumbar puncture, basic suturing/knot tying, or ultrasound. The level of fidelity that these simulators offer may vary, and it is difficult to make a general recommendation for procurement practices based on fidelity characteristics. In general, simulators with higher levels of fidelity to clinical reality are associated with progressively higher costs relative to low-fidelity models. Low-fidelity cardiopulmonary resuscitation mannequins, low-tech patient care trainers, and basic birthing mannequins may provide adequate opportunities for essential SBT. High-fidelity, full-body patient simulators with physiologic response to interventions, anatomically precise physical examination features related to pathophysiology, and advanced features, such as portability and wireless functionality, may be costly, but they provide usability that might be essential to address curricular needs. It is necessary to balance both the curricular mission and the desire to have high-fidelity resources with practical budgetary limitations and a careful consideration of the potential impact of lower-fidelity solutions on educational effectiveness. In some cases, evidence exists to guide this decision-making. In most circumstances, however, none is present, and these decisions are made on the basis of precedents established in other centers. Most centers use a balanced approach and maintain an inventory of simulation devices of varying levels of complexity and fidelity (Table 8.1).

In addition to actual device costs, associated costs for the adjunct equipment required for implementation of the simulator(s) within a curriculum must be considered. For example, successful implementation of an SBT curriculum for anesthesiology requires a difficult airway cart, an anesthesia machine, and a defibrillator, in addition to a full-body high-fidelity patient simulator. Complex, high-fidelity equipment necessitates the purchase of maintenance warranty contracts, and these ongoing costs must be anticipated. In addition, numerous smaller costs related to setup of the simulation environment, consumables (e.g., sutures, intravenous bags, catheters),

Table 8.1 Basic inventory of simulation devices exclusive of simulated tissue models, actual medical equipment, and standardized patients (actors)

Benchtop part-task trainers
Airway simulator, adult (2)
Airway simulator, pediatric (1)
Airway simulator, neonatal (1)
Part-body trauma skills simulator (1)
Central venous catheter insertion trainer, ultrasound capable (1)
Breast ultrasound and puncture trainer (1)
Phlebotomy/IV access trainer (1)
Lumbar puncture trainer (1)
Thoracentesis trainer, ultrasound capable (1)
Laparoscopic skills training
Virtual reality laparoscopic skills simulator (1)
Videoscopic box trainer (2)
Patient simulation
High-fidelity adult manikin patient simulator (2)
High-fidelity neonatal manikin patient simulator (1)
Full-body birthing simulator (1)

and materials required for preparation and assessment of learners exist. In addition, actual medical equipment, such as surgical instruments, ultrasound machines, defibrillators, and intravenous infusion pumps, may be required to complete the materials list for some simulations. With careful planning and experience, management of these issues becomes possible within the curriculum development and implementation process.

Learning Management Infrastructure

Given the full range of activities that will occur in a simulation center, a method is necessary for managing information pertaining to scheduling of learners and learning resources (e.g., simulators, rooms), as well as the information generated as the result of simulation sessions. The scale of this effort must be appreciated, even for a small center. A variety of options are available to accomplish this learning management, ranging in sophistication from simple pen-and-paper methods to a commercially available Learning Management System (LMS) whose software is developed specifically for simulation center information management. The major advantage of a commercial solution is the ability to integrate all aspects of the education process into a single platform (Table 8.2).

Although potentially a costly budget item, a sophisticated LMS can be an invaluable tool for curriculum implementation, performance assessment, and research within and across institutions. Irrespective of how information is managed within the center, evidence of learning should be maintained through AV capture records, assessment tools, feedback forms, and learner portfolios.

CURRICULUM DEVELOPMENT

The importance of educationally sound, curricular-based activities for all learner groups cannot be overstated. Although a full treatment of curriculum development is beyond the scope of this chapter, a few important considerations must be mentioned. For a complete discussion of educational principles related to SBT, please refer to chapter 5 (Educational Principles in Simulation).

Defining Mission and Learner Groups

The simulation center leadership can define an overarching mission based on ambitious educational outcomes like educational innovation, effective teamwork, improved patient safety, and increased efficacy in health care. In the final analysis, however, most centers exist to improve health care provider effectiveness through education in the form of clinical experience, in which simulation can successfully substitute for elements of actual patient care. The categories of learners (e.g., undergraduate nursing students, surgical interns, the entire labor and delivery team) to whom this education is directed is the most important determinant of what occurs in the center (Table 8.3).

Curricula cannot be developed without a clear sense of what learner groups will use the center and what their teachers want them to achieve.

Needs Assessment

Curriculum development ought to be based on a formal needs assessment process, taking into account the requirements of both individuals and the larger organization.[14] The needs of individual learners, groups of learners within departments or divisions, entire institutions, or even geographical regions may be taken into account when developing curricula. A needs assessment can be accomplished based on information derived from clinical, academic, or simulated environments. It can be gathered from global assessments or direct feedback from faculty. Often,

Table 8.2 Simulation center learning management system functions

- Facilitate assembling elements of curricula
- Deliver curricular materials to learners
- Schedule learners and center resources
- Capture and archive audio-visual simulation events
- Assess performance
- Provide database functionality

Table 8.3 Examples of simulation center curricular areas based on learner group

LEARNER GROUP	CURRICULAR ACTIVITY	RESOURCES
Surgical resident (PGY 1-2)	Central venous catheter (CVC) insertion	CVC insertion part-task model Bedside ultrasound machine CVC insertion kit
Undergraduate nursing student	Pressure ulcer prevention	Full-body patient simulator
NICU fellow Pediatric chief resident	Respiratory arrest in a neonate	High-fidelity neonate patient simulator Neonatal airway part task trainer Neonatal airway cart NICU code cart
Medical unit nurse	Rapid response team activation	High-fidelity adult patient simulator
Radiology resident (PGY 2-3)	CT suite anaphylaxis event	High-fidelity adult patient simulator Code cart
Surgical physician assistant	Basic laparoscopic skills training	Virtual reality laparoscopic trainer

a combination of information gathering is applied to the needs assessment process.

Curriculum Design and Implementation

Knowledge of baseline comprehension and skill in individuals or groups, and a careful definition of the skill, competency, or behavior that must be modeled, allow the educator to define specific goals and related objectives for training. Careful development of goals and objectives for all educational activities is the best basis for effective curriculum design.

Early in the development of the simulation center at Baystate Medical Center, a template approach to curriculum design was adopted. The responsibility of setting goals and objectives, as well as contribution of content, was assigned to the user group leadership. The standardized organization of the template allowed simulation center staff to design the specific simulation activity in collaboration with the educator who originated the template request. This template request would typically include the requests for specific simulators and associated materials to run the simulation.

For simulation-based curricula, effective implementation requires that a lesson plan be defined, describing what the learner will encounter. Elements of this plan might include the simulation environment setup, simulator device programming or preparation (e.g., programming a case on a computer-driven full-patient simulator, configuring difficulty levels on a virtual reality task trainer), educator and/or facilitator preparation, briefing and debriefing methods, and provision of any assessment methodology to be used. Examples of these types of plans, developed specifically for simulation training, can be found in the American College of Surgeons—Association of Program Directors in Surgery (ACS-APDS) Phase I (basic skills), Phase II (advanced skills), and Phase III (team training) curricula.[15]

Arguably, a curriculum in high-fidelity patient simulation is more complex and intimidating to implement than curricula for focused technical skills. Starting with highly scripted simulation events and gaining experience running a few scenarios well is the best strategy prior to moving on to more advanced approaches. With experience, using the simulation as a dynamic tool to challenge the learner becomes much easier. It is important for center staff to pilot the implementation of such simulations with education faculty prior to their rollout to designated learner groups. During this rehearsal phase, educators may define areas that require modification. In addition, these pilot projects allow all staff the opportunity to understand their roles in the simulated learning activity. It is also important for the educational team to pre-brief prior to each simulation, in order to solidify expectations and inject some flexibility into the simulated experience (e.g., to determine whether events will be modified in response to a learner need identified during the simulation, or whether the course of action will remain as scripted, without tailoring to identified learner strength, deficit, or unexpected event). Any structured assessments should be objectives-driven and should be reviewed with learners during post-simulation debriefings.

Just as important as skill in delivering the simulation, center staff and educators using the center must gain skill related to immediate post-simulation debriefing. The effectiveness of the simulation in providing a meaningful educational experience is largely determined by the quality of the debriefing. The center must provide an appropriate environment for debriefing, either in a classroom with access to an A-V record of the event, or in the simulation suite at "the bedside." Debriefings should be conducted in a learner-centric manner, thus stimulating a reflective process in learners that achieves review and new insights into the experience and addressing key elements defined in the curricular objectives.

Using the center as a means to deliver a good team training experience in simulation offers an opportunity to align SBT with numerous health care quality initiatives and to garner institutional support. At Baystate Medical Center, such alignment has resulted in SBT related to disruptive behavior, patient handoffs, disclosure of adverse events, and preoperative time-out checklists.

OPERATIONAL CONSIDERATIONS

Ongoing operation of a simulation training site requires processes for oversight and quality control, management of the operational budget, centralized scheduling, and frequent review of improvement standards set by governing bodies in order to optimize center use and learner benefit.

Scheduling

Scheduling of simulation center activities must be well organized to avoid conflicts or last-minute competition for resources. Although self-scheduling is possible through some LMS products, at Baystate Medical Center, schedule management is restricted to a limited group of individuals to optimize good service and to allocate resources flexibly. Scheduling on a recurring basis for specific departments or facilitators is conducive to orderly usage, but it is not always possible. Centralized scheduling maintains order, ensures accurate time allotment for setup and take-down, and avoids chaotic situations during particularly busy periods.

Oversight and Quality Control

Oversight of SBT should occur at multiple levels. Although strategic decision-making can be managed by a qualified center director, a well-constituted steering committee allows the director to clearly articulate strategy in the context of the center's existing activities to those with oversight of financial and infrastructure planning. A means of reviewing curriculum quality by both examination of educational outcomes and reevaluation of goals and objectives should be an integral part of a new simulation center's educational infrastructure. At Baystate Medical Center, this review process is assigned to a specific committee with representation from the center's major user groups. This committee also has an oversight function for operational-level planning. Initiatives that might affect multiple programs, such as a health care quality initiative to encourage hand washing, for example, require the broad oversight of implementation that such a committee can provide. Inclusion of education experts (e.g., doctoral-level educator[s]), and a member representing the institution's health care quality agency, broadens the scope of material that this committee can cover.

Operational Budget

An operational budget should be anticipated each fiscal year, based in part on review of the prior year's center costs and projection of any increases that might be associated with the expansion of current or initiation of new programs. An operational budget will typically cover items below a threshold cost for a capital budget. It typically covers environmental or moulage materials, medical supplies, device warranty contracts, office supplies, new furniture, and professional development for simulation center staff (e.g., travel for training). Grants, philanthropic support, and tuition fees for CME courses or outside user bookings may also provide funds to offset operational costs.

Threats to Success

Success in establishing and sustaining a simulation center effort requires buy-in from learners, as well as from clinical, administrative, and educational leadership. The best way to ensure success, which to a great extent is in the control of simulation center staff, is to deliver an outstanding educational product. Problems with buy-in jeopardize the success of the center's efforts and are best addressed by the concerted engagement of the person(s) in question. Lack of progress in improving quality, lack of leadership, and, ultimately, lack of vision are the greatest threats to center success.

Although a space that is too small or hampered by flawed design can be described as a threat, it is better described as a limitation, since it rarely diminishes the quality of education for activities that can be accommodated, provided all other requirements are in place. Budgetary constraints, particularly in the operational budget, can similarly be described as a limitation, requiring available resources to be used to best effect. Rather than focus on the quality of the educational process, some institutions have made the error of devoting substantial chunks of fiscal resources to extravagant devices or a multitude of simulators that go unused due to lack of interest or need, or for the lack of a high-quality curriculum.

Even with an outstanding center, one potentially fatal threat to success is improper treatment of learners. Adversarial and shame- or blame-based encounters must be avoided by simulation center staff and clinical area leadership. Lack of safety and privacy for learners may threaten user compliance to a significant and sometimes irreversible extent.

CONCLUSION

Future Developments

The future promises to bring numerous changes to simulation centers and the educational products they must deliver. Against a turbulent health care policy backdrop, an evolving vision for simulation-based education, with a growing emphasis on mandated usage to meet externally imposed training or certification requirements, is present. The technical state-of-the-art in simulation will also evolve, and new tools will appear to meet the changing training mission. Most importantly, changes in medical care (i.e., the very things that are to be simulated) are driving changes in the simulation-based methods used and the content that must be delivered. The status quo will be further challenged by advances in simulator fidelity, by immersive virtual environments, and by screen-based patient simulation. With wider implementation, a more uniform experiential learning playing field can be delivered to a larger array of learners in medical education. Such a situation is in stark contrast to the traditional learning, based primarily on random opportunity in the actual patient care environment. The extent to which these efforts can be shown to be effective will determine the magnitude of health care resources that will be diverted to simulation-based education in the future. Simulation educators, therefore, must take advantage of opportunities to conduct research aimed at making SBT more evidence-based.

REFERENCES

1. Johnson KA, Sachdeva AK, Pellegrini CA. The critical role of accreditation in establishing the ACS Education Institutes to advance patient safety through simulation. *J Gastrointest Surg.* 2008;12:207–209.

2. Qayumi K. Centers of Excellence: a new dimension in surgical education. *Surg Innov.* 2006;13:120–128.

3. Sachdeva AK, Pellegrini CA, Johnson KA. Support for simulation-based surgical education through the American College of Surgeons-accredited education institutes. *World J Surg.* 2008;32:196–207.

4. American Board of Surgery. General requirements for the General Surgery Qualifying Exam. Accessed December 1, 2011, at http://home.absurgery.org/default.jsp?certgsqe

5. Residency Review Committee for General Surgery. ACGME program requirements for graduate medical education in surgery. Accessed December 1, 2011, at http://www.acgme.org/acWebsite/RRC_440/440_prindex.asp

6. Tofi NM, White ML, Grant M, et al. Severe contrast reaction emergencies: high fidelity simulation training for radiology residents and technologists in a children's hospital. *Acad Radiol.* 2010;17:934–940.

7. Mendiratta-Lala M, Williams T, de Quadros N, et al. The use of a simulation center to improve resident proficiency in performing ultrasound-guided procedures. *Acad Radiol.* 2010;17:535–540.

8. Dawson S. Procedural simulation: a primer. *Radiology.* 2006;241:17–25.

9. Desser TS. Simulation-based training: the next revolution in radiology education. *J Am Coll Radiol.* 2007;4:816–824.

10. Patel AA, Gould DA. Simulation in interventional radiology training and evaluation: a paradigm shift is on the horizon. *J Vasc Interv Radiol.* 2006;17:S163–S173.

11. Dunn W, Coltvet G, Belda T, et al. From the ground up: simulation center building blocks—creating a simulation center. Accessed December 1, 2011, at www.mayo.edu/simulationcenter

12. Meier A. Running a surgical education center: from small to large. *Surg Clin North Am.* 2010;90: 491–504.

13. Haluck RS, Satava RM, Fried G, et al. Establishing a simulation center for surgical skills: what to do and how to do it. *Surg Endosc.* 2007;21:1223–1232.

14. DaRosa DA, Bell RH. Graduate surgical education redesign: reflections on curriculum theory and practice. *Surgery.* 2004;136:956–974.

15. American College of Surgeons Division of Education, ACS—APDS Surgical Skills Curriculum for Residents. Accessed December 2, 2011, at http://elearning.facs.org (requires setup of Moodle account).

SECTION 3

APPLYING SIMULATION IN RADIOLOGY

9

Basic Skills: Seldinger Technique and Post-Puncture Hemostasis

LEONARD R. BOK AND HECTOR FERRAL

THE SELDINGER technique and subsequent modifications of the technique are key components in many vascular and nonvascular interventional procedures.[1–3] It is used routinely for arteriograms of many types, as well as for percutaneous drainage of fluid collections, as in percutaneous nephrostomies, gastrostomies, biliary drainages, and abscess drainages in the abdomen, pelvis, and chest. This chapter focuses primarily on using the Seldinger technique in vascular access (i.e., via vascular puncture of a blood vessel), but the principles apply to its use in other percutaneous procedures (e.g., abscess or fluid collection drainage). Currently, the Seldinger technique is not incorporated into commercially available vascular simulators (e.g., virtual reality endovascular trainers). Nonetheless, it is critical that this key technique for many interventional procedures be included in simulation-based training (SBT). Likewise, hemostasis at the vascular access site is not addressed in high-fidelity vascular simulator curricula at this time, but it too should be integrated into a SBT program.

The current commercially available vascular simulator devices generally use a simulated vascular sheath through which the trainee operator places the selected catheter to begin the simulation (Figure 9.1). Luboz et al[4] have described a simulator combining two haptic devices, including a virtual needle for vessel puncture and another for catheter and guidewire manipulation. The development of high-fidelity simulators for teaching the Seldinger technique may occur in the future; at this time, however, the Seldinger technique and its modifications appear to be amenable to SBT using part-task trainers.

It follows logically that part-task SBT can be applied to achieving hemostasis at the close of a vascular procedure. Post-puncture hemostasis techniques will be discussed at the end of this chapter.

Instructor and trainee feedback has indicated that part-task training may be helpful to teach some procedure-related tasks that are frequently taken for granted. The selection and maintenance of all material supplies during the procedure can be effectively

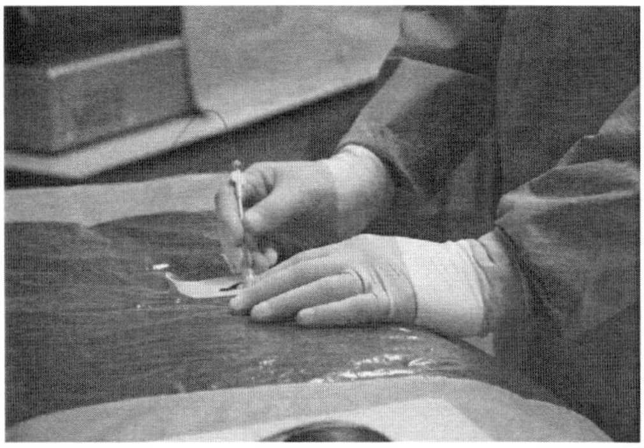

FIGURE 9.1 Endovascular high-fidelity simulator with sheath in place. Guidewire and catheter insertion. Photo courtesy of Vladimir Kiselov, MD.

taught using a mock-up and display of the angiographic room set up. Representative samples of the supplies and devices used in interventional procedures form the basis for the demonstration-simulation room discussed and illustrated in this chapter (Figure 9.2).

The Seldinger technique and hemostasis are routine but critical portions of vascular procedures that require a high level of both cognitive and technical skill for safe practice. As with sterile technique and knot tying, more complex procedures in interventional radiology (IR) and other subspecialties of radiology cannot be safely and properly performed without the knowledge and technical ability to perform fundamental tasks, including the Seldinger technique, the management of a guidewire, and the safe achievement of hemostasis.

In SBT, reliance on the use of high-fidelity simulation, but without sound curricular content, runs the risk of the training and simulators transforming into expensive computer games with limited lasting educational value. The goal of introducing part-task demonstrations and other forms of SBT into a training curriculum is to improve the efficiency and effectiveness of the overall training and to allow deliberate practice within the context of a relevant curriculum, under the direction of content experts. The demonstration of SBT should be accompanied by relevant teaching materials. Such teaching can take the form of a computer module, computer-based slide presentation, printed handout, video or live demonstration, supervised practice, or other format, as the educator deems appropriate. Pre- and post-tests following SBT are very useful for providing metrics to track the progressive development of procedural skills. An observational checklist conducted in person or by video review can be used to confirm and document skill acquisition, as well as to provide formative feedback. Observation and scoring can be performed real time or based upon video recording.

THE SELDINGER TECHNIQUE

Didactic material for any SBT activity focusing on the Seldinger technique should include some background regarding the knowledge and skills needed to successfully perform the procedure. The following paragraphs contain an example of such educational content:

> *Sven Ivar Seldinger described a technique for vascular access and placement of intravascular catheter in 1953. This method and its modifications, including micropuncture technique, are all in the tradition of "Seldinger technique." The*

(A) (B)

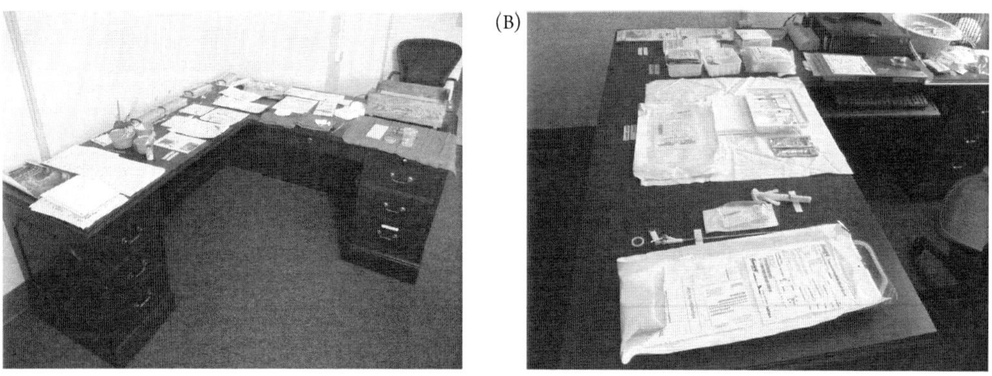

FIGURE 9.2 (A) Radiology simulation-demonstration laboratory. Photo courtesy of Luis Serrano, MD. (B) Radiology simulation-demonstration laboratory. Photo courtesy of Luis Serrano, MD.

technique is performed while constantly observing strict sterile procedure, since the skin, subcutaneous tissues, and vascular system are entered externally by needle and catheter. The Seldinger technique consists of three key maneuvers. First, percutaneous puncture of the artery or body cavity is performed. For femoral vascular access, it is critical that the puncture be performed below the inguinal ligament to avoid nondetectable retroperitoneal or intraperitoneal bleeding after catheter removal, which, in extreme circumstances, can be fatal. Second, the careful placement of a flexible tip guidewire is introduced through the needle into the artery, vein, or cavity, with the subsequent removal of the needle over the guidewire. Third, careful serial vessel or cavity dilation to the catheter size is performed, if necessary, followed by placement of the vascular sheath and/or catheter over the guidewire. Originally, the Seldinger technique was described utilizing palpation of the common femoral artery anterior to the femoral head for guidance. In the technique, a "double-wall puncture," is done with an 18 gauge needle with stylet without bevel (to minimize the risk of subintimal passage of the guidewire). The needle is then advanced through both anterior and posterior walls of the artery. The stylet is removed, and the needle is withdrawn into the vessel lumen until pulsatile blood return is seen. A soft tip "J" (i.e., curved) or soft tip straight guidewire is advanced gently through the needle into the vessel utilizing haptic (i.e., tactile) sensation to avoid passing the guidewire subintimally. This haptic element is difficult to teach with many currently available commercial simulators.

As equipment has developed, 18 and 19 gauge single-wall puncture needles became widely used in many institutions. Subsequently, micropuncture technique has been commonly used. Micropuncture technique is essentially a serial Seldinger technique beginning with a 21 gauge vascular puncture needle, through which an 0.18 inch guidewire is passed; the needle is removed, and a coaxial micropuncture sheath is placed over the microwire. After removal of the inner stiffener catheter, this micropuncture sheath will accept a standard 0.32, 0.35, or 0.38 inch guide. Over this wire, serial vessel dilators or the vascular sheath can be placed, and the selected vascular catheter can then be inserted through the sheath. Real-time ultrasound guidance can be used to supplement (or replace) manual/tactile or fluoroscopic guidance of the arterial puncture, particularly in obese extremities or in the case of the barely palpable pulse.

The primary options for SBT for skill development in the Seldinger technique include traditional apprenticeship with the trainee learning on a patient under close supervision; the use of a physical or animal model; or the use of an appropriate simulation device. Tactile sense is a key aspect of interventional radiology. As noted previously, Luboz et al[4] have described a prototype simulator that combines two haptic devices for vessel puncture with a virtual needle and catheter and guidewire manipulation. Other investigators are also working on haptic feedback devices.[5] Although SBT is not yet fully validated, it is increasingly accepted that patient safety is improved through simulation-based surgical training and that SBT is relevant to radiology.[6,7] It is therefore considered appropriate to begin the integration of simulation into radiology residency curricula.

A key step in creating a complete simulation of the Seldinger technique or other procedure is the performance of a task analysis. Johnson et al[9] describe the importance of physical and cognitive task analysis in interventional radiology. They point out that cognitive task analysis can be very time-consuming. For example, analyzing 1 hour of focused expert work may require on the order of 30 hours of analysis by a trained cognitive task analyst.[8] Johnson et al have analyzed five key interventional procedures: arterial puncture, nephrostomy, venous access, biopsy (ultrasound or computed tomography [CT] guided), and percutaneous transhepatic cholangiogram. The analysis documents can be very helpful to others who wish to simulate and teach any of these tasks.

Sheena Johnson of the University of Liverpool has created a task analysis for arterial puncture that is 20 pages in length, with 101 steps and 24 decision-making points. Other step-by-step task descriptions and decision protocols are graciously supplied on the Collaborators in Radiological Interventional Virtual Environments (CRaIVE) website (www.craive.org.uk) for anyone's use, as long as the authors are acknowledged.[9] The use of this website, dedicated to cognitive task analysis in IR, when used with appropriate local variations can save an institution vital time and resources in comparison to an effort that starts such an analysis from scratch.

Knowledge of supplies, equipment, steps, and decision points is essential in the training of novices.

The Dreyfus Five-Stage Model of Skill Acquisition recognizes that the journey from novice to expert passes through numerous phases and that it is sometimes difficult for the novice to learn directly from an expert because the novice needs to start with a list of steps, whereas the expert often approaches the situation more holistically and without the use of an explicit list.[10,11] Thus, cognitive task analysis is vital to the development of a meaningful curriculum for any simulation-based teaching.

Given the current absence of availability of a high-fidelity simulator for the Seldinger technique, low-fidelity methodology has been utilized. At Louisiana State University Health Sciences Center in New Orleans (LSUHSC-NO), a radiology department room has been designated the radiology simulation demonstration laboratory. Low-fidelity demonstrations and simulators have been developed and implemented in this room. Practical, inexpensive displays of equipment packs and instruments used in ultrasound and CT-guided interventional procedures are presented for both individual and group teaching and learning sessions. Simple devices are available for part-task simulated training and practice under direct vision for the Seldinger arterial puncture and vascular sheath placement, using femoral artery–sized clear plastic tubing. A high-fidelity vascular simulation laboratory elsewhere on campus is utilized for SBT of endovascular catheter procedures (Figure 9.3).

Didactic materials are available for the resident trainees. They include a chapter on the Seldinger technique and its modifications, and diagrams of the femoral head as it would be seen fluoroscopically with the location of the femoral vessels marked on it. Compact SBT demonstration models provide a visual display for understanding and learning the evolution of the Seldinger technique. These models demonstrate the double-wall vessel puncture (i.e., the classic Seldinger technique), the single-wall puncture, the micropuncture, and the intravascular placement of a vascular sheath (Figures 9.4–9.7).

Various guidewires and vascular catheters are available for examination and learning. The differences between the trocar technique and the Seldinger technique for drainage of fluid collections with percutaneous catheters are discussed and demonstrated. The classic methods of achieving vascular puncture site hemostasis with manual compression are presented to trainees. A vascular puncture site closure device is available for instruction and examination.

Residents are oriented to this room early during the first vascular interventional rotation and are encouraged to return to the room periodically to familiarize themselves with the techniques and supplies as their clinical exposure and knowledge increases. Trainees are encouraged to explore these models and physically place the needle, guidewire, or micropuncture devices in this nonthreatening, visually enhanced environment remote from actual patient procedures. This curriculum component is in constant development.[12]

Other approaches to vascular access simulation have been described. These include the use of commercial simulation devices that are available from

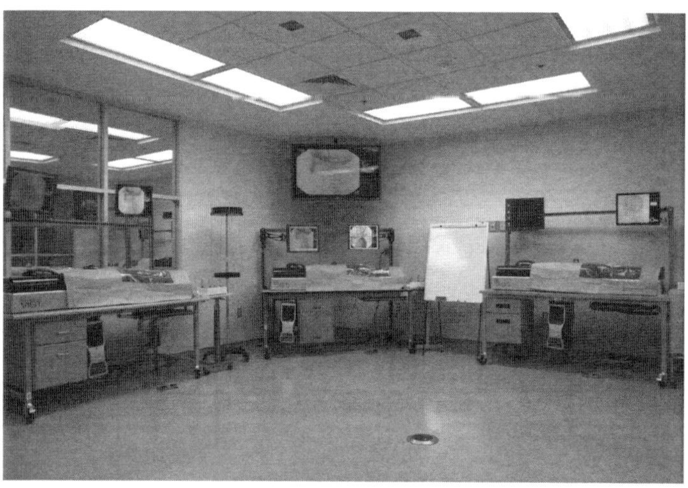

FIGURE 9.3 High-fidelity endovascular simulation laboratory. Photo courtesy of Vladimir Kiselov, MD.

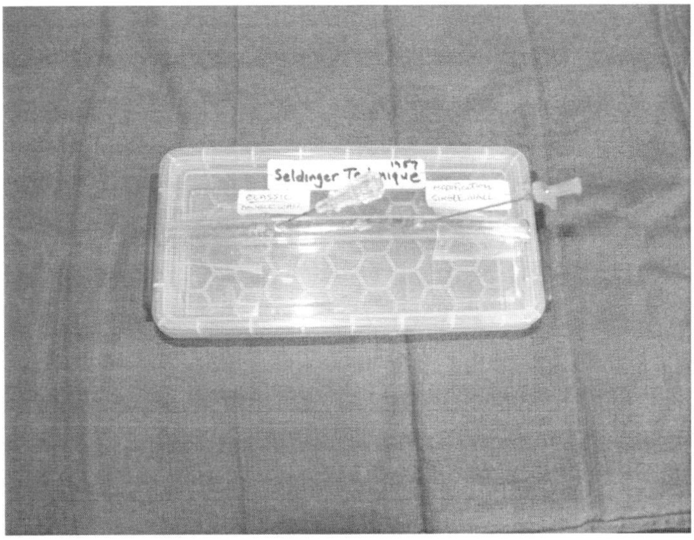

FIGURE 9.4 Simple demonstration device: double-wall and single-wall puncture. Photo courtesy of Leonard R. Bok, MD.

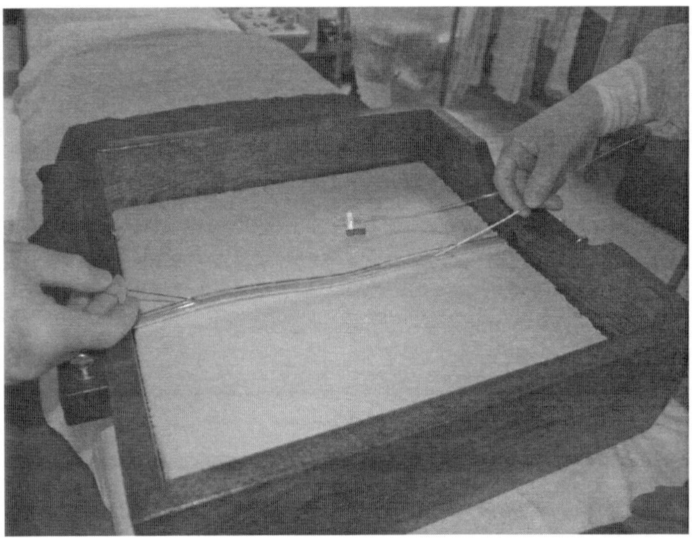

FIGURE 9.5 Part-task simulation device for practicing the Seldinger technique by a trainee with instructor. Photo courtesy of Luis Serrano, MD.

a variety of manufacturers for internal jugular vein puncture, femoral arterial and femoral venous puncture, and peripheral venous puncture for central venous catheter placement.[13–15]

POST-PUNCTURE HEMOSTASIS

Traditionally, at the completion of an infrainguinal procedure utilizing the Seldinger technique, hemostasis is achieved using manual pressure at the femoral artery over the puncture site. Pressure is typically held for 10–15 minutes or as long as necessary to achieve hemostasis.[3] This basic approach can be taught by diagrams or direct mannequin demonstration. Close supervision is required for the novice trainee performing this hemostasis technique on patients until a consistently high skill level is achieved. Refractory or recurrent bleeding at the puncture site requires a repeat of manual compression until hemostasis is achieved. Occasionally, with

(A) (B)

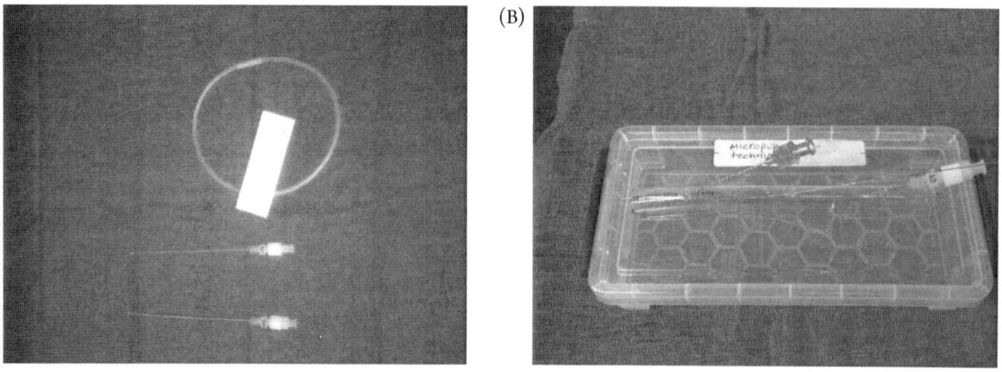

FIGURE 9.6 (A) Micropuncture set. Photo courtesy of Leonard R. Bok, MD. (B) Micropuncture demonstration. Photo courtesy of Leonard R. Bok, MD.

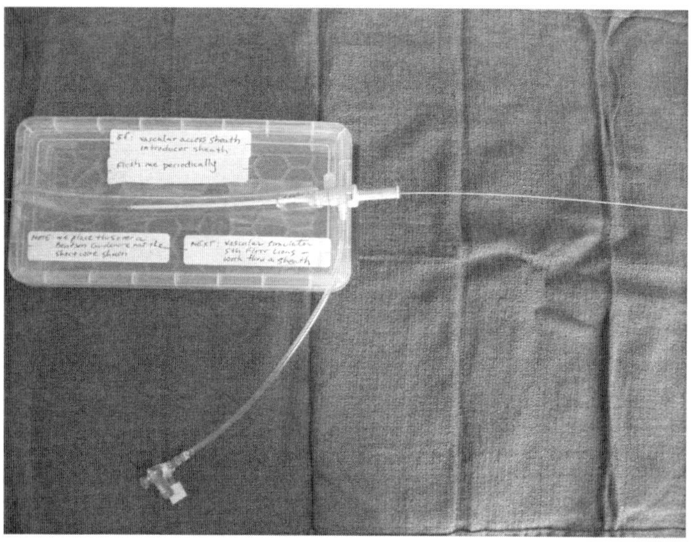

FIGURE 9.7 Vascular sheath demonstration. Photo courtesy of Luis Serrano, MD.

refractory hemostasis, particularly in hypertensive patients, a 5–10 pound sandbag is placed for 1–2 hours over the puncture site. During and at frequent time intervals after compression at the puncture site, arterial pulses distal to the puncture site (e.g., dorsalis pedis and posterior tibial foot pulses) are palpated or assessed by ultrasound to assure intact blood flow. In the past, when large-caliber catheters were utilized, a pressure dressing was sometimes applied over the puncture site after arterial compression, and the patient was kept flat in bed for 6–12 hours. Procedures are now frequently performed on an outpatient basis using smaller 4 and 5 French catheters. Typically, a latex bandage or a thrombin-assisted bandage is placed on the puncture site, and the patient is kept at bed rest for shorter periods of time, on the order of 6 to 8 hours. Outpatients with hypertension and those travelling considerable distances to home following arteriogram require careful assessment before discharge from hospital.

Vascular puncture site closure methods and devices can be placed into at least four categories. They include manual compression, suture, collagen plug, and clip.[16] A number of hemostatic devices are available from a variety of manufacturers, including Perclose (Abbott Laboratories, Abbott Park, Illinois), Angio-Seal (St. Jude Medical, Inc., St. Paul, Minnesota), and Starclose (Abbott Laboratories, Abbott Park, Illinois). In appropriate circumstances, with a normal femoral artery and the absence of hypertension, placement of these devices can be useful in facilitating early patient

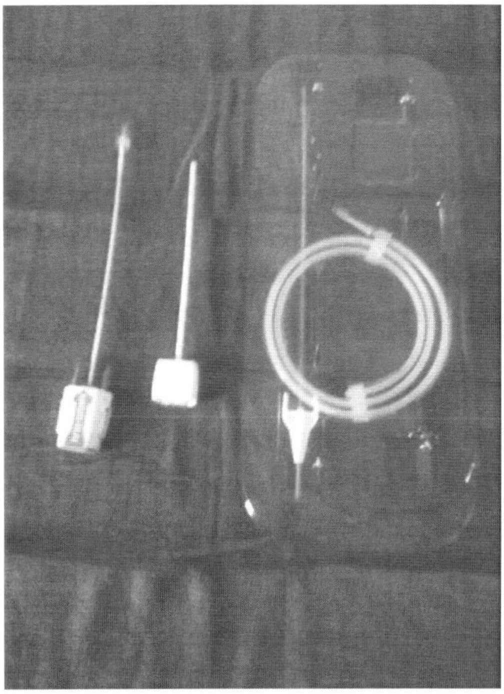

FIGURE 9.8 Arterial puncture site closure device (Angio-Seal™, St. Jude Medical). Photo courtesy of Leonard R. Bok, MD.

ambulation, typically within approximately 2 hours after the completion of the procedure. The use of a closure device can be taught by didactic instruction, demonstration, and part-task training with supervision and subsequent individual practice before the device is used in a patient procedure. At LSUHSC-NO, the radiology simulation demonstration laboratory has a display of a puncture site closure device (Figure 9.8).

A simple demonstration device is employed by manufacturers of closure devices to assist procedure operators in understanding and practicing the device deployment. Such a device could be made from materials, such as plastic tubing found in a hardware store, for use in a radiology simulation demonstration laboratory.

CONCLUSION

In summary, the Seldinger technique and post-puncture hemostasis are critical fundamental skills needed for successful completion of complex IR tasks and procedures. Although high-fidelity simulators currently lack curricular components for teaching these important basic skills, they can be learned via part-task SBT. Given that the demonstration and simulation of procedures and parts of procedures prior to trainee attempts at performance on patients can potentially improve patient safety, the quality of medical care, and the efficiency of teaching and learning complex skills, SBT of the Seldinger technique and post-puncture hemostasis should be integrated into radiology residency curricula.

REFERENCES

1. Seldinger SI. Catheter replacement of the needle in percutaneous arteriography: a new technique. *Acta Radiol.* 1953;39:368–376.

2. Seldinger S. Catheter replacement of the needle in percutaneous arteriography; a new technique [Reprint]. *Am J Roentgenol.* 1984;142:5–7.

3. Bok L, Ferral H, Bjarnason H. Access Techniques and Hemostasis. In: Ferral H, Bjarnason H, Qian Z, eds. *Synopsis of Castaneda's: Interventional Radiology*. Philadelphia: Lippincott, Williams and Wilkins; 2000:19–26.

4. Luboz V, Hughes C, Gould D, et al. Real-time Seldinger technique simulation in complex vascular models. *Int J CARS.* 2009;4:589–596.

5. Vidal F, Chalmers N, Gould D, et al. Developing a needle guidance virtual environment with patient specific data and force feedback. Paper presented at CARS 2005.

6. Satava R. Emerging trends that herald the future of surgical simulation. *Surg Clin N Amer.* 2010;90:623–633.

7. Becker GJ. Simulation and the coming transformation of medical education and training. *Radiology*. 2007;245:7–9.

8. Johnson S, Healey A, Evans J, et al. Physical and cognitive task analysis in interventional radiology. *Clin Radiol.* 2006;61:97–103.

9. CRaIVE—Collaborators in Radiological Interventional Virtual Environments. Accessed December 2, 2011, at http://hpv.cs.bangor.ac.uk/CRaIVE/projects.php

10. Batalden P, Leach D, Swing S, et al. General competencies and accreditation in graduate medical education. *Health Affairs.* 2002;21:103–111.

11. Dreyfus S, Dreyfus H. A five-stage model of the mental activities involved in directed skill acquisition. Berkeley: University of California, Operations Research Center; 1980:1–18.

12. Gould D, Kessel A, Healey S, et al. Simulators in catheter-based interventional radiology: training or computer games? *Clin Radiol.* 2006;61:556–561.

13. Dong Y, Suri HS, Cook DA, et al. Simulation-based objective assessment discerns clinical proficiency in central line placement: construct validation. *Chest.* 2010;137:1050-1056. [Epub January 8, 2010.]

14. Mahne A, Driavid V, Landmesser S. Interventional radiology simulation lab: initial experience with US-guided right internal jugular central venous catheter placement. AUR Annual Meeting April 2011. Paper SS01–09.

15. Blue Phantom. Accessed December 2, 2011, at www.bluephantom.com

16. Hamel W. Femoral artery closure after cardiac catheterization. *Crit Care Nurs*. 2009;29:39–46.

10

Basic Skills: Knot-Tying

NABEEL A. ARAIN AND DANIEL J. SCOTT

SURGICAL EDUCATION has evolved immensely since the apprenticeship model was introduced by William Halsted.[1] Knot-tying is a fundamental surgical technique used to achieve proper closure of a wound site or to secure drains or catheters. Basic principles of knot-tying must be taught and used to ensure proficiency in procedural techniques, as well as appropriate quality in patient care.

The scope of knot-tying should not be confined only to the field of surgery and related subspecialties. Knot-tying is an essential basic technical skill that is often practiced in other disciplines such as interventional cardiology, family medicine, emergency medicine, and interventional radiology. Acquiring this basic skill, therefore, can be of great value to all practitioners involved in technical tasks requiring any form of suturing or knot-tying, from minor surgical procedures to complex interventional procedures that require closure of access sites.

Although knot-tying might at first be considered a relatively easy basic skill to acquire, to tie a knot properly in reality is actually quite a technically complex and difficult task to accomplish. A recent study published in the *International Journal of Obstetrics and Gynecology* demonstrated that approximately 45% of gynecology residents were unable to tie knots securely and up to 15% of knots had to be classified as dangerous (i.e., the knots were not secure).[2] This study not only demonstrated the necessity for formal training in knot-tying, but it uncovered the potential consequences related to technical skill development in training programs lacking a formal knot-tying curriculum. Based on these findings, the authors of this study instituted a knot-tying curriculum and documented that knot-tying skills, including knot security, significantly increased after additional training.[2] Such improvement related to formal training in suturing and knot-tying has been demonstrated time and again.[3–5]

Developing, enhancing, and ultimately mastering one's knot-tying skills certainly will affect the reliability and security of the knot. Furthermore, the quality of the knot itself is of much greater importance than the actual technique employed to create it, as demonstrated by a recent study analyzing the daily routine in operation theaters. In it, the authors found that the reliability of surgical knots does not primarily depend on the intraoperative situation, but rather on the operating surgeon's skill.[6]

A considerable variation in knot-tying techniques exists among health care practitioners; for example, variation can be found between knots tied by different surgeons and even between knots tied by the same individual on different occasions.[7] In the absence of any evidence of the superiority of one particular technique (i.e., one- vs. two-handed ties), continuing education should focus on the quality of the knot and should perfect the details of the particular technique selected. In addition, speed in tying knots may result in less than perfect placement of the strands if proper technique is not used. Special attention should therefore be given to the security and quality of knots, rather than simply the speed in which the knot is tied. Training programs that emphasize proper technique and consistency can improve not only the quality of the knots but also patient care.[6]

BASIC ASPECTS OF KNOT-TYING AND SUTURING

There are several important principles and aims of knot-tying (Table 10.1).[8]

First and foremost is the ability of the practitioner to tie a *square knot*. This means laying down the knots in a flat and untwisted fashion, such that successive knots abut one another tightly. Tying a knot squarely is the critical maneuver for achieving knot security (i.e., where the knot will not unravel or slip). Thus, tissue may be appropriately approximated without concerns for disruption due to tension or movement. When tissue is under tension, successive knots may have a tendency to slip. Two options exist to overcome this problem. A surgeon's knot may be used for the first throw; this knot is constructed by wrapping the suture tail around the needle strand

Table 10.1 General principles of knot-tying

1. The completed knot must be firm, and so tied that slipping is virtually impossible. The simplest knot for the material is the most desirable.

2. The knot must be as small as possible to prevent an excessive amount of tissue reaction when absorbable sutures are used, or to minimize foreign body reaction to nonabsorbable sutures. Ends should be cut as short as possible.

3. In tying any knot, friction between strands ("sawing") must be avoided as this can weaken the integrity of the suture.

4. Care should be taken to avoid damage to the suture material when handling. Avoid the crushing or crimping application of surgical instruments, such as needle holders and forceps, to the strand except when grasping the free end of the suture during an instrument tie.

5. Excessive tension applied by the surgeon will cause breaking of the suture and may cut tissue. Practice in avoiding excessive tension leads to successful use of finer gauge materials.

6. Sutures used for approximation should not be tied too tightly because this may contribute to tissue strangulation.

7. After the first loop is tied, it is necessary to maintain traction on one end of the strand to avoid loosening of the throw being tied under any tension.

8. Final tension of final throw should be as nearly horizontal as possible.

9. The surgeon should not hesitate to change stance or position in relation to the patient in order to place a knot securely and flat.

10. Extra ties do not add to the strength of a properly tied knot. They only contribute to its bulk. With some synthetic materials, knot security requires the standard surgical technique of flat and square ties with additional throws if indicated by surgical circumstances and the experience of the surgeon.

*Adapted from University of Pennsylvania Surgery: http://www.uphs.upenn.edu/surgery/dse/medicalstudents/basicknot.html#prin.

two times, and it aims to increase friction in order to hold the first throw in place as the second throw is configured. Alternatively, a *slip knot* may be used by constructing two throws in the same direction while the needle strand is held tautly; this allows the first two knots to slide down the needle strand (hence the name "slip knot"), and abut the tissue firmly.

Knot-tying can be accomplished by either the *two-handed* or *one-handed* technique. Either technique can be readily applied to any surgical or interventional procedure; the choice is left to the preference of the operator. The two-handed technique is considered somewhat simpler and involves holding the needle strand in one hand as the tail is wrapped using the other hand to form successive throws (see simulation-based exercises below for additional information). The one-handed technique allows the surgeon to hold an instrument (i.e., needle driver) in the free hand while throwing knots with the other. Essentially, one hand is used to form the knots by wrapping the suture tail with index or middle finger manipulations (see simulation-based exercises below for additional information).

Alternatively, when suture length needs to be conserved, as in the placement of multiple skin closure sutures, an *instrument tie* may be used. This technique involves wrapping the needle strand over the needle driver and grasping the tail with the instrument; the knot may then be tied and successive throws may be performed. Instrument tying allows the use of a very short tail and thereby allows placement of several knots using a single strand.

Another important aspect of good suturing technique is avoiding a "seesaw" motion, or the sawing of one strand down over another during formation of the knot; such motion may weaken the suture material to the point of fraying or breaking, thus undermining the strength of the material and the security of the knot. If the two ends of the suture are pulled in opposite directions using uniform rate and tension, this problem may be avoided.[8] Careful attention should also be taken to avoid damage to the suture material when it is handled, especially when grasping the material with instruments, as this may inadvertently weaken the integrity of the material. Excessive tension should not be applied, as this will potentiate breakage of the suture and cutting of the tissue.

Suture selection is another key component. In general, multifilament or braided sutures are somewhat easier to handle and tie compared to monofilament sutures, which can be slippery and have a tendency to fray or break more easily, especially if handled with instruments (i.e., during instrument tying). One touted advantage of monofilament suture, however, is a lack of interstices where bacteria may reside. In clinical practice, both multifilament and monofilament sutures may be used in a broad range of applications with excellent and equivalent results. For multifilament sutures, the nature of the material and the braided or twisted construction provide a high coefficient of friction, and the knots may be easier to keep in position as they are laid down, especially if tissues are under tension.

Unlike multifilament sutures, monofilament sutures have a relatively low coefficient of friction, resulting in a greater tendency for the knot to loosen during successive throws. As a result, the suture should be held tautly as successive throws are laid down. Furthermore, monofilament sutures often possess the property of *memory*. Memory is the tendency of a suture not to lie flat, but to return to a given shape set by the material's extrusion process or the suture's packaging.[9] In other words, monofilament sutures may bow, coil, or position themselves in somewhat awkward locations, making knot-tying difficult. "Teasing out the memory" is a technique whereby the suture strand is grasped manually and stripped, in order to eliminate bowing or coils in an effort to straighten the material into a linear configuration. This technique may help eliminate difficulties associated with monofilament sutures.

Depending on the suture material type, the appropriate number of knots and tail length may vary. Generally, a minimum of three square knots is required for multifilament suture, such as silk, polyester, or polyglactin (e.g., Vicryl™). Most experts recommend at least four square knots, if not more, for monofilament suture, such as polypropylene (e.g., Prolene™), nylon, poliglecaprone (e.g., Monocyrl™), or polydioxanone (e.g., PDS™). A tail of at least 2–3 mm is appropriate for multifilament suture, whereas a tail of about 1cm may be more appropriate for monofilament suture.

Suture size or diameter is indicated by a conventional rating system. The smaller the number, the larger the suture; for instance, a 2–0 suture is larger than a 4–0. The suture size should be matched to the appropriate use. Larger sutures, such as 0, may be required for robust tissues such as the deep fascia of the abdominal wall. Very fine sutures, such as 4–0 or 5–0 may be required for delicate suturing, such as in a facial incision closure. Due to the characteristics of the material, larger sutures may require additional knots and slightly longer tails to ensure knot security, especially for monofilament sutures, due to their low friction coefficient. Beyond the minimal appropriate requirements, additional knots or longer tail lengths are generally not helpful and increase bulk, potentially compromising wound healing if materials are placed within a body cavity or subcutaneously.

Additionally, a variety of needle types exist. A *tapered needle* has a fine point to foster easy penetration of soft tissues but does not have any cutting surfaces, thus ensuring a very tight fit between the suture material and the needle hole. These needles may be especially well suited for vascular and intestinal suturing, but they also have applicability to subcutaneous tissues, such as fascia or fat. *Cutting needles,* in contrast, are designed for easy penetration of more resilient tissues, such as skin. As such, they are manufactured with both a sharp, fine point, as well as with faceted edges along the course of the needle, which act as cutting edges as the needle passes through the tissue.

Similar to suture size, the needle size should be matched to the specific use. Larger needles, such as a CT-1, CT-2, CTX, or TP-1, are well suited for closure of large bites of tissue, whereas smaller needles, such as SH, CV-1, CV-2, PS-1, or PS-2, are well suited for finer tissues. Needles may also be manufactured in *curved* or *straight* (e.g., Keith needle) configurations. The needle shape should be matched to the use at hand and selected according to the preference of the practitioner. With any needle type, appropriate technique should be used to follow the contour of the needle and minimize extraneous (i.e., lateral or vertical) forces so that tissue trauma may be minimized.

TRAINING STRATEGIES FOR TECHNICAL SKILLS

An optimal training strategy for any skill acquisition program must ensure that the subject has sufficient knowledge of *what* to do, *why* to do it, and *when* and *where* to do it. It is also important that the learner know what *not* to do, as it may be quite troublesome to unlearn bad habits once they have been formed. These goals can be achieved in several ways, including through books, journal publications, videos, lectures, and interactive seminars.[10] Central to the acquisition of technical skills such as suturing and knot-tying, however, is the opportunity to practice the necessary skills.

Over the past several decades, simulation-based education has made much progress to afford such practice. Numerous methods may be used, including the use of animal, cadaver, inanimate, or virtual reality models, and they are readily applicable to a wide variety of learners and disciplines. Advancements have been made not only from a simulation technology standpoint, but also from the standpoint of the science of simulation. These methods have met with great success in education for residents, and also for medical students, allied health professionals, and even practicing physicians.[11,12]

Several aspects regarding training deserve discussion. For a curriculum to be effective and meaningful, the content must be carefully determined. Traditionally, creating effective content can be accomplished through a needs assessment of the targeted learner group. Often, it also involves obtaining expert opinion regarding those skills that are relevant and necessary for the clinical task at hand. Simulators can be used to replicate the manual skills that are required to perform an actual procedure. Reliable metrics that accurately measure performance are also needed, such that ongoing feedback (i.e., formative assessments), as well as final evaluations (i.e., summative assessments) may be provided. Once the curricular content is chosen and suitable manual skill exercises with accurate metrics are designed, an appropriately structured practice regimen is necessary.[9]

Deliberate, distributed, and proficiency-based practice plays an important role in developing expertise through simulation-based training. *Deliberate practice* refers to the concept that expertise is acquired through carefully structured training that motivates the learner to refine skills in a goal-oriented fashion, in which practice is separated from actual performance.[13] In other words, various critical aspects of performance are defined and practiced repetitively during dedicated training sessions in order for skills to be mastered and subsequently applied during performance of actual procedures.

Another effective educational methodology is *distributed practice.* Distributed practice is a technique whereby the trainee distributes the training efforts over numerous sessions that are relatively short in duration. By contrast, the more commonly used technique is *massed practice,* whereby skills are practiced for long duration over fewer practice sessions. Distributed practice is consistent with psychomotor learning theories that stipulate that humans more robustly acquire skills using this method.[14] For example, fatigue is avoided if sessions are limited to no more than 1–1.5 hours at a time and to no more than one or two sessions per day. Additionally, by spacing sessions out over weeks to months, the consolidation of skill acquisition is facilitated, whereby neural networks have sufficient time to foster cognitive integration and internalization of the necessary components to successfully perform a task.[14] Compared to massed practice, distributed practice results in superior skill acquisition and retention.[14]

Proficiency-based training is also an important concept that has evolved considerably over recent years and has been successfully applied to simulation for development of technical skills. In contrast to arbitrary training durations, such as a fixed number of hours or set number of repetitions, proficiency-based training stipulates that tasks should be practiced until a suitable level of performance is achieved. This strategy maximizes curricular effectiveness and efficiency. If a learner has had prior extensive experience or acquires skills rapidly due to expertise in other related disciplines, only a small amount of practice may be required to reach an expert level of performance. In this case, proficiency is achieved with a small time commitment, thereby minimizing ineffective allocation of training and educational time. On the other hand, if a learner requires an extensive amount of practice, this opportunity is afforded until proficiency for the requisite skill set is verified. Thus, regardless of the amount of training that is needed for any given individual, all trainees complete a given curriculum with a level of performance that has been deemed suitable. Additionally, by providing learners with a performance-derived training endpoint, motivation is enhanced and goal-oriented practice is afforded, both key components of adult-based learning.[15] This latter aspect seems especially beneficial in the context of maximizing learning and curricular effectiveness.

Metrics play an essential role in providing feedback. In particular, metrics regarding errors are especially useful. The whole point of training is to improve performance, make performance consistent, and reduce errors. One of the major values of simulators is that they allow the trainee to make mistakes in a consequence-free environment before he or she ever performs a procedure on an actual patient. By identifying errors during simulation-based training, learners can determine what they have done wrong, correct their mistakes, and achieve suitable performance. Accordingly, learners will not be prone to repeating these same mistakes when performing procedures on actual patients.

Feedback is fundamentally important to assist adult learners in achieving their educational goals. Proctors may provide invaluable feedback to enhance learning. Manpower resources, however, may be limited, thereby constraining the amount of faculty-provided feedback available. Feedback for basic technical skills may also be provided by video tutorials that demonstrate both correct performance strategies and pitfalls. Such educational techniques may be especially useful if error avoidance strategies are demonstrated. Video tutorials may be quite effective when combined with self-directed learning and practice, and they can overcome the significant cost hurdles associated with providing direct faculty feedback.[16]

KNOT-TYING AND SUTURING SIMULATION

Numerous reports have been published regarding the acquisition of knot-tying and suturing skills.[6,10,16–21] However, methods and training practices vary widely, and very little standardization exists. Moreover, prior reports have failed to incorporate deliberate, distributed, and proficiency-based practice. Accordingly, our simulation team designed a structured curriculum for basic open knot-tying and suturing that meets these criteria. Although our program was designed for surgery residents entering their internship year, the content of this curriculum is suitable for any level of trainee, of any discipline, who is in need of these basic suturing skills.

Our program is highly structured and includes 12 tasks that use cost-effective, commercially available simulation models combined with objective criteria of time- and error-based metrics (Table 10.2 and 10.3).

Our curriculum consists of an orientation session in which trainees view the video tutorials of all 12 tasks that demonstrate the correct method for each task, as well as critical error avoidance strategies. These videos are available free of charge on our website.[22]

Under proctored supervision, each trainee completes one repetition of each of the 12 tasks (Figures 10.1–10.4).

These performances are scored, and this score serves as a baseline measure of skill (i.e., pre-test score) and is useful in documenting the educational benefit of the curriculum by evaluating the amount of objective improvement following training (Figure 10.5).

Table 10.2 Task descriptions and expert proficiency levels

TASK 1: PALM NEEDLE DRIVER	
Model	Suture board
Description	Grasp 5 mm colored segment on thin single rubber tubing by opening and closing (three full clicks) the needle driver held by palming only and perform the maneuver five times
Errors	Nonclosure, accuracy, instrument drop, non-palming
Cutoff time (seconds)	60
Expert proficiency score	53 (7 seconds with no errors)
TASK 2: KNOT-TYING, NO TENSION, TWO-HANDED	
Model	Suture board
Description	Tie a 46 cm 2-0 silk ligature around 5 mm colored segment on thick single rubber tubing using only a two-handed technique, three square knots, time starts with tie in place, not crossed, one end in each hand
Errors	Accuracy, gap, slippage, breakage
Cutoff time (seconds)	60
Expert proficiency score	50 (10 seconds with no errors)
TASK 3: KNOT-TYING, NO TENSION, ONE-HANDED	
Model	Suture board
Description	Tie a 46 cm 2-0 silk ligature around 5 mm colored segment on thick single rubber tubing using only a one-handed technique, three square knots
Errors	Accuracy, gap, slippage, breakage
Cutoff time (seconds)	60
Expert proficiency score	50 (10 seconds with no errors)
TASK 4: KNOT-TYING, UNDER TENSION, 2-HANDED, SURGEON'S KNOT	
Model	Suture board
Description	Tie a 46 cm 2-0 silk ligature around 5 mm colored segments to approximate thick double rubber tubing set using only a two-handed technique, surgeon's knot then two squares (three knots total)
Errors	Accuracy, gap, slippage, breakage
Cutoff time (seconds)	60
Expert proficiency score	47 (13 seconds with no errors)

(*continued*)

Table 10.2 (continued)

TASK 5: KNOT-TYING, UNDER TENSION, TWO-HANDED, SLIP KNOT	
Model	Suture board
Description	Tie a 46 cm 2-0 silk ligature around 5 mm colored segments to approximate thick double rubber tubing set using only a two-handed technique, slip knot on first two throws then two square throws (four knots total)
Errors	Accuracy, gap, slippage, breakage
Cutoff time (seconds)	60
Expert proficiency score	45 (15 seconds with no errors)
TASK 6: KNOT-TYING, UNDER TENSION, ONE-HANDED, SLIP KNOT	
Model	Suture board
Description	Tie a 46 cm 2-0 silk ligature around 5 mm colored segments to approximate thick double rubber tubing set using only a one-handed technique, slip knot on first two throws then two square throws (four knots total)
Errors	Accuracy, gap, slippage, breakage
Cutoff time (seconds)	60
Expert proficiency score	45 (15 seconds with no errors)
TASK 7: SUTURING, INTERRUPTED, SIMPLE	
Model	Suture board
Description	30 cm, 3-0 undyed Polysorb on tapered needle, pass needle through two inked targets for simple interrupted suture, instrument tie surgeon's knot then two squares (three knots total)
Errors	Accuracy, gap, slippage, breakage, non-palming, needle loading
Cutoff time (seconds)	120
Expert proficiency score	102 (18 seconds with no errors)
TASK 8: SUTURING, INTERRUPTED, HORIZONTAL MATTRESS	
Model	FLS Penrose drain
Description	30 cm, 3-0 undyed Polysorb on tapered needle, pass needle through four inked targets for horizontal mattress suture, instrument tie surgeon's knot then two squares (three knots total)
Errors	Accuracy, gap, slippage, breakage, non-palming, needle loading

(continued)

Table 10.2 (Continued)

TASK 9: SUTURING, INTERRUPTED, VERTICAL MATTRESS	
Expert proficiency score	89 (31 seconds with no errors)
Model	FLS Penrose drain
Description	30 cm, 3-0 undyed Polysorb on tapered needle, pass needle through four inked targets for vertical mattress suture, instrument tie surgeon's knot then two squares (three knots total)
Errors	Accuracy, gap, slippage, breakage, non-palming, needle loading
Cutoff time (seconds)	120
Expert proficiency score	89 (31 seconds with no errors)
TASK 10: SUTURING, RUNNING, SIMPLE	
Model	Dasie model
Description	46 cm, 3-0 nylon on a cutting needle, model oriented perpendicular to bench edge, instrument tie surgeon's knot then three squares (four knots total) at each corner, pass the needle through 22 inked targets to perform simple running suture, tie to loop at end, cut tails <1 cm
Errors	Accuracy, gap, slippage, breakage, non-palming, needle loading
Cutoff time (seconds)	600
Expert proficiency score	435 (2'45" [165 seconds] with no errors)
TASK 11: SUTURING, RUNNING, SUBCUTICULAR	
Model	Dasie model
Description	46 cm 4-0 undyed monofilament on a cutting needle, model oriented horizontal to bench edge, no inked targets, anchoring stitch in the first corner with instrument tie surgeon's knot then three squares (four knots total), pass needle through subcuticular layer to perform running closure, and complete using an Aberdeen (pull through the loop) knot (four throws), cut tails flush
Errors	Gap, breakage, non-palming, needle loading, tails
Cutoff time (seconds)	600
Expert proficiency score	396 (3'24" [204 seconds] with no errors)

(*continued*)

Table 10.2 (Continued)

TASK 12: SUTURING, INTERRUPTED, SUBCUTICULAR	
Model	Dasie model
Description	Any length 3-0 nylon on a cutting needle, model oriented parallel to bench edge, 1.5cm long full-thickness incision in the model (no inked targets), place a single buried subcuticular suture in a vertical fashion (perpendicular to the incision) with an instrument tie (surgeon's knot then three squares [four knots total]), cut tails flush with the model surface
Errors	Gap, breakage, non-palming, needle loading, tails
Cutoff time (seconds)	120
Expert proficiency score	87 (33 seconds with no errors)

Table 10.3 Task descriptions and expert proficiency levels

TASK	CUTOFF TIME (SECONDS)	PROFICIENCY SCORE*
1 Palm needle driver	60	53 (7 seconds, no errors)
2 Two-handed knot tying without tension	60	50 (10 seconds, no errors)
3 One-handed knot tying without tension	60	50 (10 seconds, no errors)
4 Two-handed knot tying with tension, surgeon's knot	60	47 (13 seconds, no errors)
5 Two-handed knot tying with tension, slip knot	60	45 (15 seconds, no errors)
6 One-handed knot tying with tension, slip knot	60	45 (15 seconds, no errors)
7 Simple interrupted suturing	120	102 (18 seconds, no errors)
8 Interrupted horizontal mattress suturing	120	89 (31 seconds, no errors)
9 Interrupted vertical mattress suturing	120	89 (31 seconds, no errors)
10 Simple running suturing	600	435 (165 seconds, no errors)
11 Subcuticular running suturing	600	396 (204 seconds, no errors)
12 Subcuticular interrupted suturing	120	87 (33 seconds, no errors)

*Score = Cutoff time – Completion time – (10 × sum of errors)

Trainees are oriented to the expert performance levels for each task, which serve as the proficiency-based training goals. The trainees are allowed 2 months of self-practice, during which time they are expected to practice all tasks until the proficiency levels are achieved on at least two consecutive repetitions. During this time, they have free access to the video tutorials. This practice has proven effective in very efficiently limiting requirements and logistics for personnel resources. Upon request, additional resident or faculty mentoring is afforded. Score sheets help keep track of the progress of each learner and can be tracked by the education coordinator on a weekly basis.[22] The sheets are kept in the skills laboratory and are filled out by learners after each repetition. Learners who are not adequately progressing

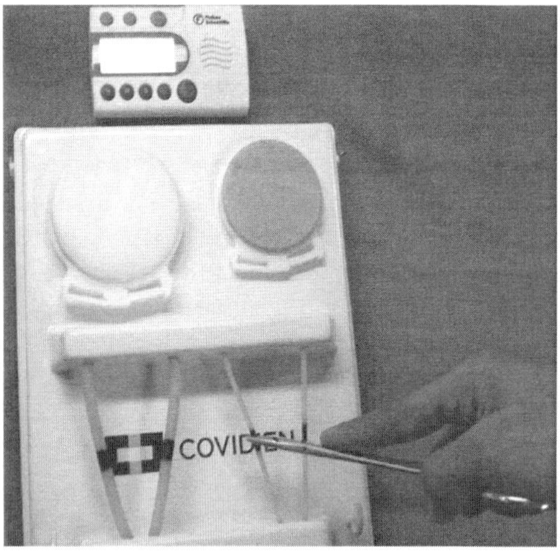

FIGURE 10.1 Task 1 (Palm Needle Driver) is performed by grasping the marked segments of a single thin rubber tube on the suture board.

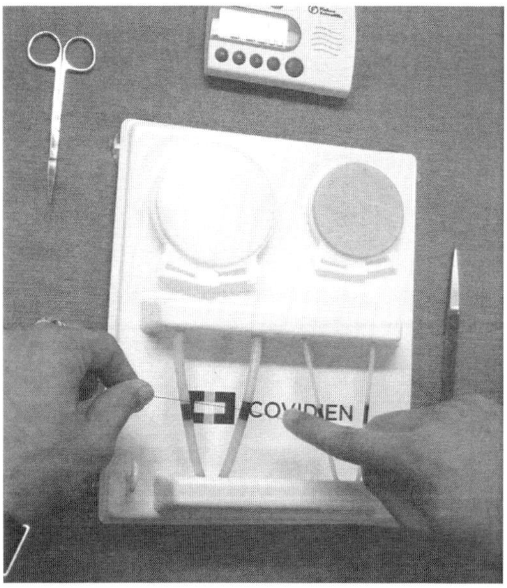

FIGURE 10.2 Tasks 2 through 6 use a suture board with marked segments of tubing to facilitate one- and two-handed knot-tying.

through the curriculum in a timely fashion are sent numerous reminders by e-mail and electronic pages. Additionally, individual tutoring is arranged as needed. Participation is ensured through the support of our residency program director.

Once trainees have documented completion of the proficiency-based training, a one-on-one proctored post-test is conducted that consists of performing one

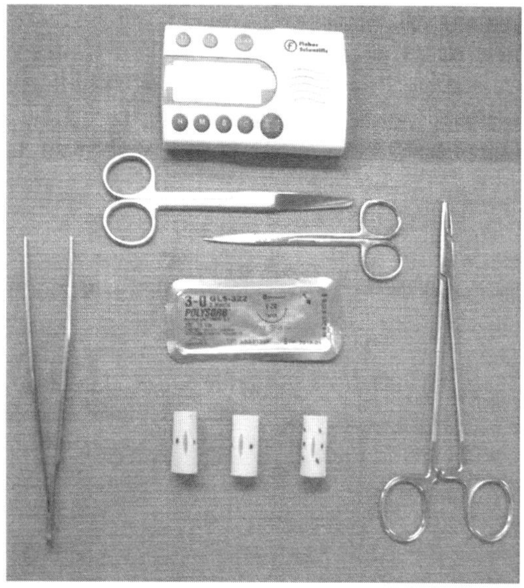

FIGURE 10.3 Tasks 7 through 9 use a slit Penrose drain to facilitate interrupted suturing.

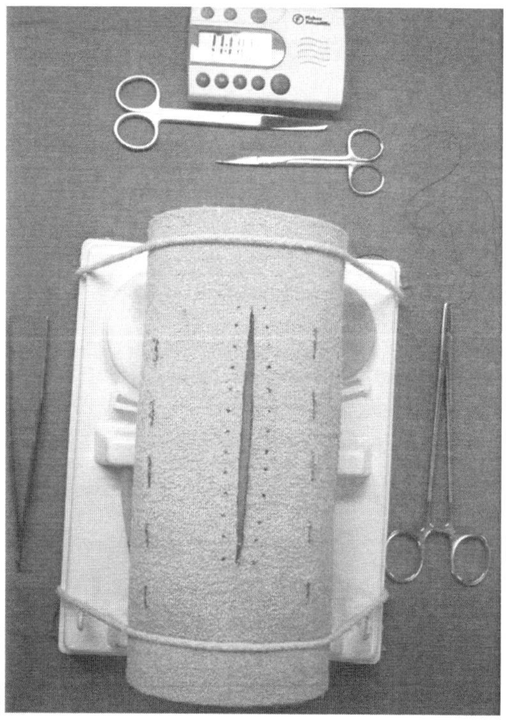

FIGURE 10.4 Tasks 10 through 12 use a laminated fabric model to facilitate continuous and interrupted subcuticular suturing.

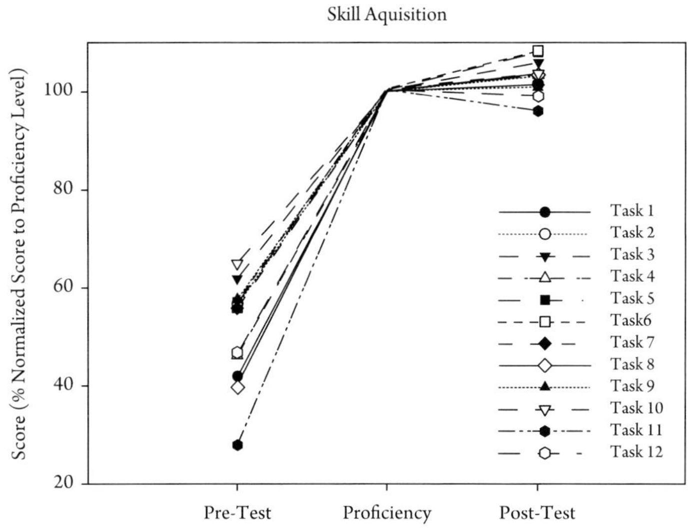

FIGURE 10.5 Trainee pre- and post-test scores were significantly different according to composite scores and for all 12 tasks scores (p <0.001 for all comparisons); normalized scores are shown graphically, and 100% corresponds to proficiency.

repetition of each task without warm-up. This strategy is used to evaluate effectively the degree of skill acquisition internalized by the learner and to verify that adequate practice has been performed. The learners are not expected to achieve full proficiency levels at post-testing. Rather, our experience has shown that if a learner achieves a score of at least 80% of the proficiency level, then adequate skill acquisition has been achieved. If needed, remediation in the form of additional required practice is prescribed.

The 12 tasks used for this curriculum are designed to teach instrument handling, two-handed ties, one-handed ties, placement of a surgeon's knot, placement of a slip knot, interrupted suturing, and continuous suturing (Table 10.2). All of these exercises use inexpensive, commercially available materials, including suture boards (Syneture, Covidien, New Haven, Connecticut), Fundamentals of Laparoscopic Surgery (FLS) Penrose drain models (www.flsprogram.org), and laminated fabric models (Dasie International, Elora, Canada). Scoring is performed on a real-time basis by either a proctor (i.e., pre-test and post-test) or by the trainee (i.e., during practice), and consists of the objective measures of time to completion and defined error rates (Table 10.3).

This curriculum has proven robust and effective. At our institution, the curriculum has been used successfully for 5 consecutive years. Our research has confirmed construct validity for each of the 12 tasks, indicating that the exercises effectively measure the skills that they aim to evaluate and teach.[16,17] This aspect was demonstrated by finding significant differences in performance between novices and experts, thus establishing the validity of using expert levels as training goals. Moreover, training to expert levels has been universally feasible for our trainees. In our initial implementation study, we documented that all 37 postgraduate year 1 (PGY1) surgery residents completed the curriculum over the first 3 months of their internships. On average, they performed 141 ± 80 repetitions (range, 52–513) and required 12.7 ± 5.3 hours of practice (range, 6.9–37.1).[16,17]

The variability in the amount of training required to reach proficiency underscores the value of the proficiency-based curriculum. As seen in our study, even in a homogenous class of surgery interns, a wide variation in baseline skills and rates of skill acquisition was present (Figure 10.5). Nonetheless, all trainees completed the curriculum and demonstrated an excellent level of ultimate performance. Moreover, the curriculum was extremely cost-effective, requiring only $776 in materials to train 37 residents over 376 hours.[16,17]

SPECIFIC KNOT-TYING SKILLS FOR INTERVENTIONAL RADIOLOGISTS

The simulation exercises described above are highly relevant for interventional radiologists as this curriculum teaches the fundamental aspects of basic knot-tying and suturing techniques. For drainage catheters, a simple interrupted suture may be placed in the skin, followed by several wraps of the suture tails around the catheter, with subsequent knots placed to hold the catheter in position securely. For skin closure of small to even large incisions, several of the techniques described are appropriate. Using absorbable suture, an interrupted or running buried technique may be quite useful, as this obviates the need for subsequent suture removal and provides excellent cosmesis. For larger openings under tension, a horizontal or preferably a vertical mattress suture may be used. Although completion of all 12 skills would give a radiologist a wide range of basic knot-tying and suturing skills beneficial to an interventionalist practice, learning at least one knot-tying technique (e.g., two- vs. one-handed tying) and to place interrupted sutures would be a minimal requirement.

SCRUBBING AND ASEPTIC TECHNIQUE FOR OPERATIVE PROCEDURES

To avoid contamination of the sterile field and potential infectious complications, appropriate preparation and technique are paramount. This is especially important when indwelling catheters or other foreign bodies are being placed or left within the patient. Surgical site infections (SSIs) are the third most common nosocomial infection and are responsible for longer hospital stays and increased costs to the patient and hospital.[23] By utilizing aseptic technique, SSIs can be drastically reduced in frequency.

Scrubbing is required for any individual who will come into contact with the sterile field or sterile instruments and equipment. This procedure requires use of a long-acting, powerful, antimicrobial soap on the hands and forearms for a longer period of time than used for typical handwashing. Institutional policy usually designates an acceptable minimum length of time required. The Centers for Disease Control and Prevention recommend at least 2 to 5 minutes of scrubbing.[23] Thorough drying is essential, as moist surfaces invite the presence of pathogens. Such drying must be done using a sterile towel. Contact with the faucet or other potential contaminants should be avoided. An important principle of aseptic technique is that fluid, a potential mode of pathogen transmission, flows in the direction of gravity. With this in mind, hands are held below elbows during the surgical scrub and above elbows following the surgical scrub. Despite this careful scrub, bare hands are always considered potential sources of infection, although this practice is highly effective in decreasing the microbial load on the skin.[23]

Any time an interventional procedure is performed, aseptic technique must be used. In addition to physician scrubbing, the patient should be appropriately prepped. If hair removal is necessary, it should be done at the time of procedure, using clippers as opposed to razors. The skin should be widely prepared using standard disinfectants, such as iodine, alcohol, or chlorhexidine gluconate solutions. The operative field, as well as the instrument table, should be sterile draped to ensure that contamination does not occur. The team must be vigilant to also ensure prevention of contact between any part of the sterile field and any other surfaces that are not sterile.

As with knot-tying, scrubbing and prepping techniques can be mastered using simulation-based curricula incorporating focused, distributed practice to predefined proficiency levels. Such training allows learners the opportunity to learn from breaks in sterility without risk to the patient (i.e., the development of SSIs). Through such simulation-based training, aseptic principles and techniques can become second nature for learners, allowing for their proper application in the clinical environment.

CONCLUSION

Knot-tying and suturing are basic technical skills with important applications in multiple medical specialties including radiology. Proper technique in performing these skills is essential for adequate knot security, and, consequently, quality of care. In radiology, learning at least one knot-tying technique (e.g. one- or two-handed tying) and simple interrupted suturing are minimal requirements. Simulation-based training is well suited for teaching knot-tying and suturing. In order to be most effective, such training should incorporate deliberate, distributed practice until proficiency-driven endpoints are achieved. By adhering to such principles, educators can ensure standardized quality in knot tying and suturing, enhancing patient care.

REFERENCES

1. Scott DJ. Patient safety competency, and future of surgical simulation. *Simul Healthc.* 2006;1:164–170.

2. Ind TE, Shelton JC, Shepherd JH. Influence of training on reliability of surgical knots. *BJOG*. 2001; 108:1013–1016.
3. Summers AN, Rinehart GC, Simpson D, et al. Acquisition of surgical skills: a randomized trial of didactic, videotape, and computer-based learning. *Surgery*. 1999;126:330–336.
4. Nousiainen M, Brydges R, Backstein D, et al. Comparison of expert instruction and computer-based video training in teaching fundamental surgical skills to medical students. *Surgery*. 2008;143:539–544.
5. Jensen AR, Wright AS, Levy AE, et al. Acquiring basic skills: is a faculty mentor really needed? *Am J Surg*. 2009;197:82–88.
6. Fischer L, Bruckner T, Muller-Stich BP, et al. Variability of surgical knot tying techniques: do we need to standardize? *Langenbecks Arch Surg*. 2010;395:445–450.
7. University of California, San Diego, Department of Surgery. Accessed December 2, 2011, at http://plasticsurgery.ucsd.edu/Portals/0/Knot_Tying_Manual[1].pdf
8. University of Pennsylvania Surgery. Accessed July 19, 2010, at http://www.uphs.upenn.edu/surgery/dse/medicalstudents/basicknot.html#prin
9. Schaverien MV. Development of expertise in surgical training. *J Surg Educ*. 2010;67:37–43.
10. Gallagher A, Ritter E, Champion H, et al. Virtual reality simulation for the operating room: Proficiency-based training as a paradigm shift in surgical skills training. *Ann Surg*. 2005;241:364–372.
11. Naylor RA, Hollett LA, Valentine J, et al. Can medical students achieve skills proficiency through simulation training? *Am J Surg*. 2009;198: 277–282.
12. Stefanidis D, Sierra R, Korndorffer J, et al. Intensive continuing medical education course training on simulators results in proficiency for laparoscopic suturing. *Am J Surg*. 2006;191:23–27.
13. Ericsson KA. Deliberate practice and the acquisition and maintenance of expert performance in medicine and related domains. *Acad Med*. 2004;79:S70–S81.
14. Moulton CA, Dubrowski A, Macrae H, et al. Teaching surgical skills: what kind of practice makes perfect? *Ann Surg*. 2006;244:400–409.
15. Knowles MS, Holton III EF, Swanson RA. *The Adult Learner*, 5th edition. Woburn, MA: Butterworth-Heinemann; 1998.
16. Scott DJ, Goova MT, Tesfay ST. A cost-effective proficiency-based knot-tying and suturing curriculum for residency programs. *J Surg Res*. 2007;141:7–15.
17. Goova MT, Hollett LA, Tesfay ST, et al. Implementation, construct validity, and benefit of a proficiency-based knot-tying and suturing curriculum. *J Surg Ed*. doi: 1931–7204/08, 10.1016/j.jsurg.2008.04.004
18. Sanders CW, Edwards JC, Burdenski TK. A survey of basic technical skills of medical students. *Acad Med*. 2004;79:873.
19. McMahon DJ, Chen S, Maclellan DG. Formal teaching of basic surgical skills. *Aust NZ J Surg*. 1995;65:607.
20. Lossing AG, Hatswell EM, Gilas T, et al. A technical skills course for first-year residents in general surgery: A descriptive study. *Can J Surg*. 1992;35:536.
21. Beard JD, Jolly BC, Newble DI, et al. Assessing the technical skills of surgical trainees. *Br J Surg*. 2005;92:778.
22. University of Texas Southwestern Center for Minimally Invasive Surgery. Accessed July 19, 2010, at http://www.utsouthwestern.edu/utsw/cda/dept48035/files/264752.html
23. Mangram A, Horan T, Pearson M, et al. Guideline for prevention of surgical site infection,. *Infect Cont Hosp Epidemiol*. 1999;20:247–278.

11

Basic Skills: Biopsies—Core Biopsies and Aspiration Biopsies

LEONARD R. BOK AND HECTOR FERRAL

IMAGE-GUIDED BIOPSY techniques have been in use since at least the 1920s[1] and have been applied to virtually all locations in the body. Several imaging modalities have been used for image-based guidance in these procedures including X-ray fluoroscopy, computed tomography (CT), ultrasound (US), magnetic resonance imaging (MRI), and recently, positron emission tomography-computed tomography (PET-CT). The skill set for each of these techniques is varied. Simulation-based training (SBT) in image-guided biopsy techniques requires complete physical and cognitive task analysis for each technique.[2] Subject matter (i.e., content) experts, educational specialists, and psychological professionals are necessary for the development of the procedural task analysis. The Collaborators in Radiological Interventional Virtual Environments (CRaIVE) website provides expert guidance in structuring techniques.[3] Once a technique is developed, efficient and effective uses of the method are skillfully designed. The ultimate goal is the validation of the SBT and the metrics provided in the use of the technique to ensure its utility as an educational and skill development tool.[4]

SIMULATION-BASED TRAINING IN PERCUTANEOUS BIOPSY

Certain percutaneous biopsy procedures can be performed without the need of image guidance and are amenable to training using part-task simulators.[5] For example, superficial soft tissue lesions, palpable breast masses, and palpable thyroid nodules have traditionally been biopsied without image guidance. Initial SBT of learners in percutaneous biopsy without image guidance has several advantages. First, it allows the trainee to master the basic technical skills involved in percutaneous biopsy through deliberate practice prior to taking on the additional learning challenge of image guidance. Second, it allows the trainee the opportunity to become familiar with commonly used biopsy devices prior to the introduction of imaging technology. Finally, it allows the learner to focus on core skills involving basic requisite medical knowledge and haptic elements (i.e., sensation of touch and feel) of needle passage through different tissues. This instruction and expert demonstration in all elements of diagnostic needle biopsies prepares the trainee for individual SBT using deliberate practice of biopsies of various organs utilizing CT and/or ultrasound guidance[6] (see chapter 25, Simulation-Based Training for Ultrasound and Computed Tomography–Guided Interventional Procedures). In this manner, the learner can incorporate, practice, and master the imaging elements once the biopsy techniques have been understood and mastered.

An SBT program in percutaneous biopsy techniques must be incorporated into a carefully developed curriculum[3–5,7] (see chapter 7, Building and Incorporating Simulation into a Radiology Residency Program Curriculum). One structure for such a training curriculum could include an initial pretest followed by a didactic component (e.g., expert level lecture, computer-based slide show presentation, or online module), the SBT in percutaneous biopsy itself, and a concluding post-test. Such a curriculum in percutaneous biopsy would optimally cover materials and techniques, as well as procedure planning, risks and benefits, and informed consent. It would include a practical demonstration of all equipment and supplies used in needle biopsy procedures. Finally, it would emphasize that this procedure depends upon cooperation and teamwork between the referring clinical team, the radiologist, and the pathologist in order to set realistic expectations and optimize results.

Ideally, SBT would be outcomes-based (i.e., proficiency-driven), distributed over time, and structured around deliberate practice of the skills being taught. Thus, a trainee's mentored initial performance and formative feedback would be followed by repeated deliberate practice of mentor targeted skills by the trainee. In this manner, training would be individualized according to each learner's skill level. Additionally, the period of training would vary for each learner, since the deliberate practice would continue until the trainee had attained a predetermined level of proficiency in the training task. Such proficiency would be assessed via post-training assessment of both procedural knowledge and technical skill. Methods of assessment would include multiple-choice questions, checklist scoring, and global performance rating. Analysis for proficiency of procedural technical skills can be performed by evaluating trainee performance of the procedure using either direct instructor observation or videotape review. Results can be maintained to catalogue evidence of proficiency in the demonstrated skills.

A simple simulation-demonstration laboratory is present in the department of radiology at the Louisiana State University Health Sciences Center in New Orleans (LSUHSC-NO). It is equipped with sample interventional procedure supplies that enable trainees to become familiar with the necessary materials before participating in SBT and subsequent supervised patient procedures (Figures 11.1–11.3). This laboratory also allows trainees to perform basic simulated tasks, such as vessel needle puncture and the

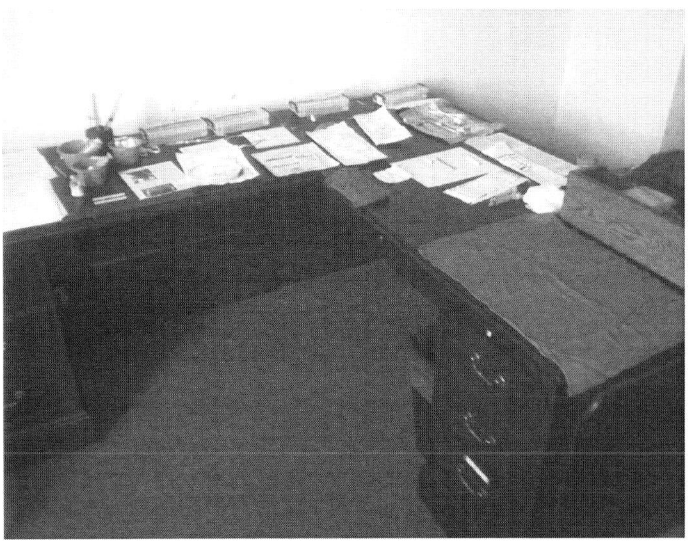

FIGURE 11.1 Small demonstration/simulation laboratory with sample supplies for interventional procedures.

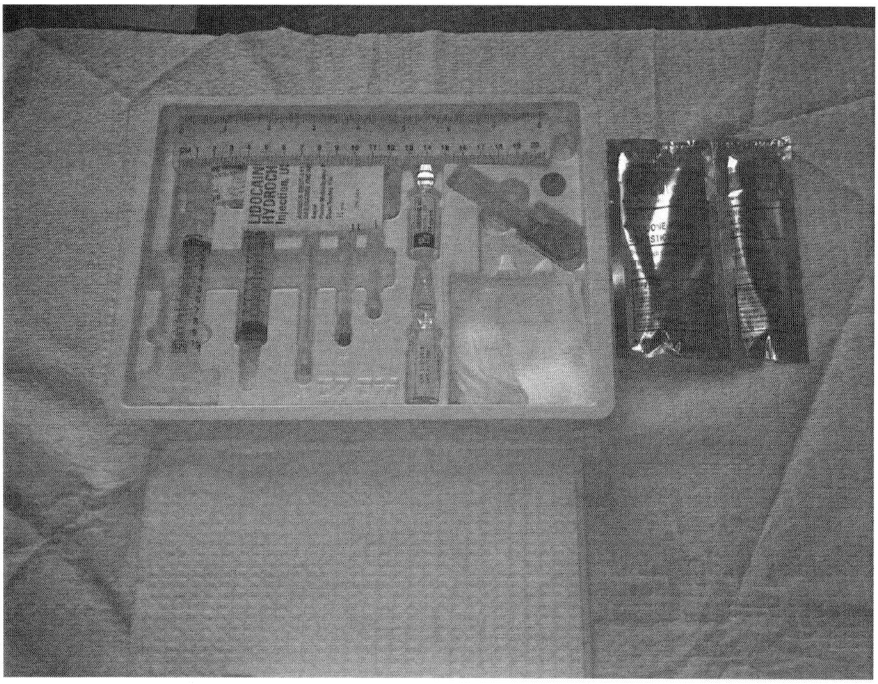

FIGURE 11.2 Sample biopsy tray.

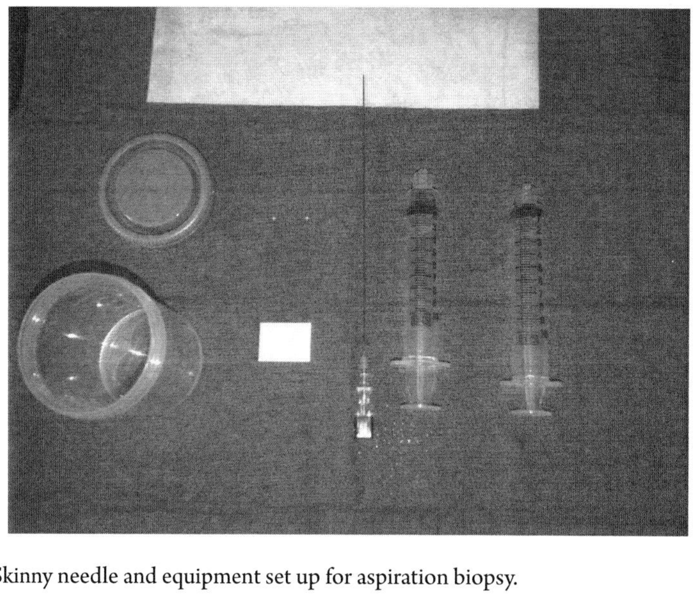

FIGURE 11.3 Skinny needle and equipment set up for aspiration biopsy.

insertion of a vascular sheath and catheter, in simple part-task training devices. The fully equipped Russell C. Klein, MD, Center for Advanced Practice is utilized for comprehensive endovascular SBT (Figures 11.1 and 11.2). Trainees have reported that the preliminary "hands-on" demonstrations are useful in increasing confidence when beginning SBT. The overall goals of increased patient safety with improved procedural skills, and the effectiveness of the training methods, will require a cohesive curriculum with specified goals and objectives, as well as validated outcome measurement tools.

Biopsy needles can be classified according to function: *cutting (core) needles*, which obtain a core sample of tissue for histopathologic evaluation; and *aspiration needles*, which obtain an aspirate of cells that can then be prepared for cytological evaluation.[8] Needles are also classified by size: *small-caliber* (i.e., 21–25 gauge "skinny needles"); *medium-caliber* (i.e., 18–20 gauge); and *large-caliber* (i.e., 16 gauge or larger). Recently, in an effort to decrease biopsy procedural morbidity, a trend toward the use of small- or medium-gauge needles, when reasonably possible, has occurred.[8] Examples of commonly used cutting and aspiration biopsy needles include the Chiba, Turner, Franseen, Madayag, Greene, and Westcott varieties.[9] As part of the SBT experience, the trainee should have an opportunity to practice with a variety of biopsy needles, in order to become familiar with each one's use (Figure 11.3).

Aspiration biopsy is performed utilizing a gentle to-and-fro motion with simultaneous gentle syringe suction, with the needle inserted at the tissue target site.[8] Commonly, the operator applies gentle suction with a 5–10 cc syringe but avoids applying excessive suction that draws blood into the needle, thereby contaminating the cell aspirate and rendering cytologic diagnosis difficult or impossible. The manual skills of tissue aspiration biopsy can be learned via deliberate practice utilizing simple models such as bologna, other meats, fruits, or vegetables, which are all readily and inexpensively available in the grocery market (Figures 11.4 and 11.5).

The simple cutting needle has a sharp tip that can cut a tissue core when advanced to the tissue target site. The core biopsy needle (e.g., the Tru-Cut soft tissue biopsy needle) has a slotted inner stylet that is advanced to the target site and an outer stylet that is then advanced over it. Core biopsy needle varieties

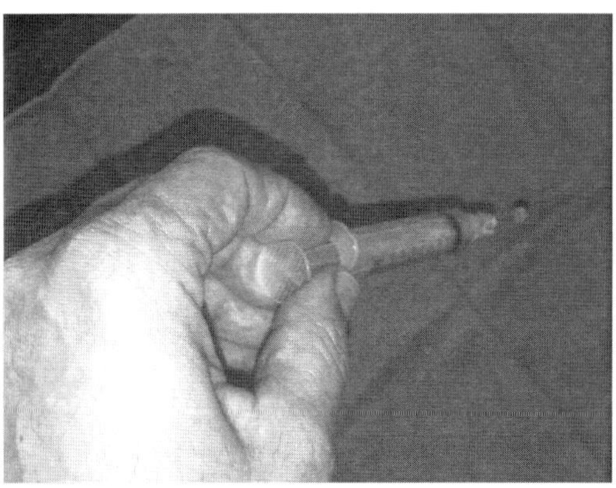

FIGURE 11.4 Practicing simulated aspiration biopsy with skinny needle.

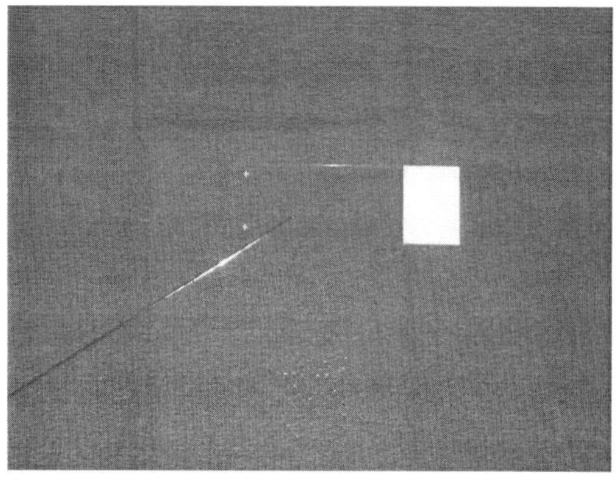

FIGURE 11.5 Practicing placing aspirate on microscopic slide for smear preparation.

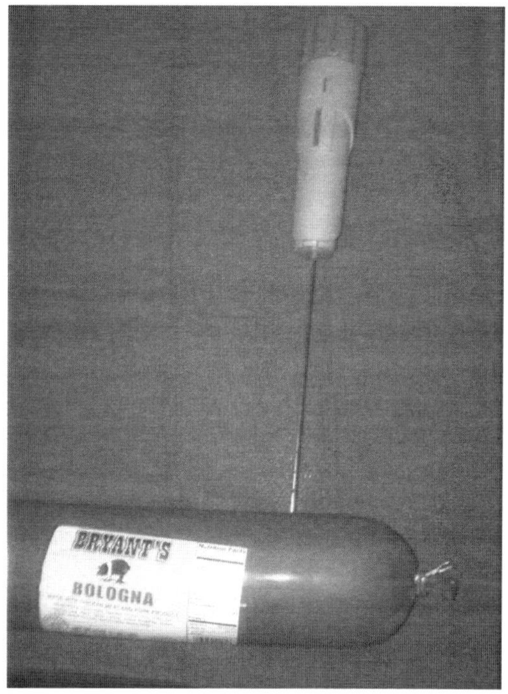

FIGURE 11.6 Practicing core biopsy with simple bologna model.

include both manual and automated (i.e., spring driven). Core biopsy techniques can be learned using deliberate practice on simple, inexpensive models such as meats, vegetables (e.g., eggplant or onion), or fruits (e.g., orange, apple, or melon). A technique variation is the use of a guiding stylet along which the cutting needle is placed. This allows multiple core biopsy samples to be taken with only one puncture site in the simulated skin and target organ, and it can be practiced via SBT (Figures 11.6–11.8).

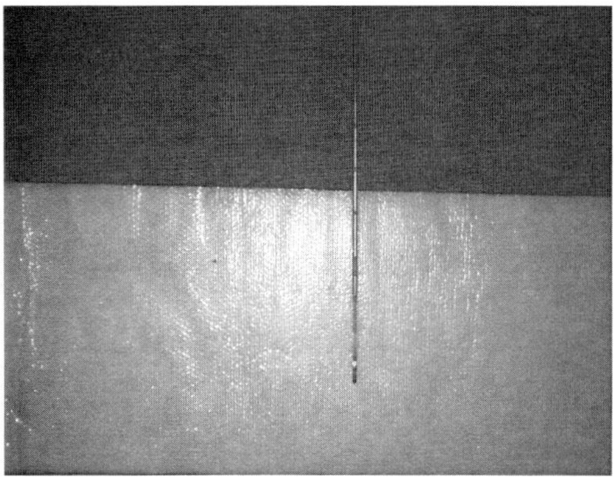

FIGURE 11.7 Practicing rolling core biopsy on Telfa pad.

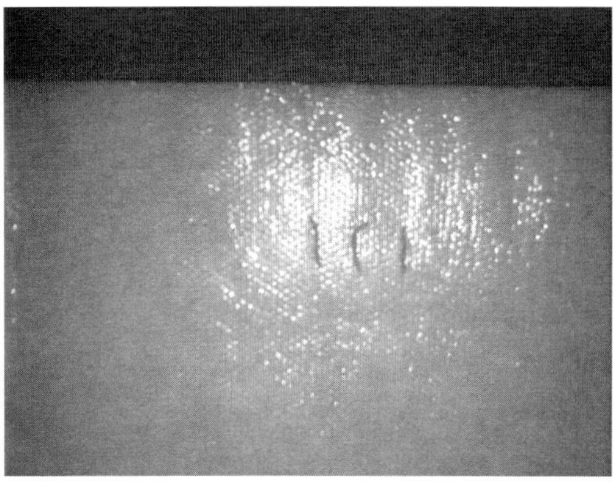

FIGURE 11.8 Three practice bologna tissue cores placed on Telfa pad.

CONCLUSION

Demonstrations of interventional procedure equipment and supplies and SBT have increasing utility in graduate medical education.[10,11] Both can be used to good effect in teaching percutaneous needle biopsy techniques. Patient safety and quality of care are of paramount importance for all interventional procedures. Hence, the use of a proficiency-based curriculum in percutaneous biopsy technique, combined with validated methods of SBT, can be the basis for successful outcomes-based training in this important basic skill. In fact, validated SBT techniques and metrics in percutaneous biopsy techniques can form a basis for long-term maintenance of competence during and following residency training in this key skill, thus helping to enhance patient safety in interventional procedures.

REFERENCES

1. Moulton J, Leoni S, Worth S. Percutaneous image-guided biopsy. In: Baum S, Pentecost M, eds. *Abrams' Angiography: Interventional Radiology*. Philadelphia: Lippincott, Williams & Wilkins; 2006:257–279.
2. Johnson S, Healey A, Evans J, et al. Physical and cognitive task analysis in interventional radiology. *Clin Radiol.* 2006;61:97–103.
3. CRaIVE—Collaborators in Radiological Interventional Virtual Environments. Accessed July 8, 2011, at http://hpv.csbangor.ac.uk/CRaIVE/projects.php
4. Gould D, Patel A, Becker G, et al. SIR/RSNA/CIRSE Joint Medical Simulation Task Force strategic plan executive summary. *J Vasc Interv Radiol.* 2007;18:953–955.
5. Dawson S. Procedural simulation: a primer. *Radiology.* 2006; 241:17–25.
6. Ericsson K, Drampe R, Tesch-Romer C. The role of deliberate practice in the acquisition of expert performance. *Psychol Rev.* 1993;100:363–406.
7. Patel A, Gould D. Simulators in interventional radiology training and evaluation: a paradigm shift is on the horizon. *J Vasc Interv Radiol.* 2006;17: S163–S173.
8. Moulton J, Leoni S, Worth S. Percutaneous image-guided biopsy. In: Baum S, Pentecost M, eds. *Abrams' Angiography: Interventional Radiology*. Philadelphia: Lippincott, Williams & Wilkins; 2006:257–279.
9. Silverman S, Segal D. Abdominal biopsies. In: Kandarpa K, Machan L, eds. *Handbook of Interventional Radiologic Procedures.* Philadelphia: Wolters Kluwer-Lippincott Williams & Wilkins; 2011:516–526.
10. Satava R. The revolution in medical education—the role of simulation. *J Grad Med Educ.* 2009;Dec:172–175.
11. Becker, G. Simulation and the coming transformation of medical education and training. *Radiology.* 2007;245:7–9.

12

Interprofessional Team-Based Training

DEBORAH GARBEE, LAURA BONANNO, KENDRA BARRIER, AND JOHN T. PAIGE

INEFFECTIVE TEAMWORK and poor communication among health care providers can decrease the quality of patient care and potentially lead to poor patient outcomes. Consequently, many prominent national organizations have made team training among health care professionals a priority. For example, the Institute of Medicine (IOM) has established the ability to work in interdisciplinary teams as one of its core competencies for health care professionals.[1] Additionally, the Joint Commission has recognized the role of poor communication in the root cause of sentinel events,[2] and, as a result, has emphasized the importance of team training in its own publications.[3] Finally, the Agency for Healthcare Research and Quality (AHRQ) has sponsored research aimed at defining the current relationship between medical teamwork, team training, and patient safety.[4]

Poor teamwork has been shown to impact negatively on patient outcomes. For example, Mills et al[5] demonstrated that failure in coordination and communication among teams in the surgical intensive care unit led to higher mortality rates and longer lengths of stay. Consequently, improving team-based skills among health care professionals has taken on increasing importance. The Joint Commission has even included improving the effectiveness of communication among caregivers as one of its 2010 National Patient Safety Goals.[6] Fortunately, team-based skills can be taught.[7] In fact, team training is an ideal tool when utilized to improve patient safety and reduce medical error, especially since teams make fewer mistakes when every member of a team is aware of each teammate's responsibilities.[4] High-fidelity simulation-based training (SBT) is particularly well suited for team-oriented training because it provides the opportunity for teams to work together in treating low-frequency, high-risk events in an immersive, safe learning environment without consequences to patients.[8] Furthermore, integration of SBT into academic institutions can promote effective teamwork and communication skills prior to entry into the health care field. Finally, SBT allows for repetition of practice, so that human response becomes automatic in an emergency situation.

This chapter focuses on the use of simulation in promoting interprofessional team training. First, it will provide an extensive review of the state of the science related to team function and training, including the current role of SBT. Later, it will provide an example of the implementation of high-fidelity SBT of interprofessional teams by discussing the experience at Louisiana State University Health Sciences Center, New Orleans (LSUHSC-NO) in training interprofessional student teams. Finally, it will discuss potential applications of such team training in the field of radiology.

TEAMWORK IN CLINICAL PRACTICE

The IOM and Teamwork

In its 1999 ground-breaking report on patient safety, *To Err Is Human: Building a Safer Health System*,[9] the IOM identified that preventable medical errors exacted significant tolls. Human error was identified as a key factor leading to unfavorable patient outcomes. In particular, work environments and factors related to health care professionals' fatigue, stress, and poor communication were found to be associated with the greatest number of potentially serious mistakes, often occurring during high-stress and crisis events.[10] Since patients rely on health care professionals for their safety and well-being, errors also were recognized as costly in terms of loss of trust in the health care system by patients and diminished satisfaction by both patients and health care professionals.[10]

To Err Is Human identified five critical conditions for creating a safe health care system that promotes best practices while maintaining quality health care environments. They included providing leadership, respecting human limits in process design, *promoting effective team functioning*, anticipating the unexpected, and *creating a learning environment*.[10] In 2003, the IOM published *Health Professions Education: A Bridge to Quality*.[1] In it, the IOM stated that "the goal of health professional education should be outcome-based education…"[1] and that these outcomes should be guided by five core competencies: the provision of patient-centered care, *work in interdisciplinary teams*, the employment of evidence-based practice, the application of quality improvement, and the utilization of informatics.[1] These IOM recommendations to deliver quality health care in a work environment in which patient-centered care relies on the interaction of an interprofessional team comprised of individuals from highly diverse backgrounds in terms of education, training, and experience have led to several national initiatives promoting teamwork and communication skills. Examples of national organizations currently advocating team training include the Committee on Quality of Healthcare in America, the AHRQ, the Accreditation Council for Graduate Medical Education (ACGME), the Association of American Medical Colleges (AAMC), the National Quality Forum (NQF), the Joint Commission, and the Centers for Medicare and Medicaid Services (CMS).[11]

Current Teamwork Climate

Unfortunately, teamwork in health care is far from adequate. The current research on team function and performance in health care suggests that health care teams are more "groups of experts" rather than "expert teams."[12] That is, members tend to favor *multiprofessional* over *interprofessional* collaboration and interaction,[13] thereby fostering friction among professions and promoting the "silo mentality" well known to clinicians working in the industry.[14] This mentality contributes to the alienation of each profession from the other, making effective teamwork nearly impossible. For example, operating room (OR) staff "tribalism" has been implicated as an important reason for the ambivalent attitude of many surgical teams to the use and implementation of the surgical time-out.[15] Less appreciated, but equally important in terms of its perpetuation, is the silo mentality's role in the so-called "hidden curriculum" that is so influential in shaping health profession students' attitudes and behaviors in medicine. Haldet and Stein[16] have demonstrated that certain premises within the culture of medicine lead to the adoption of assumptions detrimental to effective team function. For example, the cultural belief that "hierarchy is necessary" fosters the attitude that nurses and junior medical staff should not question senior doctors, thus impeding communication and impairing team function. To make matters worse, Wear and Skillicorn[17] have demonstrated that faculty members' perception of the impact of the hidden curriculum on students may in fact be opposite to what actually occurs. Consequently, role modeling thought to be positive and beneficial by the faculty may in fact be perceived in a negative manner by the students themselves. Finally, in a review of the literature, Reese et al[18] found that nursing and medical programs rarely include interdisciplinary or collaborative educational experiences in their curricula, thus making team training of students nearly impossible. Gettman et al[19] found a similar problem for residents, noting that, other than on-the-job training, structured learning opportunities for residents in surgical training programs to learn effective teamwork, effective communication, and laparoscopic principles are limited.

Mishra et al[20] have noted that poor communication and teamwork can lead to adverse events in the operating room and that teaching teamwork skills may reduce surgical error. Furthermore, lack of teamwork among emergency department personnel has been found to be a leading contributor to closed claim cases in the emergency department.[21] Mazzocco et al[22] have shown that poor surgical teamwork correlated with higher complication rates and increased mortality among patients. More recently, Andersen et al,[23] in a qualitative semi-structured interview study of cardiac resuscitation instructors, revealed that dysfunctional team dynamics, such as rigid hierarchies and poor workload distribution and communication, can negatively impact cardiac resuscitations. Taken together, these examples demonstrate that teamwork in current clinical practice is inadequate and that further team training is necessary. As Rosen et al[24] have noted: "Teamwork is central to safety in health care as it is often the interactions of health care workers that produce effective or ineffective performance."

The Science of Teamwork: Definitions, Models, and Concepts

The AHRQ's Core Curriculum for Patient Safety characterizes a team as consisting of two or more people with an identified leader and members with designated responsibilities, all of whom function interactively toward a common goal.[25] The team has accountability as a unit. In health care, the focus of the team is to provide the highest standard of patient care. When the same people are always working together, the team is classified as a fixed (i.e., intact) team. In situations in which people are brought together to act as a team and the individual members may never have met (or at least do not always work together), the team is classified as a nonfixed (i.e., ad hoc) team. Three challenges for health care teams have been identified: professional complexity (e.g., multiple cultural backgrounds, professional disciplines, levels of knowledge/authority, and administrative problems); personal complexity (e.g., members have different backgrounds, responsibilities, and motivations); and patient complexity (e.g., patients have a role as both team members and as the team's focus, yet they are the least familiar with the health care model).[11]

Salas et al[26] have created a theoretical model of the interrelations among the "Big Five" competencies in teamwork that includes taxonomies that most heavily affect team performance. The framework provides an understanding of the concepts, including how they occur in different team tasks and different daily situations. The supporting mechanisms, known as the *core components* of the "Big Five" model of teamwork, include team leadership, mutual performance monitoring, backup behavior, adaptability, and team orientation. The coordinating mechanisms needed to meld together the supporting mechanisms include a shared mental model, mutual trust, and open (i.e., closed-loop) communication. When the "Big Five" is implemented during team training, effective teams rely on a complex mixture of variables that include organizational support and individual skills.

Jeffries et al[27] have developed a collaborative practice model using simulation as an innovative way to teach interprofessional providers and/or students how to work together to deliver care in real-world clinical practice. The model reveals the knowledge, skills, and critical thinking practices of all disciplines, thus fostering an appreciation of all contributions of team members and helping to create a safe system of care. Again, communication and collaboration are key elements: "Essentials needed for collaborative work includes responsibility, accountability, coordination, communication, cooperation, risk-taking, assertiveness, autonomy, and mutual trust and respect."[27] In this model, challenges to collaborative (i.e., effective team) practice include role ambiguity and confusion, hierarchical relationships, educational differences, gender issues, and differences in professional cultures.[27] Key benefits of their model include positive team outcomes, improved patient safety, improved patient satisfaction, and better coordination of care. In their work, the authors provided a framework for setting up a simulated collaborative practice model including design, examples, evaluation, and the implications for interprofessional teams.[27]

Baker et al[4] have demonstrated that team-based competencies can be divided into categories based on the knowledge, skills, and attitudes (KSA) classification. Knowledge competencies include abilities such as awareness of environment (i.e., situational awareness), shared understanding of goals and tasks (i.e., shared mental model), and familiarity with team members' roles and responsibilities (i.e., role clarity). Skill competencies typically include monitoring of each other's performance (i.e., cross-monitoring), flexibility and adaptability, supporting and backing up team members (i.e., back-up behavior), team leadership, conflict resolution, closed-loop communication, effective information exchange, and feedback. Finally, attitudinal competencies include a shared vision and orientation to team functioning (i.e., team cohesion and interaction) and a collective belief regarding overall team efficacy (i.e., team orientation and mutual trust).

According to Frankel et al,[28] "effective teamwork and communication skills are cornerstones of safe, reliable, and high-quality health care." Clearly, team-based KSAs are critical for effective team function. Baker et al[7] have gone so far to argue that team-based KSAs are essential for organizational-level effectiveness, since high-reliability organizations (HROs) cannot exist without efficiently functioning, highly reliable teams. High-reliability organizations, by definition, are institutions that operate in complex, hazardous environments, yet, over long periods of time, make few mistakes.[27] The hypercomplexity of a HRO is manifest in its having various levels, systems, and hierarchies for success.[27] These hierarchies are differentiated and have clear roles.[27] Furthermore, HROs are characterized by having many decision-makers, a high degree of accountability, and frequent feedback with tight coupling across levels related to task interdependence.[27] Finally, HROs possess a performance-oriented generative organizational culture in which failure is embraced, opportunities for improvement are constantly sought, and root causes are actively investigated.[29] Such a work environment is characteristic of a culture of safety that helps to foster resiliency in times of failure and allows HROs to function effectively in times of crisis.[30,31] Without highly reliable teams, such resiliency and adaptability could not occur.

The team-based KSAs used to promote highly reliable team function are also referred to as *non-technical skills* (NTS). For example, communication, leadership, and situational awareness are behavioral markers that focus on the interpersonal skills of the team to improve safety and ensure effective team function. According to Jeffries et al,[27] communication influences synergistic decision-making of separate and shared knowledge, skills, and critical thinking when delivering care. Further, negative team factors, poor planning, a lack of support by the creator, and communication gaps lead to communication breakdown among team members. Competing priorities and goals among team members, failure to compromise with conflicting goals, and poor coordination of activities are main factors leading to fragmentation. Aspects of team functioning that can cause communication gaps include situations in which members have different interactive styles (e.g., hierarchical, egalitarian, or other), are focused on a single task (e.g., tunnel vision patient care, jargon, task-centered vs. patient-centered), or the chain of command is unclear.[11] As Leonard et al[32] point out: "Effective communication that creates a well understood plan of care greatly reduces the chances of inevitable error becoming consequential and injuring patients."

Effective leadership requires the establishment of a strong shared mental model. Typically, a shared mental model is used by effective teams to achieve a mutually agreed upon goal in the safest possible manner. In this situation, clear roles and responsibilities exist, clear values and a shared vision are present, and strong leadership in the team with a flattened hierarchy are evident. Taken together, these characteristics create a trusting environment in which team members feel safe to "speak up" when they have a safety concern.[11,32] The team then engages in a cycle of feedback that builds a strong sense of "collective trust" and confidence, allowing members to cooperate and coordinate. When the team has a shared mental model, performance outcomes are optimal. As Sundar et al[33] comment: "To work effectively together, team members must also possess appropriate knowledge, skills, and attitudes, such as monitoring each other's performance, knowledge of their own and their teammates' responsibilities, and a positive disposition toward working in a team."

Situational awareness is a critical component in decision-making for medical practitioners. According to Wright et al,[34] it can be thought of as an internal mental model of the current state of an individual's environment. "Situational Awareness is defined as a person's perception of elements in the environment, comprehension of that information, and the ability to project future events based on this understanding."[32] It is the ongoing dialogue that keeps team members up to date with what is happening and how they will respond if the situation changes.[32] When NTS are deficient, team function can deteriorate as a result of human limitations. Limited memory capacity, the effects of stress and fatigue, the risks associated with distractions and interruptions, and the limited ability to multitask ensure that even a skilled, experienced provider will make mistakes.[32] Thus, the importance of team training in NTS/team-based KSAs becomes apparent, since they can improve such important features of team function as decision-making, situational awareness, and interpersonal communication.[35]

TEAM TRAINING STRATEGIES AND TOOLS

Crisis Resource Management (CRM)

The complex, dynamic industry of commercial aviation has conducted training of pilots and crew members in team-based KSAs for decades. Such training arose from research indicating that aircraft accidents were often the result of a crew's failure in NTS (i.e., effectively managing resources) rather than technical mistakes. The term *crew* (originally *cockpit*) *resource management* (CRM) came from a collaboration between the National Aeronautics and Space Administration (NASA) and the U.S. military that conceptualized a new type of training to address this lack of resource management in crisis situations.[36] From its start, aviation-based CRM training has relied heavily on simulation-based techniques to mimic in-flight emergencies to hone pilots' NTS and technical skills. This strategy of team training has helped transform the commercial airline industry from an accident-prone method of travel to one of the safest means of transportation in the world.

In 1987, Gaba et al[37] first adapted the principles of CRM to health care by creating a simulation-based curriculum for anesthesiology known as Anesthesia Crisis Resource Management (ACRM). After the inception of the curriculum, an initial review of videotapes of the experiments and simulations, along with personal anesthesia expertise, identified gaps concerning several critical aspects of decision-making and crisis management. Reasons that the gaps existed and strategies to close the gaps were also identified and evaluated. Key points were identified regarding decision making and cognition. They include knowing the environment, anticipating and planning next steps, using all available information and cross-checking, preventing or managing fixation errors, and using cognitive aids.[37] In addition, the following key points regarding teamwork and resource management were also emphasized: exercising leadership and followership, calling for help early, communicating effectively, distributing the workload, and mobilizing all available resources for optimal management.[37]

From the earliest simulations done in the operating rooms with investigators role playing as other team members, the ACRM training has adhered to principles of aviation-based CRM. Over the years, Gaba has noted that, in order to possess effective teamwork skills, teams should undergo two approaches that are complementary methods to improve decision-making and teamwork skills. First, each discipline/profession should go through single-discipline (i.e., crew-based) training that includes comprehensive teaching and practice in the integrated use of technical, cognitive, and behavioral skills in managing crises relevant to their domains. Once this training is completed, each discipline/profession should go through combined team (i.e., interprofessional) training that allows for more natural team interactions and reinforces understanding across disciplines.[36]

Crew resource management teaches learners to use all available resources, information, equipment, and people to achieve optimum patient outcomes. It is now employed in multiple fields of health care as a team training strategy to promote high reliability. As Rudy et al[38] have observed: "CRM has evolved as a training methodology for preparing health care professionals to perform in high-stress, life-threatening crises through the application of concepts such as leadership, communication, assertiveness, decision making, and team performance."

Team Strategies and Tools to Enhance Performance and Patient Safety (TeamSTEPPS™)

TeamSTEPPS™ is a training package that capitalized on the Department of Defense's (DoD) expertise in medical and nonmedical team performance and the AHRQ's extensive research in the fields of patient safety and health care quality. It is a flexible, evidenced-based teamwork system designed for health care facilities and providers to improve patient safety through enhanced communication and other teamwork skills.[39] It is designed to improve the quality, safety, and efficiency of health care by improving communication and other teamwork skills. The design has three continuous phases: assessment; planning, training, and implementation; and maintenance. Each phase incorporates keys actions: (1) set the stage, (2) decide what to do, (3) make it happen, and (4) make it stick.[40] Four competency areas encourage situational awareness and communication by all members of the team and foster mutual respect among team members, regardless of their roles. They are: team leadership, situational monitoring (i.e., mutual performance monitoring), mutual support (i.e., back-up behavior), and communication.[39] These skills lead to important team outcomes by helping teams to adapt to care plans, develop positive attitudes toward and appreciation of the benefits of team work, and provide safer, more reliable, and more efficient care.[40]

TeamSTEPPS™ has been employed worldwide in diverse health care environments in an attempt to improve team function and effectiveness. For example, its implementation at a Level 1 Trauma Center in the United States improved important process measures, including time to the computed tomography (CT) scanner, time to endotracheal intubation, and time to the OR.[41] In South Australia, its implementation at a mental health facility resulted in an improvement in event reporting, organizational learning, and staff KSAs related to teamwork and communication.[42] It has even been combined with SBT to optimize learning.[43] Its advent has been a way to promote the development of HROs in health care and to serve as a national framework to conduct team training.[7]

Team Training Tools

Both CRM and TeamSTEPPS™ offer learners a variety of tools to enhance individual team member's NTS and, in doing so, overall team function. For example, the *repeat-back technique* of communication helps to "close the loop" between team members, thus ensuring that information conveyed by the sender is understood by the receiver. Another frequently taught communication tool is the acronym *SBAR* (Situation, Background, Assessment, and Recommendation), in which the conveyer of information uses a structured format to communicate with the receiver of information. Its predictable structure addresses key items including the "situation (i.e., what's going on with the patient?), background (i.e., what is the clinical background/context?), assessment (i.e., what do I think the problems is?), and recommendation (i.e., what do I do to correct this?)."[32] It is a very effective technique to bridge differences in communication styles (e.g., between nurse and physician) and to help everyone "get on the same page" (i.e., create a shared mental model).

Tools to assist with assertiveness are also taught in team training. Assertiveness training has created a cultural change in health care that encourages respect for each team member and broadens a team's situational awareness. Often, such assertiveness is hindered by the lack of a shared mental model or the presence of a rigid hierarchical team structure. A key factor in safety is being able to express concerns politely and persistently, as well as being competent and team-centered. Assertiveness, however, should not be confused with being aggressive, hostile, tyrannical, confrontational, ambiguous, or ridiculing; it's about what's best for the patient.[11]

The *two-challenge rule* assists with assertiveness by setting guidelines for challenging a professional opinion or action and encouraging team members whose initial assertions are ignored to express their concern at least twice to ensure they have been heard.[40] It is an effective nonconfrontational way of asserting a team member's concern. Key steps include: (1) getting the person's attention, (2) expressing concern, (3) stating the problem, (4) offering a solution, and (5) obtaining agreement. If failure to respond occurs on the part of the person being approached, a team member is to assume loss of situational awareness.[32] A team member makes two such challenges before seeking help from someone at a higher level.

Another tool for increasing assertiveness is the use of critical language as accepted red flags. For example, the use of "CUS words" creates a clearly agreed upon communication model that helps avoid the natural tendency to speak indirectly and deferentially. CUS is an acronym for accepted code words that convey a team member's safety concern. They include the expressions "I'm ***c***oncerned," "I'm ***u***ncomfortable," "This is un***s***afe," or "I'm ***s***cared." When employed, these words mean "We have a serious problem: stop and listen."[32]

Team briefs are another tool taught in CRM- and TeamSTEPPS™-based courses to enhance team effectiveness. A team brief takes place at the beginning of a team encounter in order to get every member at the same starting point, avoid surprises, and affect positively how the team works.[32] A team briefing clarifies roles, as well as describes plans and resources available for utilization. It is the premise for situational awareness: "During briefing, safety issues are discussed and compensatory or corrective actions are proposed. After a briefing, members of the team are asked to verify their understanding of these plans, thus cultivating the formation of a shared mental model."[33]

Team Training Using Simulation

Not surprisingly, the first computer-based simulator in health care was developed in the late-1960s at the University of Southern California by an anesthesiologist, Dr. J. Samuel Denson, and an education specialist, Dr. Stephen Abrahamson, for the purpose of training anesthesiology residents.[44] This pioneering work in computer-based simulation was taken up again in the 1980s by two groups of anesthesiologists, Drs. David Gaba and Abe DeAnda at Stanford, and Drs. Michael Good and Joachim S. Gravenstein at the University of Florida, who independently developed computer-run mannequins for training.[45] Prior to that, high-fidelity simulation (HFS) had been widely used as a teaching strategy in other industries, such as aviation, transportation, and nuclear power.[46] Currently, many different health care disciplines are utilizing SBT to improve teamwork and communication in an effort to improve patient outcomes. Examples exist in anesthesia,[37] emergency medicine,[47] pediatrics,[48] obstetrics,[49,50] surgery,[35,51] and radiology.[52]

Simulation-based training is particularly well suited for team-based training. First, core competencies from CRM and TeamSTEPPS can easily be included into it. Second, it is very conducive to interprofessional training. High-fidelity simulation interprofessional training not only introduces each profession to these critical team-based competencies, but it also introduces each profession to one another in a safe, nonthreatening environment, outside the hospital setting. In this manner, it allows each profession to learn another discipline's capabilities, strengths, and responsibilities, and it flattens the hierarchy of the team, thus creating an environment in which each participant feels free to speak up. Such interprofessional collaboration is a vital component in attaining the IOM's goal of a safe, efficient, patient-centered health care system. Finally, high-fidelity SBT provides the opportunity for participants to practice treating low-frequency, high-risk events as a team in a realistic, safe, nonthreatening learning environment to hone both technical skills and NTS without detriment to the patient.[8,18]

Currently, high-fidelity SBT has been implemented for a variety of reasons across many disciplines in health care. For example, it has been used in emergency medicine to teach and assess the Accreditation Council for Graduate Medical Education (ACGME) core competencies in emergency room residents using an eight-step process, in which each simulation scenario is a reflection of the ACGME core competencies.[47] Additionally, it has been employed to teach and evaluate medical resident's pediatric resuscitation skills,[53] as well as to identify obstetrical residents' clinical performance deficiencies during an obstetric crisis.[54] Finally, in situ (i.e., sessions located within the actual patient care setting) HFS team training has been conducted in both obstetrics[50] and general surgical[51] settings, in an attempt to foster team-based NTS.

Reese et al[18] conducted a study to investigate the use of an innovative teaching strategy using simulation to support the collaboration between nursing and medical students in an educational setting. The study evaluated the collaborative (i.e., combined medical and nursing) management of a surgical patient with complications. The study concluded that designing simulations that place medical and nursing students together is beneficial for both groups. A majority of the students indicated the interdisciplinary training prepares them for real-world situations and could reduce medical errors.[18]

Sehgal et al[55] developed a multidisciplinary teamwork training program focused on teaching teamwork behaviors and communication skills. The program included internal medicine residents, hospitalists, nurses, pharmacists, and other staff on a designated inpatient medical unit at an academic medical center. This study provided students the opportunity to practice working together in a crisis situation in a safe, nonthreatening simulation environment. Such training will ultimately not only benefit the students, but their future patients as well.

Abrahamson et al[56] tested a new protocol for cardiac arrest in a patient with severe acute respiratory syndrome (SARS). The protocol included the use of HFS and teamwork training of health care workers. In this study, the following conclusions were made:

- HFS was proved to be a valuable tool in evaluating a new treatment protocol in a rapidly evolving crisis.
- Scenario-based simulation training was resource intense.
- Simulation was suited to teamwork training for disaster management.
- Simulation training, when used for uncommon events, should be done in both the teaching arena and the actual patient environment.

Wayne et al[57] have noted that the use of simulation technology has great potential to shape medical education, certification, licensure, and quality of care. Simulation has been demonstrated to be effective to achieve, measure, and maintain trainee skill in performing various clinical procedures. The authors conducted a retrospective case–control study of cardiac arrest teams using internal medicine residents. Medical records of Advanced Cardiac Life Support (ACLS) events were reviewed to assess adherence with ACLS response quality indicators. The study included medical residents who all received traditional ACLS education. The study compared second-year residents who also received an educational program that included deliberate practice of ACLS scenarios using a human patient simulator and third-year residents who were not trained using simulation. The effects of SBT on the quality of ACLS care provided were evaluated. The study concluded that a simulation-based educational program significantly improved the quality of care provided by residents during actual ACLS events.[57] Similarly, Gettman et al[19] found that teamwork, intraoperative communication, and laparoscopic skills of urology residents improved with the use of HFS in a simulated operating room. In other words, HFS was effective in assessing and teaching ACGME core competencies related to intraoperative communication, teamwork, and laparoscopic skills.

The Role of Debriefing in Simulation-Based Training

Effective debriefing is critical for learning and retention of team-based competencies in high-fidelity SBT. In fact, Gaba et al[37] considered debriefing sessions as the most important component of ACRM. Debriefing should take place after the teamwork and communication training session, critiquing both team dynamics and what occurred. Every effort should be made by the facilitator to foster an atmosphere of mutual trust and comfort in expressing constructive criticisms without placing blame or making personal attacks on other participants. Attention is drawn to common errors that could potentially interfere with optimal patient care. Participants are encouraged to focus on possible solutions and ways in which positive behaviors and actions can favorably impact patient outcomes.[38]

In nursing, the terms clinical judgment, clinical reasoning, diagnostic reasoning, and critical thinking are used interchangeably. *Clinical judgment* is the term most commonly used. According to Tanner,[58] "clinical judgments are more influenced by what the nurse brings to the situation than the objective data about the situation at hand." In clinical situations, the context is important. Nurses use a variety of reasoning patterns such as analytic processes, intuition, narrative thinking, and reflection to develop clinical reasoning.[58] Tanner's Clinical Judgment Model is used as a guide for debriefing after simulation. Key components of the model include: (1) noticing (i.e., getting an initial grasp), (2) interpreting (i.e., using analytic, intuitive, and narrative faculties), (3) responding (i.e., taking action to get outcomes), and (4) reflecting (i.e., reflecting on action and clinical learning).[58]

Debriefing serves to strengthen clinical judgment and the application of knowledge. Although team training focuses on team behaviors and not medical management, nursing often looks at the skills and nursing management in a simulation as well. Reflection occurs with simple plus/delta charts to reflect on what went well and what needs improvement. Decker et al[59] promoted clinical judgment in undergraduate nursing students through the use of concept maps after simulations and cause-and-effect diagramming, in a process the authors call *SAM RIOT*. The acronym stands for student assessment model (SAM) and root, impression, outcome, and treatment (RIOT).[59]

Measurement of Team Behaviors in Simulation-Based Training

Four main methods for simulation-based team training measurement exist: event-based measurement, behaviorally anchored rating scales, behavioral observation scales, and self-report measures.[47] A multifaceted approach to assessment is best. In medical simulations, evaluation and measurement of outcomes of interprofessional simulation-based education can be based on the Simulation Module for Assessment of Resident Targeted Event Responses (SMARTER) methodology.[47] The SMARTER methodology consists of eight steps that encompass a simulation in its entirety. The first step is to look at core competencies and, in the second step, develop learning objectives and measurement tools. In the third step, the clinical context and scenario are chosen. The fourth step defines the knowledge, skills, and attitudes necessary for the scenario. The fifth step creates triggers or critical performance indicators that must be managed. In the sixth step, target responses for each critical event that are observable and thus measurable are identified. For the seventh step, measurement tools and/or checklists are selected. Last, in the eighth step, a scenario script for how the simulation will unfold is developed, and decision pathways and responses anticipated.[47]

One of the first behavior-based evaluation tools came from the aviation industry and was called *line operation safety audits* (LOSA).[21] Issues to consider with behavior-based assessment tools include the unit of assessment, identification of team skills, method of assessment, rater reliability, and rater training.[21] The Observational Teamwork Assessment of Surgery (OTAS) assesses technical and interpersonal skills. Task and team behaviors are assessed in five dimensions: cooperation, coordination, leadership, monitoring, and communication.[60] Another frequently used measure in surgery is the Anaesthetists' Non-Technical Skills (ANTS) tool, which assesses the skill categories of task management, team working, situation awareness, and decision-making.[61] Originally designed to assess performance in the domain of anesthesia, it has been followed by other specialty-specific measures like the Non-Technical Skills for Surgeons (NOTSS) tool.[62] Finally, the Operating Room Teamwork Assessment Scales (ORTAS) assesses NTS using three scales: preoperative briefing and preparation, individual team-based behaviors, and overall team effectiveness.[63] The second scale is designed as a multisource rating scale for both individual and peer-based assessment. Hence, this tool can be used as an observer-based, peer-based, and/or self-assessment measurement.

Frankel et al[28] developed the Communication and Teamwork Skills (CATS) assessment tool as a global measure of behavior-based assessments. Subscales include the domains of cooperation, situational awareness, coordination, and communication.[21] In addition to the frequency of a behavior, its quality is also rated using a three-point scale: observed and good, variation in quality, and expected but not observed.[28] Using CATS, it can become difficult to differentiate between individual and team performance. This fact illustrates that global observer-based measures can be fraught with bias and error.[47]

As part of an obstetrical safety initiative, the Clinical Teamwork Scale (CTS) was developed.[64] It contains 15 items measuring five domains (i.e., communication, situational awareness, decision making, role responsibility, and patient-friendliness) on a 0–10 scale. Unlike the CATS tool, which is completed by trained observers,[28] the CTS is designed for overall evaluation by group members.

Like the CTS, the Mayo High Performance Teamwork Scale (MHPTS) is completed by participants to assess both the effectiveness of training and to encourage self-reflection on the simulation experience.[65] The Emergency Response Performance Tool (ERPT), on the other hand, is an observer-based assessment tool in which targeted tasks are timed. It was developed to assess behaviors in an ACLS ventricular tachycardia simulation.[66]

In nursing, one simulation-specific model to guide simulation is the Nursing Education Simulation Framework.[67] Frequently, clinical reasoning models guide simulation in nursing[58,68] or skill-based assessment tools.[69] The Simulation Design Scale (SDS) and Satisfaction and Self-Confidence Scale were developed by the National League for Nursing.[18,70]

The above-mentioned tools are just a few of the many assessment instruments in the process of being developed to assess individual- and team-based behaviors in SBT. Depending on its method of assessment (e.g., behaviorally anchored, self-reported), each tool has strengths and weaknesses that should be taken into account when choosing the best one for a particular SBT situation.

INTERPROFESSIONAL STUDENT HIGH-FIDELITY SIMULATION-BASED TEAM TRAINING AT LSUHSC-NO

Planning, Implementation, and Evaluation

The authors were privileged to be a part of three separate interprofessional student HFS team training projects. Although the methods used for each project were similar, the scenario setting and the student composition for each one was different. The first project involved team training in a mock OR setting. The second involved training in a simulated emergency department. The third project was designed around an intensive care unit (ICU) environment.

Although planning for interprofessional team-based training scenarios can be challenging, the rewards that come from working with an interprofessional team of educators are manifold. Given the disparities in the schedules of the various schools within a health sciences center, a large component of the planning phase of interprofessional student team training hinges on coordination of schedules.

Planning for interprofessional simulations is a necessity. The establishment of a purpose, learning objectives, outcomes, and/or research questions for the simulation aids in guiding activities. Once these items have been addressed, selecting scenarios with sufficient fidelity, trigger events/cues to action, and relevance to meet these objectives is the next step. Once scenarios are selected, a list of supplies must be drafted. Supplies should include both expensive (e.g., part-task simulator for intravenous access) and inexpensive (e.g., intravenous catheters) items needed to create a sense of realism (i.e., fidelity) for the scenario. By creating a realistic environment with realistic equipment, participants will "suspend disbelief" that the scenario is not real. In our experience, it was easier to plan for and ensure the availability of expensive items, as they were critical to the scenario, but the smaller, inexpensive items such as syringes, needles, patient charts, and defibrillator pads, were often forgotten. It is highly recommended to conduct a trial of the simulation scenarios (i.e., a pilot running) to allow their refinement prior to their initiation with targeted participants.

Implementation—the actual conduct of the simulation—is frequently the enjoyable part of any project because investigators and participants tend to enjoy the simulation-based teaching/learning experience. Preparations for every simulation, however, are needed. Depending on the scenario setting, highly technical environments, such as an OR, require additional setup time, often 30 minutes to 1 hour. Setup time decreases as experience increases. In addition, setup time decreases if you are able to store supplies in or adjacent to the rooms used for the SBT. Institutional Review Board (IRB) approval is required prior to implementation if any research is related to the simulation-based project.

Proper evaluation is paramount to ensure the effectiveness of the simulation-based experience. In selecting appropriate evaluation methods and measures, one should review carefully the goals, outcomes, and/or research questions involved in the SBT. The lowest levels of measurement are participant satisfaction and self-confidence assessments. Knowledge can be measured with checklists or specific tools. Finally, demonstrating translation of learning to the clinical setting involves more complex methods of measurement.

The ICU interprofessional student HFS team training project conducted at LSUHSC-NO provides a good example of the critical steps needed for planning, implementing, and evaluating an SBT program. In its planning phase, its purpose was defined as the evaluation of the efficacy of utilizing the principles of the Crisis Resource Management (CRM) model for interdisciplinary team training with preprofessional medical, nursing, and physical therapy students from the Schools of Medicine, Nursing, and Allied Health within the Health Sciences Center. The goals of the training were to improve students' individual communication and team-based skills and to improve students' overall interprofessional teamwork as a unit. The proposed outcomes were that students would have increased teamwork competencies by self-rating and trained observer rating, and that students would retain teamwork and communication skills taught through simulation as demonstrated by mean scores equal to or greater than mean scores 5 months earlier. Since the possibility of general dissemination of the knowledge gained from this experience existed, IRB approval was obtained before starting the program.

An atrial fibrillation and a tension pneumothorax scenario were selected for the team training. These scenarios required students to work as a team to manage the patient crisis using their knowledge, skills, and attitudes to diagnose and treat properly the patient's condition. Supplies were ordered and assembled in anticipation of the simulations. Importantly, observers were taught key definitions for team-based behaviors and trained to identify team-based competencies using a video of a simulated code in the OR setting. Observers then used the ORTAS and CATS scales to rate the video-taped performances and to calibrate responses with each other in order to establish reliability and consistency in rating.

A pilot training session was conducted to identify problems and refine the scenarios accordingly. Room setup time was approximately 30 minutes (Table 12.1). It was explained to the students that the project was educational research with IRB approval, and they were given an opportunity to opt out of the research portion of the simulation; no students requested this option. The students were then oriented to the simulation room and introduced to each other and the study team. Ground rules were established: treat the simulation as if it were real, treat the study team as "ghosts" (i.e., ignore them), and treat the experience like Vegas (i.e., "what happens here..."; maintain confidentiality concerning comments and the scenarios themselves).

The atrial fibrillation scenario began with the undergraduate nursing students doing an assessment on the simulated "patient" at the start of their shift, followed closely by a physical therapy student entering the room to transfer the patient to a chair bed. Immediately following the transfer, the patient

Table 12.1 Setup for intensive care unit high-fidelity simulation team training project

High-fidelity human patient simulator
Computer
Chair bed
Crash cart
Code drugs
Foley catheter
NG tube
Laryngoscope
Endotracheal tube
LMA tube
14 g needle
Chest tube
Pleurovac
IV start kits
IV Jelcos
IV tubings
IV fluids
10 cc syringes

Table 12.2 Key questions asked during post-scenario debriefing for the intensive care unit project

During debriefing:
- How do you think the team performed?
- What went well; what went not so well?
- What do you think is needed for a good team?
- What could you do differently to improve teamwork?
- Have you been in a code in the hospital?
- Describe a good code. What made it good?
- Describe a bad code. What made it bad?

During debriefing wrap-up:
- What are you going to work on next time?
- What will you work on in the clinical setting?
- What if the physicians are difficult with you?

At the end of second simulation debriefing:
- Was this simulation useful? How?
- Was it helpful to do it two times?
- How was it helpful?
- What would you change?

began complaining of shortness of breath. As the patient's condition worsened, the nurses and physical therapists in the simulated ICU setting could choose to call for help. This help consisted of nurse anesthesia students in the ICU who were making preoperative rounds and/or medical students making patient rounds. Trained observers documented each incident of a team or communication skill on the CATS assessment tool. At the end of the scenario, students rated their teamwork and communication behaviors using the Modified ORTAS (i.e., the ORTAS without its first scale) and MHPTS, while trained observers rated the behaviors with the Modified ORTAS. Debriefing ensued after all assessments were complete, with an emphasis on team-based behaviors instead of technical skills or medical management (Table 12.2). The pneumothorax scenario was conducted using the same methods. Teamwork behaviors were highlighted in the debriefing (Table 12.3).

Approximately 5 months after the first round of scenarios given during the fall semester of the school year, students were invited to participate in two additional scenarios to assess retention. The same two scenarios were used, as well as the same

Table 12.3 Team-based behaviors highlighted in debriefing

Teamwork:
- Roles, role clarity
- Mental rehearsal
- Stating a plan

Anticipation:
- Anticipatory response
- Cross-monitoring,
- Back-up behaviors

Open communication:
- Introduce yourself, use names
- SBAR
- Repeat-back, closed-loop communication

Team orientation

Shared mental model:
- Situational awareness
- Thinking aloud

Resource management:
- Equipment as a resource
- Each other as resources

Leadership:
- Flattened hierarchy

methods. Some students did not realize that the scenarios were identical to those given during the fall semester. This fact speaks to the realism of the simulation experience.

Data were entered into SPSS for analysis. Paired samples t-tests were conducted between the first scenario, atrial fibrillation, and the second scenario, tension pneumothorax. Comparisons were done on fall semester data, spring semester data, and between simulation 2 (i.e., the final scenario) in the fall semester and simulation 1 (i.e., the first scenario) in the spring semester. Preliminary findings suggested that although some decrease in mean scores occurred initially in the spring semester, the overall scores increased with additional training. Findings suggest the benefit of repeat training in teamwork skills using interprofessional student HFS team training.

Paige[71] has "proposed the '5P' approach [to implementation], which attempts to group potential challenges into 5 major categories: finding a patron, developing a plan, locating a place, assembling the appropriate people, and choosing effective products." Based on the experience with interprofessional students obtained from endeavors like the ICU project, suggestions for conducting simulation are presented in Table 12.4.

Ethics

Prior to implementation, IRB approval was obtained. The main concern was the use of students as participants. The majority of investigators taught these students. Human subject protections were included in the IRB application that outlined methods to protect confidentiality and noncoercive student recruitment.

Benefits

Students commented that they enjoyed the simulations and interactions with other professions, (i.e., evidence of Kirkpatrick[72] level 1 training effectiveness). More importantly, as suggested by the preliminary analysis of the data, statistically significant increases in mean scores on team-based behaviors following interprofessional team training in the ICU setting were observed (i.e., evidence of Kirkpatrick level 2 training effectiveness).

Challenges

The primary challenge in implementing the ICU project was to resolve scheduling conflicts for both participants and investigators. Coordinating four health profession student groups (i.e., medical, nursing, nurse anesthetist, and physical therapy students) required multiple iterations before final schedules could be obtained. A second challenge was to manage student cancelation or rescheduling at the last minute, especially in the spring semester, when many of the students were approaching graduation. For example, medical students had already successful matched into training programs and were busy establishing new places of residence, some out of town and others out of state. On the other hand, physical therapy students were arranging for year-long clinical experiences in cities across the state. A third challenge was to maintain investigator availability because of teaching commitments and academic travel requirements. Finally, data management was an ongoing challenge for this project due to the volume of data and the shortage of available statistical assistance.

IMPLICATIONS FOR RADIOLOGY

Simulation-based training is fast becoming an important issue in the field of radiology. As Desser[73] has pointed out: "The Radiological Society of North America (RSNA), the Society of Interventional Radiology, and the Cardiovascular and Interventional

Table 12.4 Suggestions for creating a successful high-fidelity simulation team training program

- Review the literature on best practices for simulation based training.
- Train with a mentor experienced in simulation education.
- Gain administrative support.
- Establish goals, outcomes, and research questions.
- Create realistic scenarios with supplies to match practice settings.
- Pilot the simulation scenario and refine methods.
- Design evaluation plans to assess goals, outcomes, and research questions.

Radiological Society of Europe have all established individual task forces and have joined together to set strategy and issue recommendations for simulation training." The ACGME used evidence from simulation-based studies to limit duty hours for residents. Advances in radiology have led to the use of various simulators, including the RSNA's Medical Imaging Resource Center, the American College of Radiology's (ACR's) Case-in-Point series, and AuntMinnie.com's "Case of the Day." Such examples provide case-based learning on a large scale. Radiology will benefit from outcome-based models that include technical proficiency and a core knowledge base. Desser emphasizes this point: "Simulation can be used for both training and assessment and is poised to meet the needs of residency and fellowship program directors and accreditation and credentialing bodies that increasingly require documentation of proficiency."[73]

Gaba and Dunn[74] wrote an editorial after Duncan et al[75] designed an SBT intervention that reduced the risk of pneumothorax after outpatient thoracentesis performed by internal medicine residents. In establishing procedural competence for thoracentesis in their study, Duncan et al used the Miller's Pyramid framework (i.e., knows, knows how, shows how, does) for clinical assessment.[75] In their editorial, Gaba and Dunn reaffirmed that "the goal of such simulation-enhanced training systems is to accelerate the learning curve of novice learners toward true competence, resulting in fewer iatrogenic events occurring in the course of training."[74] For them, SBT alone is rarely enough to ensure safe clinical practices and process improvements in health care. Instead, it must be part of a comprehensive strategy in which intensive training is coupled with system analysis, process change, and medical cultural transformation.[74] Such methodology, along with the incorporation of CRM, teamwork, and communication skills, will, in the future, become the norm for addressing many issues in clinical outcomes and safety improvement.

For the field of radiology, team-based training of members of the interventional radiology (IR) suite seems a logical first step toward incorporating SBT of teams into residency and practice. Interventional radiology can be an intensive, highly dynamic work environment, requiring the coordinated action of each member of the team for the safe, effective delivery of care. Training the entire IR staff (i.e., from attending radiologists to technicians) using HFS would provide an opportunity for members to learn and hone their team-based skills in a safe, immersive, nonthreatening learning environment. In this manner, team function could be refined. Another obvious target for team-based training in radiology is crisis management in low-frequency, high-risk encounters, such as severe intravenous contrast media reactions. High-fidelity simulation could be incorporated to allow teams and radiologists to practice interventions known to improve outcomes. Such training would provide exposure of interprofessional SBT to a wider range of practicing radiologists, since contrast media reaction is a near universal encounter across all subspecialties in radiology. Thus, team-based competencies could be introduced to a large number of practicing radiologists. Clearly, team-based training using either HFS or another simulation-based technique will play an important role in the future training of radiologists.

CONCLUSION

The literature supports interprofessional simulation-based team training as an effective method of training health care professionals of the future. Both the ACGME and RSNA support the use of simulation as standard educational practice. As other medical professions have advanced in the area of interprofessional simulation-based team training, radiology is now following suit. Radiology has the benefit of drawing on years of research in the science of simulation-based education to translate current trends in team-based training with simulation into practice.

REFERENCES

1. Greiner AC, Knebel E, eds. *Health Professions Education: A Bridge to Quality*. Washington DC: Institute of Medicine/National Academies Press; 2003.

2. Joint Commission. Sentinel Event Data: Root Causes by Event Type. Accessed June 17, 2011, at http/www.jointcommission.org/assests/1/18/SE_RootCausesEventType2004_4Q2010.pdf

3. Chatman IJ. *Medical Team Training: Strategies for Improving Patient Care and Communication*. Oakbrook Terrace, IL: Joint Commission Resources; 2008.

4. Baker DP, Gustafson S, Beaubien J, et al. *Medical Teamwork and Patient Safety The Evidence-based Relation,* AHRQ Publication No. 05-0053, Chapter 4 Medical Team Training (July 2005). Accessed October 27, 2010, at http://www.ahrq.gov/qual/medteam/

5. Mills P, Neily J, Dunn E. Teamwork and communication in surgical teams: implications for patient safety. *J Am Coll Surg.* 2008;206:107–112.

6. The Joint Commission. 2010 National Patient Safety Goals (NPSG). Accessed October 27, 2010, at http://www.jointcommission.org/PatientSafety/NationalPatientSafetyGoals/

7. Baker DP, Day R, Salas E. Teamwork as an essential component of high-reliability organizations. *Health Serv Res.* 2006;41:1576–1598.

8. Beaubien JM, Baker DP. The use of simulation for training teamwork skills in health care: how low can you go? *Qual Saf Health Care.* 2004;13:51–56.

9. Kohn LT, Corrigan J, Donaldson MS, eds. *To Err is Human: Building a Safer Health System.* Washington, DC: Institute of Medicine/National Academies Press; 2000.

10. Finkleman A, Kenner C. *Teaching IOM. Implication of the Institute of Medicine Reports for Nursing Education.* Silver Spring, MD: ANA; 2009.

11. Teamwork as a tool for patient safety. CIRCO/RMF, May 20, 2010. Accessed June 17, 2011, at http://www.rmf.harvard.edu/patient-safety-strategies/communication-teamwork/articles/taat-facilitators-guide-and-outline.aspx

12. Burke CS, Salas E, Wilson-Donnelly K, et al. How to turn a team of experts into an expert medical team: guidance from the aviation and military communities. *Qual Saf Health Care.* 2004;13 (Suppl 1): i96–i104.

13. Bleakley A, Boyden J, Hobbs A, et al. Improving teamwork climate in operating theatres: the shift from multiprofessionalism to interprofessionalism. *J Interprof Care.* 2006:20;461–470.

14. Bleakley A. You are who I say you are: the rhetorical construction of identity in the operating theatre. *J Workplace Learning.* 2006;18:414–425.

15. Gillespie BM, Chaboyer W, Wallis M, et al. Why isn't "time out" being implemented? An exploratory study. *Qual Saf Health Care.* 2010;19:103–106.

16. Haldet P, Stein HF. The role of the student-teacher relationship in the formation of physicians: the hidden curriculum as process. *J Gen Intern Med.* 2006;21:S16-S20.

17. Wear D, Skillicorn J. Hidden in plain sight: the formal, informal, and hidden curricula of a psychiatry clerkship. *Acad Med.* 2009;84:451–458.

18. Reese CE, Jeffries PR, Engum SA. Learning together: using simulations to develop nursing and medical student collaboration. *Nurs Educ Persp.* 2010;31:33–37.

19. Gettman MT, Pereira CW, Lipsky K, et al. Use of high fidelity operating room simulation to assess and teach communication, teamwork and laparoscopic skills: initial experience. *J Urol.* 2009;181:1289–1296.

20. Mishra A, Catchpole K, Dale T, et al. The influence of non-technical performance on technical outcome in laparoscopic cholecystectomy. *Surg Endosc.* 2008;22:68–73.

21. Shapiro MJ, Gardner R, Godwin SA, et al. Defining team performance for simulation-based training: methodology, metrics, and opportunities for emergency medicine. *Acad Emerg Med.* 2008;15:1088–1097.

22. Mazzocco K, Petitti DB, Fong KT, et al. Surgical team behaviors and patient outcomes. *Am J Surg.* 2009;197:678–685.

23. Andersen PO, Jensen MK, Lippert A, et al. Identifying non-technical skills and barriers for improvement of teamwork in cardiac arrest teams. *Resuscitation.* 2010;81:695–702.

24. Rosen MA, Salas E, Wilson KA, et al. Measuring team performance in simulation-based training: adopting best practices for health care. *Simul Healthc.* 2008;3:33–41.

25. Agency for Healthcare Research and Quality. Core Curriculum for Patient Safety. Accessed October 20, 2010, at http://psnet.ahrq.gov/resource.aspx?resourceID=1030

26. Salas E, Sims DE, Burke CS. Is there a big five in teamwork? *Small Group Res.* 2005;36:555–599.

27. Jeffries PA, McNelis AM, Wheeler CA. Simulation as a vehicle for enhancing collaborative practice models. *Crit Care Nurs Clin N Am.* 2008;20:471–480.

28. Frankel A, Gardner R, Maynard L, et al. Using the communication and teamwork skills (CATS) assessment to measure health care team performance. *Jt Comm J Qual Patient Saf.* 2007;33:549.

29. Westrum R. A typology of organizational cultures. *Qual Saf Health Care.* 2004;12:22–27.

30. Schulman PR. General attributes of safe organizations. *Qual Saf Health Care.* 2004;13(Suppl II): ii39–ii44.

31. McKeon LM, Oswaks JD, Cunningham PD. Safeguarding patients: complexity science, high reliability organizations, and implications for team training in health care. *Clin Nurse Spec.* 2006;20:298–304.

32. Leonard M, Graham S, Bonacum D. The human factor: the critical importance of effective teamwork and communication in providing safe care. *Qual Saf Health Care.* 2004;13(Suppl 1): i85–i90.

33. Sundar E, Sundar S, Pawlowski J, et al. Crew resource management and team training. *Anesthesiol Clin.* 2010;25:285.

34. Wright MC, Taekman JM, Endsley MR. Objective measures of situation awareness in a simulated medical environment. *Qual Saf Health Care.* 2004;13(Suppl 1):i65–i71.

35. Moorthy K, Munz Y, Adams S, et al. A human factors analysis of technical and team skills among surgical trainees during procedural simulations in a simulated operating theatre. *Ann Surg.* 2005;242:631–639.

36. Gaba DM. Crisis resources management and teamwork training in anesthesia, *Br J Anesth.* 2010;105:6–8.

37. Gaba DM, Howard SK, Fish KJ, et al. Simulation-based training in anesthesia crisis resource management (ACRM): a decade of experience. *Simul Gaming.* 2001;32:175–193.

38. Rudy SJ, Polomano R, Murray WB, et al. Team management training using crisis resource management results in perceived benefits by health care workers. *J Cont Educ Nurs.* 2007;38:219–226.

39. Clancy CM, Tornberg DN. TeamSTEPPS: assuring optimal teamwork in clinical settings, *Am J Med Qual.* 2007;22:214–217.

40. Clancy CM. Crisis resources management and teamwork training in anesthesia. *Br J Anesth.* 2007;105:6–8.

41. Capella J, Smith S, Philp A, Putnam T, et al. Teamwork training improves the clinical care of trauma patients. *J Surg Educ.* 2010;67:439–443.

42. Stead K, Kumar S, Schultz TJ, et al. Teams communicating through STEPPS. *Med J Aust.* 2009;190:S128–132.

43. Robertson B, Kaplan B, Atallah H, et al. The use of simulation and a modified TeamSTEPPS curriculum for medical and nursing student team training. *Simul Healthc.* 2010;5:332–337.

44. Denson JS, Abrahamson S. A computer-controlled patient simulator. *JAMA.* 1969;208:504–508.

45. Rodgers DL. High fidelity patient simulation: a descriptive white paper report. 2007. Accessed December 24, 2011, at http://www.scribd.com/doc/57687160/2/Development-of-Manikin-Based-Patient-Simulation-Technology

46. Rauen CA. Simulation as a teaching strategy for nursing education and orientation in cardiac surgery. *Crit Care Nurs.* 2004;24:46–51.

47. Rosen MA, Salas E, Silvestri S, et al. A measurement tool for simulation-based training in emergency medicine: the simulation module for assessment of resident targeted event responses (SMARTER) approach. *Simul Healthc.* 2008;3:170–179.

48. Brett-Fleegler MB, Vinici RJ, Weiner DL, et al. A simulator-based tool that assesses pediatric resident resuscitation competency. *Pediatrics.* 2009;121:597–603.

49. Daniels K, Lipman S, Harney K, et al. Use of simulation based training for obstetric crisis in resident education. *Simul Healthc.* 2008; 3:154–160.

50. Deering S, Rosen MA, Salas E, et al. Building team and technical competency for obstetric emergencies: the mobile obstetric emergencies simulator (MOES) system. *Simul Healthc.* 2009;4:166–173.

51. Paige JT, Kozmenko V, Yang T, et al. High-fidelity, simulation-based, interdisciplinary operating room team training at the point of care. *Surgery.* 2009;145:138–146.

52. Tofil NM, White ML, Grant M, et al. Severe contrast reaction emergencies high-fidelity simulation training for radiology residents and technologists in a children's hospital. *Acad Radiol.* 2010;17:934–940.

53. Brett-Fleegler MB, Vinici RJ, Weiner DL, et al. A Simulator-based tool that assesses pediatric resident resuscitation competency. *Pediatrics.* 2009;121:597–603.

54. Daniels K, Lipman S, Harney K, et al. Use of simulation based training for obstetric crisis in resident education. *Simul Healthc.* 2008;3:154–160.

55. Sehgal NL, Fox M, Vidyarthi AR, et al. A multidisciplinary teamwork training program: the triad for optimal patient safety (TOPS) experience. *J Gen Intern Med.* 2008;23:2053–2057.

56. Abrahamson SD, Canzian S, Brunet F. Using simulation for training and to change protocol during the outbreak of severe acute respiratory syndrome. *Crit Care.* 2006;10:R3.

57. Wayne DB, Didwania A, Fenglass J, et al. Simulation-based education improves quality of care during cardiac arrest team responses at an academic teaching hospital. *Chest.* 2008;133:56–61.

58. Tanner CA. Thinking like a Nurse: a research-based model of clinical judgment in nursing. *J Nurs Educ.* 2006;45:204–211.

59. Decker S, Moore A, Thal W, et al. Synergistic integration of concept mapping and cause and effect diagramming into simulated experiences. *Clin Simul Nurs.* 2010;6:e153–e159.

60. Undre S, Healey AN, Darzi A, et al. Observational assessment of surgical teamwork: a feasibility study. *World J Surg.* 2006;30:1174–1183.

61. Fletcher G, Flin R, McGeorge P, et al. Anaesthetists' non-technical skills (ANTS): evaluation of a behavioral marker system. *Br J Anesth.* 2003;90:580–588.

62. Yule S, Flin R, Paterson-Brown S, et al. Development of a rating system for surgeons' non-technical skills. *Med Educ.* 2006;40:1098–1104.

63. Chauvin SW, Paige JT, Yang T. Operating Room Teamwork Assessment Scales (ORTAS). Office of Medical Education Research and Services, School of Medicine, Louisiana State University Health Sciences Center, New Orleans; 2006; Revised July 2007.

64. Guise JM, Deering SH, Kanki BG, et al. Validation of a tool to measure and promote clinical teamwork. *Simul Healthc.* 2008;3:217–223.

65. Malec JF, Torsher LC, Dunn WF, et al. The Mayo high performance teamwork scale: reliability and validity for evaluating key crew resource management skills. *Simul Healthc.* 2007;2:4–10.

66. Arnold JJ, Johnson LM, Tucker SJ, et al. Evaluation tools in simulation learning: performance and self-efficacy in emergency response. *Clin Simul Nurs.* 2010;5:e35–e43.

67. Jeffries PR. ed. *Simulation in Nursing Education from Conceptualization to Evaluation.* New York: National League for Nursing; 2007.

68. Lasater K. Clinical judgment development: using simulation to create an assessment rubric. *J Nurs Educ.* 2007;46:496–503.

69. Gantt LT. Using the Clark simulation evaluation rubric with associate degree and baccalaureate nursing students. *Nurs Educ Persp.* 2010;31:101–105.

70. Kardong-Edgren S, Adamson KA, Fitzgerald C. A review of currently published evaluation instruments for human patient simulation. *Clin Simul Nurs.* 2010;6:e25-e35.

71. Paige JT. Surgical team training: promoting high reliability with nontechnical skills. *Surg Clin N Am.* 2010;90:569–581.

72. Kirkpatrick DI. *Evaluating Training Programs: The Four Levels,* 2nd edition. San Francisco, CA: Berrett-Koehler; 1998.

73. Desser TS. Simulation-based training: the next revolution in radiology education? *J Am Coll Radiol.* 2007;4:817.

74. Gaba DM, Dunn WF. Procedural risks in thoracentesis: process, progress, and proficiency. *Chest.* 2009;135:1120–1123.

75. Duncan DR, Morgenthaler TI, Ryu JH, et al. Reducing iatrogenic risk in thoracentesis: establishing best practice via experiential training in a zero-risk environment. *Chest.* 2009;135: 1315–1320.

13

Team Training and Crisis Management: Contrast Reaction Management

GAURAVI SABHARWAL AND CHIRAAG V. DHARIA

ALTHOUGH UNCOMMON, intravenous (IV) contrast media reactions are potentially life-threatening events that require prompt recognition and management by radiology residents and faculty alike.[1] Despite the widespread use of low-osmolar contrast agents and premedication of high-risk patients, every practicing radiologist eventually faces the challenge of either a moderate or severe contrast reaction. In the event of an adverse reaction, the radiologist on site must act initially as the primary medical responder, assisting in the diagnosis, treatment, and management of the patient's care until the arrival of a rapid response or code team. Adequate training, therefore, is needed to ensure the uniform, effective delivery of care by both physicians and staff in the radiology department.

BACKGROUND

Current training in the recognition and management of contrast media reactions is highly variable across radiology residency programs. It can range from dedicated hands-on experiences using essential equipment[2] to simple video presentations or lectures on the topic. In fact, formal education in the management of contrast reactions may be minimal in some programs. The need to overcome such a disparity in training is imperative.

Radiology residents and faculty are required to certify every 2 years in Basic Life Support (BLS), Advanced Cardiac Life Support (ACLS) and, for pediatric radiologists, Pediatric Advanced Life Support (PALS). The BLS and ACLS courses primarily focus on the recognition and management of emergent problems like cardiovascular shock, myocardial infarction, and stroke. Although contrast reactions are not directly addressed in these courses,[3] the skills and knowledge needed to manage such reactions are similar. Once learned, however, a progressive diminution in the retention of skills and knowledge occurs. For example, residents have demonstrated the slow loss of acquired skills following ACLS and PALS training.[4,5] Consistent, periodic training, therefore, is needed to maintain skills in the management of acute events such as contrast reactions.[3]

Simulation-based training (SBT) has been increasingly employed in resident training programs for the development, enhancement, and retention of technical skills for many medical specialities and subspecialities.[6–8] The development and availability of different models of high-fidelity computerized mannequins for this purpose has allowed the development of sophisticated scenario-based training opportunities using simulation. In fact, mannequin-based simulations can be used to create different clinical environments, such as the intensive care unit (ICU), operating room (OR), or the emergency room (ER).[9] The use of high-fidelity simulation (HFS) for SBT is increasingly used in obstetrics and gynecology, pediatrics, emergency medicine, urology, ophthalmology, laparoscopic surgery, and several other medical specialties.[6,10–17] More recently, it is also being incorporated into radiology resident training.[18]

Management of contrast media reactions is an ideal topic for high-fidelity SBT for several reasons. First, severe contrast reactions are low-frequency, high-risk events that require prompt treatment to avoid catastrophic outcomes. Simulation-based training provides a format for repetitive practice in the management of such events to maintain skills and allow for automatic responses when an actual event occurs in clinical practice. Secondly, iodinated contrast media are universally employed in radiology for all types of imaging: intravascular, gastrointestinal, intrathecal, genitourinary, biliary, mammary ductal, fistula, and arthrographic.[19] In susceptible patients, contrast reactions can occur in any of these situations, although most reactions occur with intravascular administration. Every radiologist, therefore, needs to be familiar with the clinical manifestations and therapeutic interventions for contrast reactions. Simulation-based training provides a standardized, consistent mechanism for training large numbers of radiologists in treating these potentially devastating complications. Thirdly, since initial resuscitation and management of patients with severe contrast reactions draws on many of the same skills and principles utilized in BLS, ACLS, and PALS, SBT provides an opportunity for learners to hone and reinforce critical knowledge and skills that would otherwise diminish between infrequent episodes of actual contrast reaction in the clinical environment. Finally, effective response to a severe contrast reaction requires well-coordinated team function, with clear communication and a shared mental model. Simulation-based training provides an opportunity for team training of the staff and physicians of the radiology department in a patient-safe, nonpunitive environment where team-based competencies can be taught and perfected.

Thankfully, contrast reactions are infrequent events. Adverse effects have been reported to occur in 5%–15% of patients receiving ionic, high-osmolality contrast media.[20] Low osmolality ionic and nonionic contrast media have a lower adverse effect incidence of 0.2%–0.7%.[10,21] The true incidence of fatal outcomes from IV contrast media is unknown. A conservative estimate of 1 per 170,000 administrations arises from a large Japanese study of over 170,000 injections of high- and low-osmolality contrast media.[10]

Reactions to IV contrast can be categorized as mild, moderate, and severe. Mild reactions typically involve the development of nausea/vomiting, altered taste, sweating, cough, itching, rash/hives, warmth, pallor, nasal stuffiness, headache, flushing, facial and periorbital swelling, dizziness, chills, anxiety, and/or shaking. Moderate reactions are characterized by tachycardia/bradycardia, bronchospasm/wheezing, hypertension, generalized or diffuse erythema, mild hypotension, and/or dyspnea. Finally, severe reactions are life-threatening events involving laryngeal edema, convulsions, profound hypotension, unresponsiveness, cardiac arrhythmias, and/or cardiopulmonary arrest.[19] The differential diagnosis of any potential contrast reaction includes local anesthetic toxicity, a needle- or catheter-induced event, and physiologic changes related to patient anxiety.

THE HENRY FORD HOSPITAL EXPERIENCE IN SIMULATION-BASED TRAINING IN CONTRAST REACTION MANAGEMENT

At Henry Ford Hospital (HFH), a curriculum has been developed to train all radiology residents and staff in the recognition and management of contrast media reactions. It involves pretraining assessment of baseline knowledge and skill, didactic instruction, and SBT using a variety of scenarios. A description of each aspect of this curriculum follows.

Pre-Test Assessment

An online 20-question pre-test module was created for the residents and staff radiologists to assess their preliminary knowledge of this important topic. The test consists of multiple-choice questions relating to both adult and pediatric contrast media reactions and their management. The participants must complete the pre-test before proceeding with the rest of the curriculum.

Didactic Instruction

A 2 hour detailed didactic lecture is given to all radiology residents and staff radiologists. This lecture can be presented in a lecture room, by teleconference, or by video for convenience purposes. The lecture is conducted by a staff radiologist who is actively involved in creating protocols for the prevention and management of contrast media reactions for the department. Constant references are made to the American College of Radiology (ACR) Manual on Contrast Media.[19] The lecture describes the chemical composition and differing osmolalities of the contrast media in use and the classification and symptoms of contrast media reactions and their detailed treatment. Concise summary pocket cards for quick reference are distributed to all course participants (Table 13.1).

These cards describe the premedication regimen for patients with suspected contrast allergy and reaction management protocols for patients who develop contrast reaction, as developed by the department in consultation with the hospital pharmacy. The contact number for the hospital rapid response team (RRT) is clearly listed on the pocket cards. The RRT, a special team of intensive care nurses, can be contacted by any radiology staff member to examine a patient at the first sign of deteriorating status. This action is akin to bringing the ICU to the patient's bedside. In the lecture, participants are reminded of the protocols for notifying the code team, the team of physicians, and other health care providers who respond to "code blue" situations using ACLS protocols. The contents of the radiology crash cart are discussed, and all medications, strengths, and dosages are reviewed (Table 13.2).

In particular, the indications for IV and subcutaneous epinephrine administration are emphasized. Specific attention is given to the various clinical scenarios encountered during the scenario-based training using the high-fidelity mannequin. The residents are provided with printed handouts listing algorithms designed for the management of the scenarios, which include management of bronchospasm, cardiovascular shock, laryngeal edema, panic attack, hypertensive crisis, contrast extravasation, and urticaria. These scenarios, performed in the hospital simulation center, are designed and based on Accreditation Council for Graduate Medical Education (ACGME) core competencies (i.e., patient care, medical knowledge, practice-based learning and improvement, interpersonal and communication skills, professionalism, and systems-based practice).[22]

Orientation to the Simulation-Based Training Environment

The radiology residents and staff are next given group tours of the simulation center to familiarize them with the use of all available equipment. One simulation room is arranged to represent a computed tomography (CT) scanning room. Each group is introduced to the capabilities of SimMan™ (Laerdal Medical, Wappinger Falls, New York),[23] a life-size, portable, high-fidelity patient simulator designed for use in teamwork training scenarios (Figure 13.1).

This computerized mannequin has many features including the following:

- Spontaneous respiration with variable respiratory rate
- Life-like lung, heart, and bowel sounds on auscultation
- The ability to mimic tongue edema, pharyngeal obstruction, and laryngospasm
- Palpable carotid, femoral, brachial, radial, dorsalis pedis, and posterior tibial arterial pulses that can be synchronized with electrocardiogram (ECG) or chest compressions; tactile feedback of the pulses to the computer enables the program to progress.
- Prerecorded speech and pertinent audible sounds; for more advanced simulations, real-time voice input through a microphone is available to simulate live communication.
- Dedicated software with a user interface that allows for the building of scenarios with physiologic changes and multiple alternatives in predefined settings
- A simulated patient monitor that can incorporate real-time parameters, such as vital signs, 12-lead ECG, and X-rays

Additionally, a radiology staff nurse trained in this course assists in moving the program forward. The nurse carefully listens to each command, observes the action taken by the resident, and checks it off on the computer to allow the scenario to progress.

Table 13.1 Management of iodinated contrast reactions[a]

REACTION	TREATMENT
Urticaria	• Discontinue injection if not completed. • No treatment needed in most cases. Observe patient for 30–60 minutes. • If symptomatic: diphenhydramine (Benadryl) 25–50 mg PO, IV, or IM (may cause drowsiness—caution if driving) • If severe or widely disseminated: epinephrine (1:1,000) 0.1–0.3 mg (0.1–0.3 mL) SC[b] or IM[c] and call Rapid Response Team
Facial or laryngeal edema	• O_2 6–10 L/min via mask • Epinephrine (1:1,000) 0.1–0.3 mg (0.1–0.3 mL) SC or IM, or if hypotension evident: epinephrine (1:10,000) 0.1 mg (1 mL) slow IV[d]. Repeat as needed to maximum of 1 mg. Call Rapid Response Team. • If not responsive to therapy or if obvious acute laryngeal edema, call Blue Alert Team.
Bronchospasm	• O_2 6–10 L/min via mask • Albuterol inhaler 2–3 puffs or albuterol nebulization 2.5–5 mg • If unresponsive to albuterol: epinephrine (1:1,000) 0.1–0.3 mg (0.1–0.3 mL) SC or IM, or if hypotension evident: epinephrine (1:10,000) 0.1 mg (1 mL) slow IV. Repeat as needed to maximum of 1 mg. Call Rapid Response Team. • If severe bronchospasm or if O_2 saturation <88% persists, call Blue Alert Team
Hypotension with tachycardia	• Elevate legs or Trendelenburg position • O_2 6–10 L/min via mask • Call Rapid Response Team and consider rapid IV administration of large volumes of lactated Ringer's or normal saline • If poorly responsive: Call Blue Alert Team. Epinephrine (1:10,000) 0.1 mg (1 mL) slow IV. Repeat as needed to maximum of 1 mg.
Hypotension with bradycardia	• Elevate legs or Trendelenburg position • O_2 6–10 L/min via mask • Call Rapid Response Team and consider rapid fluid replacement with lactated Ringer's or normal saline • If patient does not respond quickly to above steps: Call Blue Alert Team and consider atropine 0.6–1 mg slow IV. Repeat up to a total dose of 0.04 mg/kg
Hypertension, severe	• O_2 6–10 L/min via mask • Call Rapid Response Team
Seizures or convulsions	• Turn on side to avoid aspiration • O_2 6–10 L/min via mask • Call Rapid Response Team and consider lorazepam (Ativan) 2–4 mg IV or midazolam (Versed) 0.5–1 mg IV
Pulmonary edema	• O_2 6–10 L/min via mask • Call Rapid Response Team and consider furosemide (Lasix) 20–40 mg slow IV
Extravasation	• Check for pulse and capillary refill • Inquire about pain, tingling sensation • Elevate limb above heart level and apply cold compresses • Call plastic surgery if >100 mL or symptomatic
Air embolism	• Administer 100% oxygen and place patient in the left lateral decubitus position (i.e., left side down)

[a]Given to residents as quick reference pocket guide for use in radiology suite, [b]SC, subcutaneous; [c]IM, intramuscular; [d]IV, intravenous

Table 13.2 Crash cart medications[a]

DRUG	DOSE	ROUTE
Albuterol	2.5 mg-5 mg	MDI
Aspirin	325 mg	PO
Atropine	0.1 mg/mL	IV
Diphenhydramine (Benadryl)	50 mg/mL	IV
Diphenhydramine (Benadryl)	25 mg	PO
Epinephrine (Epi Pen)	0.3 mg/0.3 mL (1:1000 dilution)	IMThigh
Epinephrine (Epi Pen Jr.)	0.15 mg/0.3 mL (1:2000 dilution)	IM Thigh
Epinephrine	0.1 mg/mL (1:10,000 dilution)	IV
Labetalol	10 mg	IV
Methylprednisolone (Solu-Medrol)	40 mg	IV
Nitroglycerin	0.4 mg	Sublingual

[a]Note: benzodiazepines are restricted medications and not included in this box, [b]MDI, metered dose inhaler; [c]PO, per os; [d]IV, intravenous; [e]IM, intramuscular

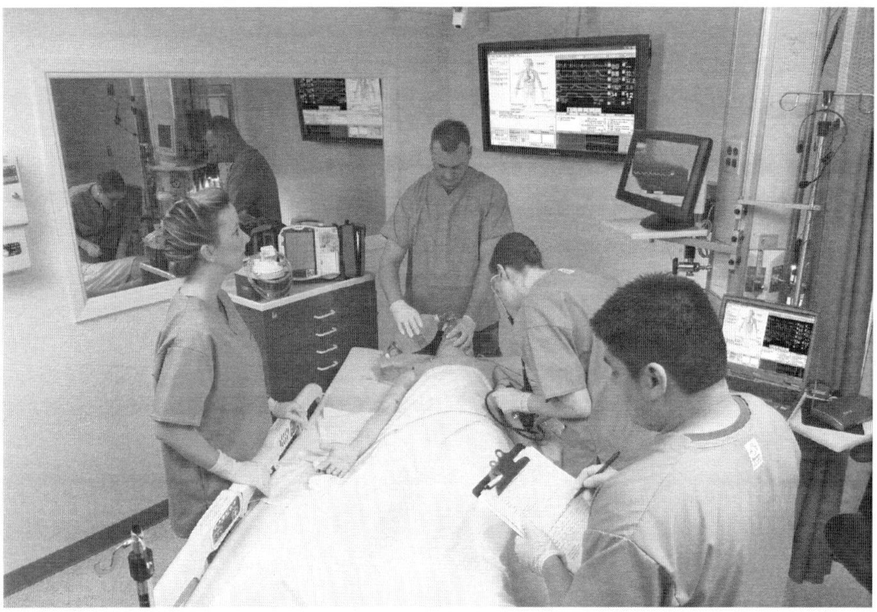

FIGURE 13.1 A scenario enactment tests the residents on the core competencies listed by the Accreditation Council for Graduate Medical Education (ACGME) (i.e., patient care, medical knowledge, practice-based learning and improvement, interpersonal and communication skills, professionalism, and systems-based practice). Photo Courtesy of Laerdal Medical.

Integrated Video Debriefing System software synchronizes video and audio obtained at the time of the simulated event with the SimMan™ log of events. This system provides assessment of individual and/or group trainee performance during the scenario-based training using high-fidelity simulation.

Scenario-Based Training Using High-Fidelity Simulation

The participants are divided into groups of four for the scenario-based training exercises. At the start of the training session, they are instructed to approach the SimMan™ as a live patient within a CT scanner. For each session, the participants are given access to all resuscitation equipment found in the CT suite, including vital sign monitoring devices, respiratory support devices, oxygen, and medications in the radiology crash cart (Figure 13.2).

For each scenario, one individual is designated as the leader. This person is primarily responsible for managing the encounter and is instructed to form a "radiology code team" by delegating assignments to the other participating team members. This leader must voice all actions in a clear, loud manner in order to ensure that the nurse assistant managing the operation of the mannequin software can advance the scenario appropriately. The scenario progresses with each appropriate action taken by the resuscitation team. If a required action is not taken by the trainees during the enactment of the scenario, the patient goes down a simulated "death spiral," in which further resuscitation is unsuccessful. In such cases, the whole scenario is restarted at the point of the missed action, in order to allow the team another opportunity to respond appropriately. After each scenario, the role of the leader is taken over by a different participant, so that each individual trainee has the opportunity to run the resuscitation and be evaluated as a team leader.

As mentioned above, seven separate scenarios reflecting varying degrees of contrast reaction have been developed for the SBT using the SimMan™ mannequin at HFH. These training exercises provide an opportunity for practicing both the medical management and the team-based response to contrast media reactions in a patient-safe, nonpunitive environment. Each scenario is described in more detail below.

PANIC ATTACK

Patient Presentation

Signs and symptoms of a panic attack include palpitations, tachycardia, sweating, trembling or shaking, sensation of shortness of breath, a feeling of choking, chest pain/discomfort, nausea or abdominal distress, feeling dizzy/unsteady/lightheaded/faint, derealization (a feeling of unreality) or depersonalization (being detached from oneself), fear of losing control or "going crazy," fear of dying, paresthesias (numbness or "tingling" sensations), chills, or hot flashes.

Scenario Introduction

The introduction is read by the designated leader to the other team members: "A 32-year-old female has just started a CT scan of the abdomen and pelvis to evaluate for intermittent chronic pain. After the scout images are acquired, the patient's heart rate increases from 80/min to 150/min. She starts to scream incessantly that she cannot breathe and is going to die. She is inconsolable. The resident is asked to assist."

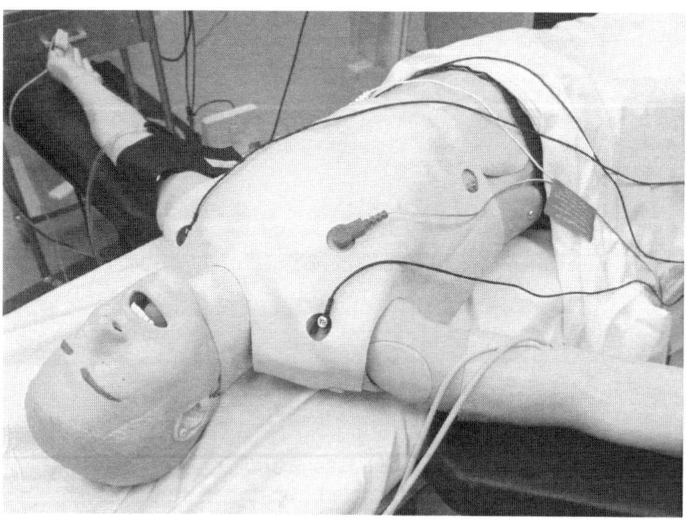

FIGURE 13.2 The SimMan™: a highly sophisticated, life-size, interactive and portable high-fidelity simulator for team training. Photo Courtesy of Laerdal Medical.

Key Management Interventions

Appropriate treatment of this patient would be to immediately remove her from the source of anxiety (i.e., the CT table), assess her using the ABCs (i.e., checking airway, breathing, and circulation), and reassure her that the environment is safe. In addition, the patient should be provided with oxygen by mask and encouraged to relax and breathe deeply. This sequence should be done while constantly checking the monitors for the patient's vital signs. In certain situations in which very rapid control of anxiety symptoms is critical, benzodiazepines are the preferred drug of choice (Figure 13.3).

Critical Performance Indicators

The designated scenario leader is expected to communicate in a clear, concise manner. If a delay in removing the patient from the CT scanner is encountered, the patient's condition worsens as she begins to hyperventilate. It is important for the resident to recognize the event as a panic attack and not a true contrast reaction, since the patient did not receive contrast before the onset of symptoms. The leader should confirm this during the patient assessment using the ABCs. The most critical action for this scenario is the removal of the patient from the CT scanner table (i.e., the offending environment that instituted the panic attack). The scenario is successfully completed when the patient says that she "feels much better."

HYPERTENSIVE CRISIS

Patient Presentation

A typical hypertensive crisis would include elevated blood pressure and the development of signs of target end-organ dysfunction, such as retinal hemorrhage, exudate, or papilledema; jugular venous distension; audible respiratory crackles or peripheral edema suggestive of heart failure; decreased level of consciousness; decreased visual fields; or focal neurologic signs suggestive of central nervous system (CNS) dysfunction.

Scenario Introduction

The introduction is read by the designated leader to the other team members: "An 88-year-old male has just completed a computed tomography angiogram (CTA) of the abdomen and pelvis for the evaluation of abdominal aortic aneurysm (AAA) graft repair. After the examination is complete, the CT technologist calls the radiology resident and states that the patient has developed an acute headache, is lightheaded, and has blurry vision. The patient's blood pressure monitor shows a systolic blood pressure of 240 mm Hg. The resident is asked to assist."

Key Management Interventions

The expected treatment for hypertensive urgency (defined as severe elevation of blood pressure *without* evidence of target organ damage) would be a

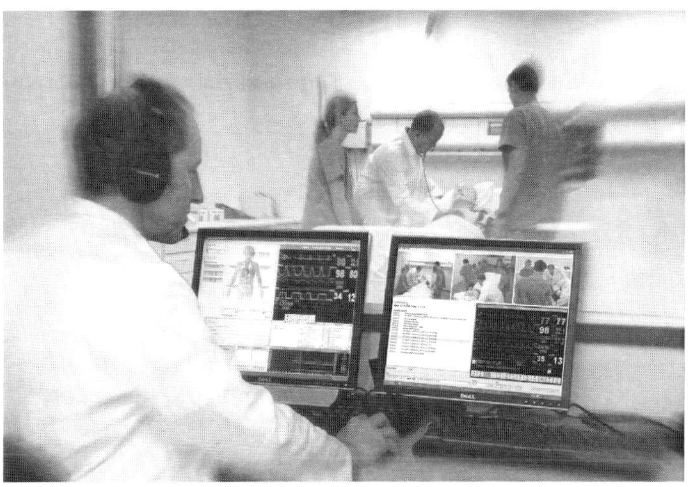

FIGURE 13.3 Simulated patient monitor with programmed 12-lead electrocardiogram and other information. A radiology nurse advances the case based on actions performed by the designated scenario leader. Photo Courtesy of Laerdal Medical.

reduction in blood pressure over a period of days to weeks. In scenarios in which target organ damage is described, the expected treatment for hypertensive crisis would be the aggressive lowering of blood pressure over minutes to hours.

Critical Performance Indicators

The designated leader is expected to request and perform frequent checks of the patient's vital signs, especially blood pressure. He or she should initiate oxygen by mask, particularly if the patient appears short of breath. During the scenario, the mannequin complains of chest discomfort. The leader must then request an ECG and another blood pressure reading. The monitors will then display elevated systolic blood pressure and a slightly decreased pulse oximetry reading. The ECG will demonstrate ST segment elevation. These new findings should precipitate instant activity by the leader and team. The leader should designate a "code team member" to summon the RRT. Oxygen is provided by mask. The leader should then designate another team member to open the radiology crash cart and administer aspirin, sublingual nitroglycerine, and a β blocker. Failure to perform any of the above critical performance indicators will result in the patient entering a simulated "death spiral." For a scenario to conclude successfully, the blood pressure must be decreased to near normal levels and the chest pain resolved. The RRT arrives and takes charge of the resuscitation at this point.

FACIAL/LARYNGEAL EDEMA

Patient Presentation

Signs and symptoms of laryngeal edema include hoarseness, dysphasia, difficulty breathing, and cough.

Scenario Introduction

The introduction is read by the designated leader to the other team members: "A 42-year-old female has just completed a CT scan of the abdomen and pelvis for the evaluation of RLQ pain. After the examination is complete, the CT technologist calls the radiology resident and states that the patient has developed progressive shortness of breath and feels something 'funny in her throat.' The resident is asked to assist."

Key Management Interventions

Expected treatment of facial/laryngeal edema involves maintaining IV access, ensuring an adequate airway, administering oxygen by face mask, obtaining vital signs, and contacting the RRT if the patient remains unstable. Epinephrine (1: 10,000) is given intravenously. The reaction should be documented in the patient care notes and on an occurrence form.

Critical Performance Indicators

The designated leader resident is expected to perform a check of the ABCs and recognize the presence of tongue swelling (Figure 13.4a and b).

During the scenario, the patient's speech is muffled and difficult to understand due to the tongue swelling. The leader should then designate one of the "code team members" to quickly summon the RRT. He should then designate another member to give oxygen by mask. He must also ensure the administration of subcutaneous epinephrine. The scenario is designed so that the patient does not respond to this subcutaneous administration of epinephrine. The leader is expected

(A) (B)

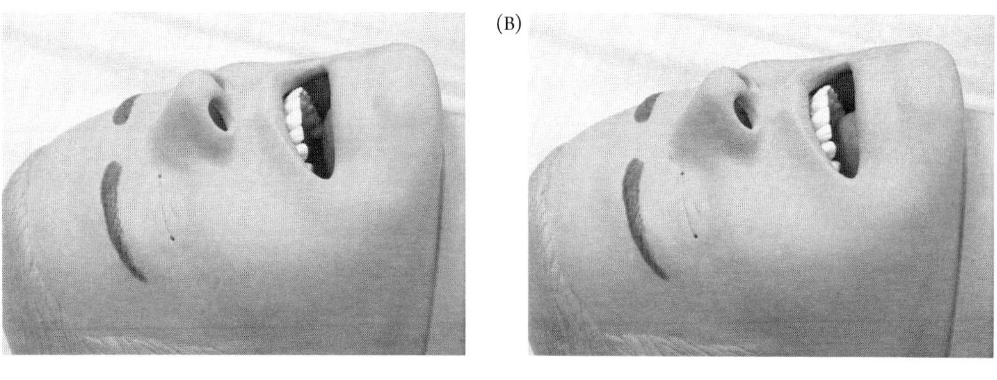

FIGURE 13.4 Evaluation of the airway should always include exploration of the mouth to exclude obstruction from swelling of the tongue. These figures demonstrate the appearance of a normal (A) and swollen (B) tongue. Photos Courtesy of Laerdal Medical.

to recognize this failure of treatment and should have obtained an IV epinephrine solution (1:10,000) or an EpiPen in anticipation of its need. The leader then has 20 seconds to administer the IV epinephrine before the simulated "death spiral" begins. The scenario finishes after the timely administration of the IV epinephrine, at which point the patient "feels much better."

CARDIOVASCULAR SHOCK

Patient Presentation

A typical presentation of cardiovascular shock includes the onset of hypotension, tachycardia, thready pulse, and diffuse pallor after receiving IV contrast.

Scenario Introduction

The introduction is read by the designated leader to the other team members: "A 71-year-old male receives IV contrast for a renal CT scan to follow-up a complex cyst noted on a recent renal ultrasound. The technologist notes the patient to be pale and lethargic. He stops the scanning and asks the resident in the CT reading room to assist."

Key Management Interventions

Appropriate treatment includes the administration of oxygen by mask, the elevation of bilateral lower extremities, immediate summoning of the RRT, and the administration of large volumes of fluids. If necessary, a "code blue" is called.

Critical Performance Indicators

Upon arrival, the designated leader is expected to perform an immediate ABC check. He should note a thready and rapid pulse, over 100/minute. He should then check a blood pressure reading. He must then designate a member of the "radiology code team" to provide oxygen by mask. Meanwhile, a blood pressure of 63/40 mm Hg is reported. The leader must designate a team member to call for the RRT and must coordinate the team to place the patient in a Trendelenberg position, start IV fluid resuscitation, and perform frequent blood pressure checks. In the scenario, the next blood pressure reading does not improve significantly. The resident should then instruct a team member to administer IV epinephrine. Following this appropriate treatment intervention, the next blood pressure reading will be 110/76 mm of Hg. The patient will then express "feeling better" and the scenario concludes.

BRONCHOSPASM

Patient Presentation

Sign and symptoms of bronchospasm can include wheezing, difficulty in breathing, and cough.

Scenario Introduction

The introduction is read by the designated leader to the other team members: "An 18-year-old male has just completed a CT scan of the chest, abdomen, and pelvis after being involved in a motor vehicle collision. After the examination is complete, the CT technologist calls the radiology resident and states that the patient has developed an acute episode of persistent wheezing. The resident is asked to assist."

Key Management Interventions

Expected treatment includes ensuring a patent airway, providing oxygen by mask, and administrating β agonist inhalers and epinephrine. The RRT should be summoned.

Critical Performance Indicators

The leader should immediately perform an ABC check. uring the scenario, the patient has a coughing spell. The resident should then designate one team member to administer oxygen by mask and instructs another member to call the RRT. Following the administration of oxygen, the pulse oximetry reading will increase. The patient's respiratory rate, however, also increases with wheezing in both lung fields. The scenario is programmed so that the patient remains symptomatic after administration of both a β agonist inhaler and/or subcutaneous epinephrine. The patient gets instant relief of his symptoms, however, with the administration of IV epinephrine. The scenario then concludes.

EXTRAVASATION

Patient Presentation

During contrast extravasation, the site may become edematous, erythematous, and tender to palpation.

Scenario Introduction

The introduction is read by the designated leader to the other team members: "A 42-year-old man is undergoing a CT angiogram of the head and neck; 90 cc of nonionic contrast is to be injected IV via a power injector. During the injection, the patient experiences sharp pain at the injection site. The injection and examination are both discontinued. The radiologist is summoned to evaluate the patient."

Key Management Interventions

Expected management of contrast extravasation includes evaluation of the site for altered tissue perfusion, inquiry into the amount of contrast extravasated, evaluation of the affected limb for change in sensation, elevation of the limb, administration of cold compresses, and, in severe cases involving tissue loss, consultation with plastic surgery.

Critical Performance Indicators

The designated leader must introduce him- or herself to the patient and explain the situation. The leader then must perform an examination of the affected injection site. This examination should include checking for capillary refill and tenderness to palpation. In addition, it should include asking the patient about any pain or "tingling" sensation. The leader must also inquire regarding the amount of extravasated contrast medium by asking the CT technologist directly the precise amount of contrast medium injected. During the scenario, the patient complains of pain and tightness at the site. The leader should instruct the patient to elevate his arm above the level of the heart and direct a team member to place some cold compresses on the site of extravasation. He then designates a team member to contact plastic surgery for consultation.

URTICARIA

Patient Presentation

Urticaria usually manifests as pruritus with the development of skin wheals.

Scenario Introduction

The introduction is read by the designated leader to the other team members: "A 45-year-old woman undergoes a CT scan of the chest to evaluate for mediastinal lymphadenopathy. During the contrast injection, she develops itching on her neck. The CT technologist asks the radiology resident to assist. The raised wheals on her neck are shown in a picture." A picture showing the appearance of skin wheals is provided to the leader and team.

Key Management Interventions

Appropriate management is based on the severity of the reaction. Mild cases are managed expectantly with close observation of the patient until resolution of symptoms. Moderate reactions are treated with diphenhydramine. Severe reactions warrant the use of epinephrine.

Critical Performance Indicators

The designated leader should introduce him- or herself to the patient and perform an examination. The leader should confirm that the contrast infusion has been stopped and perform a quick ABC check. Patient vital signs should be documented. The leader should inquire about difficulty in breathing. For the scenario, the patient has what appears to be a moderate reaction. Consequently, the leader should instruct a team member to give the patient an oral dose of diphenhydramine. The leader must explain that the diphenhydramine might cause sleepiness and inquire about a companion driving the patient home.

DEBRIEFING, FEEDBACK, AND COURSE EVALUATION

Following each scenario, the participants are given feedback by the simulation instructors regarding the treatment course and the appropriateness of actions taken during the simulation. As with all scenario-based training using HFS, the debriefing reinforces learning, and, not surprisingly, it is considered the most valuable component of this course. Scenarios can be videotaped, and the participants have the ability to review them for further insight into their reactions. They get an opportunity to review their own actions and witness their interactions as a team. Participants also complete questionnaires in order to assess the manner in which a resident prepared for the training and how the preparation related to performance on the course. This course evaluation aids in tailoring future SBT sessions. A post-test is provided to assess the knowledge gained during the SBT process. A fair comparison can be made with individual performance based on comparison of pre- and post-test scores.

CONCLUSION

Simulation-based training of contrast media reactions provides participants with practical experience in the management of these potentially life-threatening events in a safe learning environment without risk to patients. Although experienced educators may use low-fidelity models to provide the basic training, the use of HFS provides a more realistic setting for training, helping to enhance the psychological fidelity of the experience for participants who can more easily "suspend disbelief." Training with the SimMan™ mannequin can facilitate both individual and team-based training. Team-based training allows participants to practice important team-based competencies, such as communication and leadership skills. The contrast media reaction course can be integrated into the routine curriculum of the radiology residency and can help in both initial skills acquisition and the maintenance and refinement of previously acquired skills. At HFH, several factors have dictated the success of the contrast media reaction course, including distributed training (i.e., learning by repetition), matching the level of difficulty of a particular scenario to the ability of the participant involved, incorporating a variety of scenarios based on clinical encounters, and providing accurate feedback to participants during the debriefing process. The combination of these various steps optimizes the training experience and slows the deterioration of the acquired skills. By doing so, the course helps the participants in achieving the best outcomes when faced with an actual contrast medium reaction in the clinical environment.

REFERENCES

1. Krupinski EA, Patel B, Berger W, et al. Assessing radiology resident preparedness to manage IV contrast media reactions using simulation technology. *Stud Health Technol Inform.* 2009;142:139–141.
2. Echenique AM, Joseph R, Casillas VJ. Recognition and treatment of reactions to contrast media: a model for resident and faculty education employing lectures and case scenario workshops. *Acad Radiol.* 1997;4:230–234.
3. Tofil NM, White ML, Grant M, et al. Severe contrast reaction emergencies high-fidelity simulation training for radiology residents and technologists in a children's hospital. *Acad Radiol.* 2010;17:934–940.
4. Chamberlain D, Smith A, Woollard M, et al. Trials of teaching methods in basic life support : comparison of simulated CPR performance after first training and at 6 months, with a note on the value of re-training. *Resuscitation.* 2002;53:179–187.
5. Wolfram RW, Warren CM, Doyle CR, et al. Retention of Pediatric Advanced Life Support (PALS) course concepts. *J Emerg Med.* 2003;25:475–479.
6. Gettman MT, Pereira CW, Lipsky K, et al. Use of high fidelity operating room simulation to assess and teach communication, teamwork and laparoscopic skills: initial experience. *J Urol.* 2009;181:1289–1296.
7. Jacomides L, Ogan K, Cadeddu JA, et al. Use of a virtual reality simulator for ureteroscopy training. *J Urol.* 2004;171:320–323;discussion 323.
8. Le CQ, Lightner DJ, VanderLei L, et al. The current role of medical simulation in American urological residency training programs: an assessment by program directors. *J Urol.* 2007;177:288–291.
9. Kim J, Neilipovitz D, Cardinal P, et al. A pilot study using high-fidelity simulation to formally evaluate performance in the resuscitation of critically ill patients: the University of Ottawa Critical Care Medicine, High-Fidelity Simulation, and Crisis Resource Management I Study. *Crit Care Med.* 2006;34:2167–2174.
10. Katayama H, Yamaguchi K, Kozuka T, et al. Adverse reactions to ionic and nonionic contrast media. A report from the Japanese Committee on the Safety of Contrast Media. *Radiology.* 1990;175: 621–628.
11. Gurusamy K, Aggarwal R, Palanivelu L, et al. Systematic review of randomized controlled trials on the effectiveness of virtual reality training for laparoscopic surgery. *Br J Surg.* 2008;95:1088–1097.
12. Lammers RL, Byrwa MJ, Fales WD, et al. Simulation-based assessment of paramedic pediatric resuscitation skills. *Prehosp Emerg Care.* 2009;13: 345–356.
13. McLaughlin S, Fitch MT, Goyal DG, et al. Simulation in graduate medical education 2008: a review for emergency medicine. *Acad Emerg Med.* 2008;15:1117–1129.
14. Nishisaki A, Hales R, Biagas K, et al. A multi-institutional high-fidelity simulation "boot camp" orientation and training program for first year pediatric critical care fellows. *Pediatr Crit Care Med.* 2009;10:157–162.
15. Solverson DJ, Mazzoli RA, Raymond WR, et al. Virtual reality simulation in acquiring and differentiating basic ophthalmic microsurgical skills. *Simul Healthc.* 2009;4:98–103.
16. Weinberg ER, Auerbach MA, Shah NB. The use of simulation for pediatric training and assessment. *Curr Opin Pediatr.* 2009;21:282–287.

17. Robertson B, Schumacher L, Gosman G, et al. Simulation-based crisis team training for multidisciplinary obstetric providers. *Simul Healthc.* 2009;4:77–83.

18. Wang CL, Schopp JG, Petscavage JM, et al. Prospective, randomized comparison of standard didactic lecture versus high-fidelity simulation for radiology resident contrast reaction management training. *AJR Am J Roentgenol.* 2011;196:1288–1295.

19. American College of Radiology (ACR) Committee on Drugs and Contrast Media. ACR Manual on Contrast Media, Version 7. American College of Radiology 2010. Accessed June 20, 2010, at http://www.acr.org/secondarymainmenucategories/quality_safety/contrast_manual.aspx

20. Dillman JR, Strouse PJ, Ellis JH, et al. Incidence and severity of acute allergic-like reactions to i.v. nonionic iodinated contrast material in children. *AJR Am J Roentgenol.* 2007;188: 1643–1647.

21. Wang CL, Cohan RH, Ellis JH, et al. Frequency, outcome, and appropriateness of treatment of nonionic iodinated contrast media reactions. *AJR Am J Roentgenol.* 2008;191:409–415.

22. ACGME. Common program requirements: General competencies (2007). Accessed June 20, 2010, at http://www.ACGME.org

23. Laerdal Medical. Sim Man (2010). Accessed June 20, 2010, at http://www.laerdal.com/doc/7320252/SimMan.html

14

Simulation-Based Training in Intravenous Procedural Moderate Sedation/Analgesia

JAMES RIOPELLE, VALERIY KOZMENKO, AND ALAN DAVID KAYE

RECENT DECADES have seen a great increase in the administration of sedative and analgesic drugs to patients of all ages undergoing potentially uncomfortable medical tests and therapeutic procedures. In the field of radiology, such procedural sedation is most often administered by registered nurses (RNs) under supervision of the physician performing the procedure. The need to train large numbers of such nurses in the safe use of commonly utilized sedation drugs known to cause catastrophic adverse outcomes (i.e., death, anoxic brain injury, aspiration pneumonitis) has resulted in the publication of several books devoted entirely to procedural sedation for nurses, supervising physicians, or both.[1–4] Increasingly, however, academic medical centers and private corporations are now offering procedural sedation training programs that incorporate sophisticated simulation technology with the purpose of ensuring that trainees are not only knowledgeable about sedation but are also able to detect and treat drug-related complications through the recognition of respiratory and central nervous system depression and the institution of life-saving maneuvers needed to revive an apneic, comatose patient.[5]

Another essential requirement for those performing or supervising the performance of sedation is to become intimately familiar with the growing list of published standards and guidelines released by influential medical, nursing, regulatory, and accrediting organizations in the United States related to procedural sedation/analgesia (Table 14.1). The contents of the websites listed in Table 14.1 are of real educational value and include important and often very specific definitions (e.g., the difference between "moderate" and "deep" sedation) and guidelines that can determine the limits of an individual practitioner's credentialing status. Finally, a radiologist must be familiar with "RN scope-of-practice" issues as delineated in the policies of relevant state nursing boards and medical centers (e.g., the frequent requirement that an RN administering procedural sedation/analgesia hold current certification in advanced adult or pediatric life support).

Table 14.1 Published guidelines for the administration of procedural sedation/analgesia

ORGANIZATION*	GUIDELINES URL†	DATE‡
American Society of Anesthesiologists	Sedation for non-anesthesiologists http://www.asahq.org/publicationsAndServices/sedation1017.pdf	2002
	Continuum of sedation & credentialing for supervision http://www.asahq.org/publicationsAndServices/standards/20.pdf http://www.asahq.org/publicationsAndServices/standards/40.pdf	2009
	Fasting prior to elective procedures http://www.asahq.org/publicationsAndServices/NPO.pdf	1999
	Use of propofol by non-anesthesia providers http://www.asahq.org/publicationsAndServices/standards/37.pdf	2009
	Supervision of deep sedation http://www.asahq.org/publicationsAndServices/standards/39.pdf	2006
American College of Radiologists	Adult sedation http://www.acr.org/SecondaryMainMenuCategories/quality_safety/guidelines/iv/adult_sedation.aspx	2005
	Pediatric sedation http://www.acr.org/SecondaryMainMenuCategories/quality_safety/RadSafety/OtherSafetyTopics/ped-sedation.aspx	2005
American Academy of Pediatrics	Sedation http://aappolicy.aappublications.org/cgi/reprint/pediatrics;118/6/2587.pdf	2006
	Monitoring http://pediatrics.aappublications.org/cgi/reprint/118/6/2587?ijkey=dab72c1571596614bf6d4fb4ed12617d3108ed19	2006
Joint Commission	Standards PC 13.20–PC 13.40	2010

* Procedural sedation guidelines of some state nursing boards are posted on their websites; medical center policies are available through each center's Division of Administration and frequently its Division of Nursing

† Most recent revision

‡ Joint Commission for the Accreditation of Health Care Organizations; manual available in all accredited facilities and available online with paid subscription at http://www.jcrinc.com/e-dition/

The sophistication of any simulation-based training (SBT) targeting sedation nurses will depend on the resources available. Options range from low- to high-fidelity alternatives and include group-based table-top discussions, in which experts guide trainees through a mental rehearsal of the sedation process, pointing out potential trouble spots by sharing personal or second-hand stories and reviewing published reports of "near-misses" or catastrophic outcomes; role-play scenarios, in which trainees verbally demonstrate their level of understanding of pharmacologic and resuscitative principles; technical skills training, in which trainees practice on part-task models, permitting hands-on learning and the demonstration of key technical skills, such as maintaining a patent airway and applying positive-pressure ventilation; and immersive high-fidelity simulation training, in which trainees participate in carefully scripted scenarios enacted with the help of computer-driven manikins capable of nuanced response to operator interventions. As entering keywords such as "sedation training" into a standard Internet search engine will quickly reveal, many academic medical centers and several commercial medical education corporations throughout the United States already offer SBT courses in procedural sedation. The complexity of these educational activities vary from personal computer–based interactive programs to classroom-based didactic instruction combined with small-group high-fidelity SBT. The latter often requires the trainee to travel to the offering institution.

For more than a decade, it has been recognized that SBT is well-suited for teaching techniques used during procedural sedation.[6,7] One recent controlled study found enhanced learning when SBT was compared to a traditional teaching paradigm.[8] In considering the likely true value of simulation-based sedation training, it is perhaps relevant to point out the increasingly widespread adoption of SBT within the military, aerospace, automotive, and other industries.

PATIENT ASSESSMENT AND CONSENT

The purpose of the preprocedural evaluation is to identify patients at increased risk of complications from administration of respiratory and central nervous system depressant medications (i.e., apnea, airway obstruction, hypoxemia, and aspiration of gastric contents). Most hospitals have preprinted consent and assessment forms to ensure that common, important risk factors are identified (Table 14.2). Leading U.S. medical centers have also published their pre-sedation patient assessment protocols on the World Wide Web (e.g., the Harvard protocol at http://www.omed.org/downloads/pdf/publications/enews/2010/matthes_presedation_patient_assessment.pdf). Should a radiologist find the need for frequent "bail-out" deep sedation or general anesthesia from a member of the anesthesia department, it may be best to use routinely the anesthesia department's preoperative assessment and lab order forms, so that all information desired by that department is available.

Opportunities for the use of SBT for pre-sedation patient assessment include observing a trainee perform a standardized, focused preprocedural history and physical examination on a computerized manikin or standardized patient; testing a trainee's ability to identify risk factors for sedative/opioid drug-induced airway collapse and difficult mask ventilation through the use of table-top patient simulations using photographs and scripted histories; and determining a trainee's ability to adjust drug doses and interdose intervals in the presence of well-established risk factors through the use of one-on-one oral board-style questioning (Table 14.3).

As mentioned above, observing a trainee's interaction with a standardized patient (i.e., a trained actor) can also be used to determine his or her ability to customize both advice regarding preprocedural fasting time and advice concerning which routine daily medications should be taken or omitted the day of the procedure in order to maintain adequate physiologic homeostasis (Table 14.4).

Observation of a trainee interviewing a standardized patient can also be used to evaluate a trainee's ability to achieve rapport and patient trust, potentially reducing the amount of drug later required; to explain correctly issues raised during informed consent; and to ensure that the standardized patient has made arrangements for a responsible adult to drive him or her home and provide post-procedure observation and care.

An innovative SBT technique recently developed by radiologists is "test-run simulation." In it, preprocedural patient anxiety is reduced by having the patient undergo his or her simulated procedure in advance of the actual imaging scan.[9,10]

EQUIPMENT/SUPPLY SETUP

Simulation-based training can also be used to determine whether a trainee can properly and completely set up equipment and supplies for sedation, and/or notice an important deficit in a pre-ordered setup. Table 14.5 is a checklist of items that any RN administering procedural sedation should know to have immediately at hand. As such, it could be adapted

Table 14.2 Examples of risk factors for problematic procedural sedation/analgesia obtainable by history

↑ RISK OF RX-INDUCED HYPOXIA	↑ RISK OF ASPIRATION	↑ RISK OF AGITATION OR SEDATION FAILURE
Cardiac, pulmonary, hepatic or renal failure Already O_2-dependent	Reflux esophagitis	Disorientation
Extreme recent weight loss	Hiatal hernia	Chronic use of opioid/sedative Rx
Acute opioid/sedative use	Uncontrolled diabetes	
	GI obstruction	

Table 14.3 Examples of risk factors for sedation-induced hypoxia detectable on physical examination*

HEAD & NECK	BODY HABITUS	CARDIOPULMONARY	NEUROLOGICAL	OTHER
Poor mouth opening	Obesity	Wasted appearance	Stupor	Extreme age
Large tongue	Ascites	Dyspnea	Disorientation	
Short, thick neck	Pregnancy	Wheezing, rales, rhonchi		
Skin contracture	Dehydration	Already receiving oxygen		
Swelling or tumor	Distended abdomen	↓ Saturation by pulse oximetry		
↓ Neck extension				
Blocked nares				

* Modified from Rich, 2005.[11]

Table 14.4 Medications patient should take or omit prior to procedure*

TAKE	OMIT
Cardiac Rx	Oral hypoglycemic
Blood pressure Rx	Long-acting insulin preparations
Pulmonary Rx	Dietary supplements
Antacids (except particulate†)	Other Rx of low importance to homeostasis
Antiseizure medications	
Psychiatric medications	
Pain medications‡	
Any other Rx deemed essential	

* If oral, usually taken with sip of water early morning of procedure

† Maalox®, Mylanta®, Gaviscon®

‡ NB: opiates may decrease gastric emptying time

as an evaluative tool for any SBT scenario focusing on a trainee's knowledge and skill with equipment setup. Simulation-based training also allows the opportunity for trainees to demonstrate their ability to recognize the need for expert help in obtaining an airway and call for such help to come to the radiological suite in a timely manner.

PHARMACOLOGY OF MEDICATIONS COMMONLY USED DURING PROCEDURAL SEDATION/ANALGESIA

The ability of a trainee to titrate sedative/analgesic medications against procedural anxiety and discomfort can be evaluated by written test, interview technique, personal computer-based interactive programs, high-fidelity manikin-based SBT, or actual administration of procedural sedation under the supervision of a more-experienced sedation RN or clinical member of the Anesthesia Department. Tables 14.6 and 14.7 list drugs commonly used to achieve procedural sedation/analgesia and commercially available pharmacologic reversal agents for use in humans.

Apart from the use of traditional test paper- or computer-based testing, a computer-driven manikin or trained standardized patient can be used to simulate responses to medications. In the latter cases, the standard levels of the "continuum of sedation" should be included (Table 14.8).

Simulation-based training can also be used to assess a trainee's ability to recognize and trap system-based

Table 14.5 Equipment/supply setup for procedural sedation/analgesia (SSADMIT)*

System of oxygenation and positive pressure ventilation	Reliable O_2 supply (wall + back-up cylinder) Nasal cannula and O_2 mask Ambu bag
Suction equipment	Oropharyngeal suction (Yankauer) Gastric suction (e.g., 18 Fr Salem sump) Bronchial suction catheter (in case of intubation)
Airway equipment (for RN and in case of emergency conversion to general anesthesia)*	Oral airway and tongue blade Nasal airway Functioning laryngoscope and blades Stylet and Eschmann-type introducer ("bougie") Laryngeal mask airway
Drugs	Sedatives, opioid analgesics, reversal agents, code cart with drugs and defibrillator
Monitors†	Pulse oximeter (with finger and ear probes) ECG Continuous monitor of respiratory adequacy: – Continuous conversation – Pretracheal stethoscope (restricts movement) – Impedance plethysmography through ECG pads (does not detect airway obstruction with continued breath attempts) – Capnography† (recommended in all current guidelines) colorimetric CO_2 detector adequate to confirm tracheal intubation stethoscope – Can be placed on trachea to confirm apnea – For bilateral breath sound check to rule out unilateral bronchial placement of tracheal tube
Infusion	Reliable IV continuously infusing at patient-appropriate rate Easily accessible injection port Saline-filled syringe for flushing reversal drugs
Table, tape, temperature	Stable surface with restraining straps Tape to secure intravenous line, tracheal tube Warming equipment for procedure/patient prone to ↓temperature

* All equipment and supplies must be appropriately sized for the individual patient; patients who may be difficult to intubate require availability of advanced airway equipment of type specified by the team that would be summoned in case of airway emergency (e.g., anesthesiologist); this equipment may include optical laryngoscope, intubating laryngeal mask airway, emergency cricothyroidotomy kit, etc.

† Members of the anesthesia department can help with selection of monitoring equipment, which can vary greatly in quality. The pulse oximeter should be in audible mode (so that audible beep pitch and frequency continuously communicates percentage of hemoglobin saturation). Alarms must have visual and audio indicators turned on to immediately reveal to the observer's eye and ear that the value of some parameter has moved into the danger zone.

latent conditions that could lead to potentially catastrophic events. For example, a scenario could be developed to evaluate the watchfulness of a trainee for look-alike drug vials and ampoules, and the substitution of different drug strengths. (e.g., midazolam marketed in 1 mg/mL and 5 mg/mL strengths; ketamine marketed in 10 mg/mL, 50 mg/mL, and 100 mg/mL strengths.)

Table 14.6 Drugs commonly used during procedural sedation/analgesia

RX (GENERIC NAME)	RX (BRAND NAME)	TYPE	INCREMENTAL BOLUS (ADULT)*	INCREMENTAL BOLUS (CHILD)*	REVERSAL AGENT
Midazolam	Versed	Benzodiazepine	1 mg	15 mcg/kg	Flumazenil
Fentanyl	Sublimaze	Opioid	50 mcg	0.5 mcg/kg	Naloxone
Morphine		Opioid	2 mg	35 mcg/kg	Naloxone
Hydromorphone	Dilaudid	Opioid	0.2 mg	3 mcg/kg	Naloxone
Meperidine	Demerol	Opioid	20 mg	0.3 mg/kg	Naloxone
Ketamine†	Ketalar/Ketacet	Dissociative	25 mg	0.3 mg/kg	None
Propofol‡	Diprivan	Anesthetic	20 mg	0.3 mg/kg	None

* Reasonable starting increment in young, healthy, un-premedicated patient; wait 4 minutes after first dose before concluding absence of or negligible effect; flush drug into vein after each dose to avoid medication accumulation in intravenous tubing; reduce initial incremental dose by half in high-risk patients; provisionally double interdose interval in frail patients and those with known or suspected low cardiac output (who may thus exhibit a prolonged response time); increase incremental dose or shorten interdosing interval only once initially; very cautious experience with an individual patient shows that this is safe; synergism between opiates and benzodiazepine requires extra caution when drugs of both classes are used together (frequently the case).

† Can cause violent hallucinatory panic reaction if not preceded by benzodiazepine or propofol; small risk of respiratory depression when used alone; causes increased airway secretions, perhaps reduced by prior glycopyrrolate administration; easily produces general anesthesia.

‡ Classified by U.S. Food & Drug Administration as an anesthetic drug whose administration requires expertise in anesthesia; easily produces general anesthesia, airway collapse, and apnea; powerful circulatory depressant in compromised patients.[12]

Table 14.7 Pharmacologic agents useful in reversing unwanted effects of sedative/analgesic drugs

RX GENERIC NAME	RX BRAND NAME	INDICATION	INCREMENTAL BOLUS (ADULT)‡	INCREMENTAL BOLUS (CHILD)‡	SIDE EFFECTS
Naloxone*	Narcan	Opioid excess	40–80 mcg	5–10 mcg/kg	Pain, agitation
Flumazenil*	Romazicon	Benzodiazepine excess	0.2 mg	10 mcg/kg	Anxiety, seizure
Ephedrine†		Hypotension + bradycardia	10 mg	0.15 mcg/kg	Tachycardia
Phenylephrine†	Neo-Synephrine	Hypotension + tachycardia	100 mcg	1.5 mcg/kg	Hypertension
Atropine		Bradycardia	0.2 mg	20 mcg/kg	Dry mouth, fever

* Support ventilation (and, if necessary, circulation) while waiting for drug to reach central nervous system; since duration of reversal agent is less than sedation to be reversed, subsequent re-narcotization (with respiratory depression) can occur up to at least an hour after administration (2 hours observation recommended by drug manufacturer).

† Duration only a few minutes

‡ For mildly excessive sedation or respiratory depression, repeat dose × 1–5 at 2–4 minute intervals; multiply initial bolus dose of naloxone or flumazenil by 3–4 if life-threatening respiratory depression is present and positive pressure ventilation is difficult to achieve.

AIRWAY MANAGEMENT DURING INTRAVENOUS SEDATION

Perhaps no other procedural sedation technical skill set has been the focus of such intense development as airway management. Both the sedation nurse (i.e., RN) and radiologist must be competent to perform such basic life-saving airway maneuvers as:

- *Head tilt*: Extending head on neck to tighten the floor of the mouth and pull the tongue forward

Table 14.8 Continuum of sedation and appropriate response.*†

SEDATION DEPTH	SIGN(S)	APPROPRIATE RESPONSE
Minimal sedation	Normal response to voice and touch	Increase sedation dose if needed for patient comfort
Moderate sedation	Purposeful response to voice or touch	Maintain current drug dosing
Deep sedation	Blunted response to repeated or painful stimulation, potential or actual airway or respiratory compromise	Reduce rate of drug administration; focus entirely on patient breathing and circulatory adequacy; prepare to control airway and breathing; if difficulties call for emergency assistance
General anesthesia	Unresponsive to painful stimulation; respiratory and potentially circulatory compromise	Discontinue all central nervous system (CNS) depressant medications, support respiration and circulation as needed; consider reversal agent; consider summoning anesthesiologist or other emergency back-up

* Modified from Continuum of Sedation and Credentialing for Supervision (Table 1)

† The subjective nature of the transitions between these levels of CNS depression has recently been criticized[5] but no superior classification has yet been offered.

- *Jaw thrust*: Using fingers or knuckles to pull the right and left rami of the mandible straight forward from a point just below the ear; this opens the airway and also exerts a very strong painful stimulus to the exquisitely tender mandibular periosteum, often evoking vigorous spontaneous ventilation in the presence of quite deep sedation.
- *Bag-valve-mask ventilation*: Application of an Ambu-type bag-valve-mask to the patient's face to create an airtight seal around the nose and mouth, and squeezing with sufficient volume to just inflate the lungs. Success is demonstrated by the occurrence of forward chest wall movement below the nipple line with positive pressure together with fogging of the clear plastic mask on expiration.
- *Oral or nasal airway insertion*: When attempts at bag-valve-mask ventilation (together with head tilt and jaw thrust) are insufficient to cause chest wall excursion and fogging despite creation of a good mask-to-face seal
- *Laryngeal mask airway insertion*

A practitioner's skills in all these maneuvers can be greatly enhanced by participation in a course on airway management or sedation that incorporates SBT using either a part-task or high-fidelity mannikin. As such courses vary considerably in quality, it will be useful to compare the quality of any contemplated training experience against that provided at a simulation center overseen by faculty of an academic department of anesthesiology or emergency medicine, or accredited by a major national organization such as the American Society of Anesthesiologists or the American College of Surgeons. Technical skill at tracheal intubation can also be improved at such a course, although it is difficult to become truly proficient without extensive practice in patients receiving general anesthesia for elective surgical procedures under the close supervision of a clinical member of the anesthesia department.

INTRAPROCEDURAL PROBLEMS AND INTERVENTIONS

Many important adverse events that occur during the titration of sedative and analgesic drugs to maximize patient safety and comfort can be simulated to enhance training and learning prior to clinical application. If a manikin or, in some cases, a trained standardized patient is used, the ability of the trainee to perform required interventions can be evaluated. Some relatively easy-to-simulate intraprocedural adverse events related to procedural sedation and the technical and nontechnical skills related to effectively managing them are listed in Table 14.9.

Table 14.9 Examples of demonstrations of technical and nontechnical skills at handling simulated intraprocedural critical events

DEMONSTRATION OF ABILITY TO DETECT:
– hypoventilation and hypoxemia signaled by a low pitch in the beep from the pulse oximeter ± loss of capnographic waveform – loss of audible tone of pulse oximeter when distracted by other task – hypotension by noninvasive blood pressure measurement (and attempt to confirm by palpation of pulse amplitude) – disconnection of oxygen line to mask or nasal cannula (as cause of hypoxemia) – agitation/delirium (with risk of patient falling from radiology table) – stopped/blocked intravenous infusion so that administered drugs accumulate in the tubing (only to enter the patient's circulation cumulatively at a later time) – signs of internal hemorrhage (hypotension ± tachycardia) – excessive central nervous system depression NB: If continuous electroencephalographic monitoring of sedation depth (e.g., by Bispectral Index [BIS™]) is available, the ability to identify numeric ranges typically associated with sedation (65–80) versus general anesthesia (40–60).
DEMONSTRATION OF ABILITY TO DISCRIMINATE
– airway obstruction vs. apnea by capnography (both causing loss of normal repetitive square-wave pattern and replacement by straight line at bottom of screen) by noting *presence* or *absence* of attempts to breathe (as indicated by presence of intermittent chest wall motion plus inspiratory indentation of skin overlying the suprasternal notch) – true vs. artifactual respiratory crisis (the former requiring abandonment of all procedural support activity to concentrate on restoration of airway patency and effective breathing) – important ECG abnormalities (e.g., arrhythmia, asystole) vs. common artifacts (patient movement, lead disconnection) – presence of inadequate local anesthesia on the operative field (best treated by suggesting injection of additional local anesthetic solution by the radiologist) vs. anxiety or positional discomfort requiring additional sedation/analgesia
DEMONSTRATION OF THE ABILITY TO ACT EFFECTIVELY BY
– applying progressively more noxious stimulation, airway support, and positive pressure ventilation in response to occurrence of dangerously deep sedation – calling for an increase in room lighting when there is a question of cyanosis – prolonging interval between doses of sedative/analgesic medications in patients with risk factors for delayed response times (due to low cardiac output) until such time that a patient's individual pattern of response to medications has been empirically determined – performing basic airway maneuvers in the correct order – calling for airway/resuscitation back-up after application of available maneuvers has failed to restore oxygenation – responding appropriately to regurgitation (with head turn and oropharyngeal suctioning followed by consideration of Rx reversal if pharmacologically possible)

RECOVERY PERIOD

Unfortunately, the effects of even modern shorter-acting drugs do not disappear at the moment that the radiological procedure ends. Thus, a trainee should maintain a high level of alertness to the possible occurrence of complications related to sedation, even after the completion of a successful diagnostic or therapeutic procedure. In fact, once the CNS-depressive effects of sedative drugs are no longer counterbalanced by procedure-related anxiety or discomfort, a patient who was previously breathing well can become obtunded and even apneic. The timing of such an event can be delayed for up to 1 hour or more if opioid or benzodiazepine drugs have been reversed with naloxone or flumazenil, respectively. Simulation-based training of such a critical event should be included in any training session related to procedural sedation, in order to reinforce the need to continue close observation well after the completion of a procedure.

POST-RECOVERY PATIENT DISPOSITION

As alluded to above, SBT should include scenarios involving any radiology postprocedural inpatient or outpatient observation. Prolonged CNS depression from intravenous sedation/analgesia may be manifested by symptomatic dizziness, unstable ambulation, or patient inability to make logical, reasoned judgments. Delayed procedural complications may develop up to 24 or more hours after the radiological procedure. Unexpectedly prolonged CNS depression from sedation/analgesia may mask early signs of such complications. Ensuring SBT includes such scenarios helps trainees in the quick recognition and management of long-term sedation-related complications.

CONCLUSION

Radiological procedure associated sedation/analgesia can be effectively learned and practiced through the use of SBT techniques focusing on the various aspects of the sedation process (i.e., pre-, intra-, and post-sedation evaluation and management). Growing evidence in the literature suggests that such training may facilitate the consistent, safe use of sedation/analgesia in practice.[6–8]

REFERENCES

1. Kost M. *Moderate Sedation/Analgesia: Core Competencies for Practice*. St. Louis: Saunders/Elsevier; 2004.
2. Odom-Forren J, Watson D. *Practical Guide to Moderate Sedation/Analgesia*, 2nd edition. Mosby; 2005.
3. Malviya S, Naughton NN, Tremper KK, eds. *Sedation and Analgesia for Diagnostic and Therapeutic Procedures*. Totowa NJ: Humana Press; 2003.
4. Urman RD, Kaye AD. *Moderate and Deep Sedation in Clinical Practice*. Cambridge University Press. In press.
5. Green SM, Mason K. Reformulation of the sedation continuum. *JAMA*. 2010;303:876–877.
6. Farnsworth ST, Egan TD, Johnson SE, et al. Teaching sedation and analgesia with simulation. *J Clin Monit Comput*. 2000;16:273–285.
7. Hofmann N, Datz C, Schöchl H. Sedation training using a human patient simulator. *Digestion*. 2010;82:115–117.
8. Shavit I, Keidan I, Hoffmann Y, et al. Enhancing patient safety during pediatric sedation: the impact of simulation-based training of nonanesthesiologists. *Arch Pediatr Adolesc Med*. 2007;161:740–743.
9. Rosenberg DR, Sweeney JA, Gillen JS, et al. Magnetic resonance imaging of children without sedation: preparation with simulation. *J Am Acad Child Adolesc Psychiatry*. 1997;36:853–859.
10. de Amorim e Silva CJ, Mackenzie A, Hallowell LM, et al. Practice MRI: reducing the need for sedation and general anaesthesia in children undergoing MRI. *Australas Radiol*. 2006;50:319–323.
11. Rich JM. Recognition and management of the difficult airway with special emphasis on the intubating LMA-Fastrach/whistle technique: a brief review with case reports. *Proc Bayl Univ Med Cent*. 2005;18:220–227. Accessed December 2, 2011, at http://www.ncbi.nlm.nih.gov/pmc/articles/PMC1200729/
12. Woodcock, J. US Food & Drug Administration letter (Docket No. FDA-2005-P-0059) rejecting request by American College of Gastroenterology to eliminate warning labeling propofol as anesthetic agent to be administered only by practitioners trained in general anesthetic administration.

15

Simulation in Emergency Radiology and Workload Management

LEONARD R. BOK, JOHN T. PAIGE, AND ROBERT S. SITARZ

CURRENT ACCREDITATION Council of Graduate Medical Education (ACGME) guidelines require 12 months of program training before radiology residents can take call in the hospital without direct supervision. This mandate is a reflection of multiple contemporary issues in graduate medical education (GME), including concerns regarding patient safety, the introduction of competency-based residency training by the ACGME, and an increased awareness by medical educators of how the learner learns (i.e., the widespread adoption of the Dreyfus Model of Knowledge Development, delineating six distinct stages in the development of mastery with differing strategies of learning and teaching for each).[1–5] Like many other Residency Review Committees (RRCs) of the ACGME, the radiology RRC has established a somewhat arbitrary chronologic standard (i.e., 12-month minimum) as the threshold for increasing trainee responsibility in a residency.

Such a time-based standard, however, is fast becoming obsolete as the ACGME shifts to an outcomes-based (i.e., competency- or proficiency-based) residency model.[6,7] In fact, it has developed the so-call Milestones Project, in which residents will be expected to attain certain specialty-specific benchmarks or "milestones" within training to ensure that they are becoming adequately prepared to practice independently at the completion of their residency.[8,9] Milestones have already begun to be incorporated into internal medicine,[10] surgery,[11] and pediatric[12] residency training. They are even now being developed for radiology.[13] Full implementation of competency-based standards for milestones, however, will require evaluation and testing.[1,14] Creating this system is a challenging task.[15] So, we ask the question: When is a radiology resident ready for the cases and the workload of the emergency department (ED)? And how do we know that they are ready? Currently, we have a time-based standard; however, the future holds a competence-based standard.

Radiology residency programs have long attempted to answer such questions through formal and informal preparation classes, clinical experiences, and tests designed to prepare the resident for on-call ED duty and/or to determine what preparation was needed to be ready. Thus, it is not surprising that simulation of emergency radiology for both training and testing to assure that radiologists in training are ready and able to perform in this critical role has held the interest of program directors.[16–18] As in the management of contrast reactions, the treatment of life-threatening emergencies, and the application of invasive procedures, emergency call radiology is one of several key areas in radiology with a strong interest in simulation-based training (SBT) and testing.[19–22] All of these areas of radiology involve high-stress and dynamic situations, often requiring quick and accurate responses. In addition, many reflect high-risk, low-frequency events. For example, contrast reactions occur infrequently, but when they do occur, they can be life-threatening. Similarly, in emergency room coverage, high-risk conditions, such as ectopic pregnancy, testicular torsion, and other critical disorders, occur infrequently compared to the overall volume of the imaging presented to the radiologist. In fact, a number of reports on the use of simulation in high-stakes training and testing in these areas are already in the literature.[17–20] Thus, a body of shared simulation experience exists, though, as in other areas of simulation in radiology, it cannot yet rely on any fully validated approach. Thorough validation of these approaches awaits further work. That said, validation work should be done in a determined fashion.[23]

The advantages of simulation in this training and testing for emergency radiology duty seem as obvious as in the arena of aviation, which is typically credited with the origin and validation of the simulation concept. Towbin et al[24] have described a general approach to the simulation of modern picture archiving and communication system (PACS)-based radiology practice that can be tailored to preparation for on-call activity. In order to simulate on-call activity, a case mix was generated to match the difficulty and case mix seen in that institution's emergency radiology department.[25] The residents were shown 71 cases, and normal cases were excluded. Residents subsequently reported a subjective feeling that the simulator was useful.

Traditional methods of preparation and evaluation for emergency radiology call duty have included, but were not limited to, didactic lectures, cases conferences, workstation teaching, and teaching during supervised call ("mini-call"). Often, this teaching was supplemented with some form of test, usually based on a PowerPoint™ presentation with key cases or similar testing method.

Some groups, as mentioned, have tried to move beyond these traditional methods and create more fully elaborated simulated PACS environments and/or simulated emergency room/call situation environments.[25,28] The spectrum of potential simulation and assessment methods is broad. At the simple end, the PACS testing system could be loaded with the 20, 30, or 50 key diagnoses that an emergency radiologist should be able to identify despite some distracters.[28] Such SBT provides focused practice in the recognition of critical conditions encountered on ED radiology call. It does not, however, reflect the busy clinical environment in which such cases present. At the complex end of the spectrum, the ED could be studied for a set time period and the exact set of studies (made anonymous) on an emergency room PACS could be loaded on a simulated PACS. The trainee would then read these "simulated" studies while answering simulated phone calls, contrast questions, and consult requests, distractions that reflect the actual conditions of ED radiology call.[28] This style of SBT has the advantage of mimicking the actual work environment in which the trainee will operate, but it is less effective in providing repetitive, focused practice in recognizing key radiological diagnoses.

Although the approach that a particular institution chooses may depend upon access to computer power and computer support, a stepwise integration of both simple and complex SBT methods is particularly beneficial. Much like pilots train on low-fidelity simulators to learn the basics of flying a particular model aircraft before graduating to the high-fidelity simulator to practice responses to emergency situations, a radiology resident could first learn to recognize the key diagnoses related to emergency radiology on a simulated PACS before entering a simulated ED space to hone workload management skills. In this case, a PowerPoint™ presentation of carefully selected cases with multiple-choice examination would serve as a low-fidelity model with high relevance and impact with regard to key knowledge requirements. Such a model, however, would not assist in training adjustment to the affective experience in the on-call situation. On the contrary, a high-fidelity simulated emergency on-call scenario having many normal plain films and many interruptions would assist in the development of workload management skills related to the "affective" experience, but it would not be efficient or effective in imparting understanding of key knowledge elements.

If certain technical skills (i.e., the ability to perform certain procedures, such as ultrasonography or fluoroscopy) are required in an on-call situation, then SBT and testing of the particular skills in question should also be considered. They are not, however, areas of focus in the current literature related to radiology emergency room resident preparation. Consideration of knowledge, speed, affect, and skill are needed to fully simulate the on-call or emergency radiology experience. It is easier said than done, especially when trying to create an efficient learning environment. Fortunately, various frameworks in developing on-call, emergency radiology, or workflow simulations or simulators exist in the literature, as illustrated by the following examples.

Ganguli et al[19] reported on 5 years of results related to preparing residents for on-call responsibility. This program utilized a 1 month emergency radiology teaching curriculum (i.e., 25 "lectures" of approximately 45 minutes each) that was specifically based upon the American Society of Emergency Radiology (ASER) core curriculum in emergency radiology. The program was primarily focused on teaching and testing. Testing, however, was accomplished not through PowerPoint™ or paper, but through a computer-based testing system that involved "data collection" and "imaging viewing" elements. Approximately 20 selected emergency room cases were loaded onto the system. Residents then typed answers in free text. They were allowed 3.5 hours to complete the cases. Answers were scored based on a 3 point scale (range 0–2).

Ganguli et al[19] have demonstrated that, over 5 years, the participating residents consistently improved each year during their progression through residency. Interestingly, one might ask whether this approach is high on viewing-PACS-reporting fidelity, but, with a limited number of cases, low on case mix fidelity. This approach seems to choose testing of medical knowledge and workstation viewing and reporting skill over testing or training of affective or other procedural skill. This trade-off may be reasonable, especially at the early levels of training that are necessarily more concrete and less environmentally focused. This approach, however, may be less appropriate for higher-level residents who should be moving up the ladder of the Dreyfus Taxonomy[5] and Bloom's Taxonomy.[26]

Weiss et al[27] have provided interesting insight into the planning of a simulation system for ER radiology. They have recognized the parallel between the challenge and responsibility of piloting an aircraft and the challenge and responsibility of taking call in a hospital emergency radiology department, particularly any department with a Level One Trauma Center. Both are high-stakes situations. The sense of responsibility of the radiology resident physician and the supervising faculty preparing the resident to perform competently in this challenging and important environment is great.

Weiss et al[28] have argued that understanding the key use of cases is critical for the development of the simulation. They divided the development process into three parts: (1) preparation and case development, (2) development of a simulated environment, and (3) evaluation and feedback. They have proposed three possible models for SBT that optimize different aspects of simulation.

Model 1 emphasizes medical knowledge focusing on key case and image selection, with preparation of "gold standard" interpretations for later reference. This approach can utilize a clinical type PACS/dictation system but could also utilize a viewer and structured reporting interface. This model may allow greater evaluation of the resident's thought process on provocative cases, but evaluation could be potentially labor-intense for faculty.

Model 2 emphasizes the more realistic simulation of the emergency caseload experience by simply sampling a set of cases presented within a given time slot. Clinical type PACS and dictation are simulated. This type of simulation may eliminate the patient safety issues that arise in the traditional Halstead medical apprenticeship model of residency training,[28] but it will not eliminate the inefficiencies of that method, given its simple method of case selection. Evaluation of the resulting reports would be labor-intensive in the absence of the use of some type of natural language processing system. The simulation, however, would be, in one sense, "high fidelity."

Model 3 emphasizes testing. Key images relevant to the emergency setting are provided on a web page. The learner then must answer questions related to them. This format is low fidelity but provides efficient testing of medical knowledge and allows ease of comparison between residents.

In addition to resident preparation for on-call responsibilities in emergency radiology, simulation could be used as a modeling tool related to workflow and workload management in emergency radiology. Currently, such modeling has been employed to evaluate the emergency room overall[29,30] and the operating room environment.[31,32] For example, Storrow et al[31] have used simulation to investigate the impact of laboratory turnaround times on emergency department throughput and diversion rates.

Additionally, van Oostrum et al[32] have employed a simulation model to help determine the optimal size of the on-call emergency team in the operating room. Clearly, although not currently done, simulation modeling of aspects of emergency radiology workload could provide useful information regarding how to improve workflow and delivery of care. Such modeling holds future promise as a powerful tool for enhancing efficiency and safety in the delivery of care.

CONCLUSION

Computer-based simulation of the emergency radiology environment holds great promise for resident training, deliberate practice, and testing. Program goals and resources will influence how such SBT is structured. The method of integrating the on-call emergency radiology stimulation into the curriculum and verifying its overall validity will be critical. It is also critical that program goals for the curriculum and the simulation be defined. Examples of such incorporation of SBT for resident preparation for on-call duties exist in the literature and can serve as a guide for the development of curricula related to it. Finally, computer modeling of workflow and workload within the emergency radiology setting is a potentially rich source of research for improving both the efficiency and safety of radiologic care in this highly dynamic clinical environment.

REFERENCES

1. Kohn J, Corrigan J, Donaldson, eds. *To Err Is Human: Building a Safer Healthcare System.* Washington DC: National Academy Press; 2000.
2. Batalden P, Leach D, Swing S, et al. General competencies accreditation in graduate medical education: An antidote to overspecification in the education of medical specialists. *Health Affairs.* 2002;21:103–111.
3. Leach D. Changing education to improve patient care. *Qual Health Care.* 2001;10;ii54–ii58.
4. Dreyfus S, Dreyfus H. *A Five-Stage Model of the Mental Activities Involved in Directed Skill Acquisition.* University of California, Berkeley. Operations Research Center ORC 8-2; 1980:1–6.
5. Ericsson KA, Drampe R, Tesch-Romer C. The role of deliberate practice in the acquisition of expert performance. *Psychol Rev.* 1993;100;363–406.
6. Satava RM. The revolution in medical education—the role of simulation. *J Grad Med Educ.* 2009;1:172–175.
7. Accreditation Council for Graduate Medical Education. Outcomes Project. Accessed July 8, 2011, at http://www.ACGME.org
8. Nasca TJ. Where will "milestones" take us? The next accreditation system. *ACGME Bull.* 2008, Sept;3–5.
9. Accreditation Council for Graduate Medical Education. Milestones Project. Accessed July 8, 2011, at http://www.ACGME.org
10. Green M, Aagaard E, Caverzagie K, et al. Charting the road to competence: developmental milestones for internal medicine residency training. *J Grad Med Educ.* 2009 Sept;1:5–20.
11. Bell RH Jr. Overview of the milestones project for surgery. 96th Annual Clinical Congress. American College of Surgeons. 2010. Washington, DC. Accessed April 12, 2011, at http//www.facs.org/education/clinicalcongress2010/presentations/apdspanel/speaker4.pdf
12. Englander R, Hicks P, Benson B; Pediatric Milestone Project Working Group. Pediatrics milestones: a developmental approach to the competencies. *J Pediatr.* 2010;157:521–522, 522.e1.
13. Amis S. Radiology RRC Update Presentation at AUR 59th Annual Meeting, 2011. Boston, MA. Lecture Presentation.
14. Accreditation Council for Graduate Medical Education. Evaluation Toolbox. Accessed July 8, 2011, at http://www.ACGME.org
15. Bucholz E, Duncan J. Assessing system performance. *J Vasc Interv Radiol.* 2008;19:987–994.
16. Ganguli S, Pedrosa I, Yam C-S, et al. Part I: Preparing and assessing first-year radiology resident on-call readiness: *Acad Radiol.* 2006;13:764–769.
17. Yam C-S, Kruskal J, Pedrosa I, et al. Part II: Preparing and assessing first-year radiology resident on-call readiness: technical implementation. *Acad Radiol.* 2006;13:770–773.
18. Ganguli S, Camacho, M, Yam C-S, et al. Preparing first-year radiology residents and assessing their on-call responsibilities: results over five years. *AJR.* 2009;192:539–544.
19. Gaca A, Frush D, Hohenhaus S, et al. Enhancing pediatric safety: using simulation to assess radiology resident preparedness for anaphylaxis from intravenous contrast media. *Radiology.* 2007;245: 236–245.
20. Tofil N, White M, Grant M. Severe contrast reaction emergencies: high-fidelity simulation training for radiology residents and technologists in a children's hospital. *Acad Radiol.* 2010;17:934–940.
21. Dawson S, Cotin S, Meglan D, et al. Designing a computer-based simulator of interventional cardiology training. *Catheter Cardiovasc Interv.* 2000;51:522–527.

22. Patel A, Gould D. Simulators in interventional radiology training and evaluation: a paradigm shift is on the horizon. *J Vasc Interv Radiol.* 2006;17:S163–S173.

23. Ahmed K, Keeling A, Fakhry M, et al. Role of virtual reality simulation in teaching and assessing technical skills in endovascular intervention. *J Vasc Interv Radiol.* 2010;21:55–66.

24. Towbin A, Paterson B, Chang P. Computer-based simulator for radiology: an educational tool. *Radiographics.* 2008;28:309–316.

25. Towbin A, Paterson B, Chang P. A computer-based radiology simulator as a learning tool to help prepare first-year residents for being on call. *Acad Radiol.* 2007;14:1271–1283.

26. Bloom BS. *Taxonomy of Educational Objectives, Handbook I: The Cognitive Domain.* New York: David McKay Co. Inc.; 1956.

27. Weiss F, Safdar N, Vandermeer F, et al. Development of a radiology flight simulator: teaching residents to take the cockpit and fly (safely) on call. AUR 58th Annual Meeting, 2010. San Diego, CA. Scientific Poster Exhibit.

28. Rutkow IM. Moments in surgical history: William Steward Halsted. *Arch Surg.* 2000;135:1478.

29. Kolker A. Process modeling of emergency department patient flow: effect of patient length of stay on ED diversion. *J Med Syst.* 2008;32:389–401.

30. Storrow AB, Zhou C, Gaddis G, et al. Decreasing lab turnaround time improves emergency department throughput and decreases emergency medical services diversion: a simulation model. *Acad Emerg Med.* 2008;15:1130–1135.

31. Van Oostrum JM, Van Houdenhoven M, Vrielink MM. A simulation model for determining the optimal size of emergency teams on call in the operating room at night. *Anesth Analg.* 2008;107:1655–1662.

32. Sobolev BG, Sanchez V, Vasilakis C. Systematic review of the use of computer simulation modeling of patient flow in surgical care. *J Med Syst.* 2011;35:1–16.

16

Simulation in Neuroradiology

HUGH J. ROBERTSON, ROQUE FERREYRO, RICHARD FREMAUX, AND ROBERT DAWSON

RESIDENT AND fellow training in neuroradiology has traditionally been accomplished by the master–apprentice method proposed by Halsted and Flexner.[1,2] In it, progressive skills developed under the supervision of experienced clinicians for a defined time period while trainees worked directly with patients. Specialty accreditation was obtained after the training period through a comprehensive examination system. In recent years, patient referrals for invasive procedures, such as diagnostic cerebral angiography, have decreased markedly, and, as a result, suboptimal numbers of the procedures for the required training experience for residents and fellows in neuroradiology exist. This decrease is partially due to the rapid development of high-resolution computerized tomography angiography (CTA) and magnetic resonance angiography (MRA), procedures now widely accepted by referring physicians for the primary study of trauma, stroke, and cerebral vascular disease screening. In addition, other medical specialties with interest in vascular diseases have diverted some patient referrals for cerebral arteriography from neuroradiology.[3] The Institute of Medicine's 2000 report on largely preventable medical errors resulting in an annual fatality rate exceeding motor vehicle accident fatalities raised widespread public concerns of the effectiveness of medical education and the overall safety in health care.[4] Simulation-based training (SBT), combined with direct patient care, offers the promise of surpassing the traditional "master–apprentice" model of education in medicine.[1] Simulation-based training for medical students in Basic Cardiac Life Support (BCLS), Advanced Cardiac Life Support (ACLS), and lumbar puncture has been shown to be an effective educational method.[5] Successful outcomes have been reported for SBT in surgery, anesthesia, and some other specialties.[6,7] Periodic repetition of SBT has been shown to be necessary for the retention of basic knowledge and to augment acquisition of procedural skills by residents.[5] Simulation-based training for residents provides a basis for directly assessing progressive procedural skill development in a standardized, potentially unbiased environment, without risk of patient injury. Educational and simulation device capabilities must be very carefully planned and developed. A joint task force has been developed by the Society of Interventional Radiology, the Cardiovascular and Interventional Radiological Society of Europe, and the Radiological Society of North America to plan the development and validation of simulation-based techniques and devices in interventional radiology training for residents and fellows.[8] The Joint Task Force defined from the beginning 1-, 3-, 5-, and 10-year plans for the development of training standards, methods of education, simulator research and development and public awareness. Procedure-based medical specialties in the future may combine low- and high-fidelity simulation as resident training progresses and skills develop. When strict validation of SBT and appropriate simulation devices is proven, it is expected that SBT may be used to document technical proficiency for professional credentialing and recertification examinations in radiology and other procedure-based specialties.[1,3,9] A core knowledge base is expected to be acquired with SBT technical skills training. The addition of SBT to medical specialty training is expected to provide an outcomes model of proficiency, with documentation of core competencies.[1] Improved technical skills and fewer errors or complications are anticipated for SBT compared with traditional master–apprentice training.

SIMULATION AND A METHODOLOGY FOR RESIDENT TRAINING IN SELECTED INTERVENTIONAL PROCEDURES IN NEURORADIOLOGY

The SBT methodology is similar for each procedure discussed. Selected reading references are provided before the SBT, so that trainees will have some preliminary knowledge of the procedure to be discussed. The SBT begins with a didactic lecture presented by an experienced expert-level physician, directly, by video or DVD. The lecture includes the basic steps in the performance of the procedure and a detailed discussion of potential risks and complications of the procedure. This lesson is followed by a written pre-test consisting of 20 multiple-choice questions on the specific procedure. A description of the use of the simulation device(s) is given. The trainee then performs a number of simulations (e.g., three to five) as time and the resident group size permit, observed by an experienced expert-level physician proctor. The time for each simulation procedure completion, radiation dose, amount of contrast used, and number of errors are noted. In addition, procedure proficiencies are graded on a standard 5-point scale by the proctor. Metrics provided by a high-fidelity simulation device are recorded. A detailed log of each simulation performance is entered into a permanent log book. A complete log book entry is done for each trainee for the initial and subsequent simulation sessions, for each interventional procedure. After the simulation performance is completed, each resident has a written post-test of the same 20 questions in different order from the questions of the pre-test. Pre- and post-tests in subsequent SBT for the same procedure include the questions of the first tests in different order. Residents may return to the simulation laboratory by appointment to practice on the simulation device. Repeating complete SBT sessions with recorded and logged simulation and test results after a 6-week or longer interval enhances the learning and procedural skills process. Comparison of individual trainee test and simulation results over time provides evidence of knowledge and procedural skills acquisition and improvement. Each simulation session is concluded with a direct, personal, private discussion between the trainee and the physician proctor. Trainee questions are answered, and informative feedback is offered by the proctor on noteworthy errors that occurred during the SBT. The trainee's opinion is requested on the quality of the learning experience in the SBT.

Cerebral Vascular and Spine Procedural Simulation-Based Training

Currently available endovascular simulation devices are considered by the Joint Task Force to have merit, but no device has, as yet, computer-incorporated metrics that will allow validation for incorporation of the device into a regular resident training curriculum for credit for procedure training. Validation by the criteria of the Joint Task Force may allow a device to be considered for credible training curriculum use and as a subsequent component for certification of procedural proficiency.[1,3,8] Partial haptics (i.e., the touch and feel sensation experienced by the operator) are included in some endovascular simulation devices. In-depth catheter manipulation experience is currently lacking in available endovascular simulation devices,[3,10] but ongoing academic and commercial research will help to correct these deficiencies. Improved procedural performance after simulation based-endovascular, ultrasound, and team-based training has been noted in the medical literature.[11–14]

Detailed knowledge in the steps of any given procedure is necessary and should be covered in the didactic teaching given before the commencement of SBT. Samples of interventional procedure topics that should be covered follow.

Cerebral Arteriography

Here we review vascular catheterization using the Seldinger technique. Commonly used catheter types for aortic arch, selective carotid and vertebral arteriography, and superselective microcatheters and guidewires are demonstrated to the trainee(s). The principles of safe endovascular catheter use are emphasized. These include:

- A small-diameter catheter is used whenever possible. 5 French catheters are commonly used in cerebral arteriography.
- The catheter is always preceded by a flexible tip guidewire from the insertion of the catheter into the artery until the completion of all necessary selective artery catheterization. Failure to do so can result in artery wall dissection by the catheter tip. If any resistance is encountered to the passage of the guidewire, the operator must stop the advance of the wire and catheter. Contrast medium injection through the catheter is then necessary to detect or prevent dissection of the delicate endothelium of the vessel wall and to demonstrate any area of preexisting vessel wall stenosis. Use of a different flexible tip guidewire will sometimes permit the wire and catheter to pass safely beyond a stenosis.
- The catheter must be flushed at least every 2 minutes with heparinized saline flush solution (2,000–5,000 units of heparin/liter of 0.5% normal saline solution).
- The guidewire should not be cleaned with a cotton sponge since cotton fiber embolization has been demonstrated in the cerebral microcirculation. Moistened Telfa™ pads are considered safe to use to wipe down the wire.
- A guidewire that develops deformity, angulation, and/or crepitus in the deformity is fractured and must be discarded to avoid a loose intravascular wire fragment. Teflon and hydrophilic guidewire coatings are rarely a source of particle embolization to intracranial vessels. Careful, limited use of coated guidewires is recommended.
- Free flow in the catheter must always be present before any contrast medium is injected. Dissection of the vessel wall can occur if the catheter tip is occluded by contact with the vessel endothelium. A 1–2 cc test injection of contrast before a pressure or manual angiogram injection will reduce the risk of vessel wall dissection.
- A pigtail aortic arch catheter tip must be placed at least 6 cm above the aortic valve. The pigtail curve may open up with pressure injection and, if near the aortic valve, could engage a coronary artery. A large contrast volume pressure injection into a coronary artery could have disastrous consequence. A manual injection of 5 cc of contrast medium to verify the position of the pigtail catheter tip relative to the aortic valve is recommended before an aortic arch pressure injection of contrast medium.

Lumbar Puncture

A recent computed tomography (CT) brain scan is required for review by the radiologist before lumbar puncture in any patient with coincident intracranial disease, possible raised intracranial pressure, or known intracranial mass lesion to avoid risk of cerebellar tonsillar herniation with abrupt death. Lumbar subarachnoid space needle puncture is required for myelography. A diagnostic lumbar puncture with fluoroscopic guidance may be requested by a clinical service for difficult puncture in patients with scoliosis, severe obesity, or spinal canal stenosis to obtain spinal fluid specimens for laboratory study and/or spinal fluid pressure measurement. Lumbar puncture is usually not done above the L2–L3 level to avoid injury to the cauda equina and conus medullaris. A 22-gauge spinal needle is usually provided with commercial lumbar puncture tray kits. The use of larger needles increases the risk of persistent spinal fluid leak at the puncture site. A 10–15 degree bend applied to the needle tip will allow accurate needle tip placement in the center of the spinal canal with fluoroscopic guidance. An off-center, slightly oblique needle approach will allow the operator to steer the needle tip around bone obstacles to the center of the spinal canal. Lumbar spine scoliosis is corrected by positioning the patient before attempting lumbar puncture. Pads or wedge sponges are placed under the hip and iliac crest until the vertebral spinous process is midway between the pedicles at the selected puncture site on fluoroscopy. A regular direct lumbar puncture is then done. Commercial lumbar puncture simulation devices are useful for medical student and novice resident practice before attempting lumbar puncture on a patient.

Lateral C1–C2 Puncture

Magnetic resonance imaging (MRI) brain and upper cervical spine scan is recommended before lateral C1–C2 puncture, particularly to exclude preexisting Chiari 1 malformation or other causes of tonsillar herniation at the foramen magnum. A lateral needle puncture at the junction of the posterior and middle one-third of the bony spinal canal at C1–C2 level is sometimes necessary for diagnostic spinal fluid collection or myelography, when lumbar puncture is not possible. The procedure can be done with C-arm fluoroscopy, with the patient supine, or alternatively, by using a horizontal fluoroscopy unit, with the patient in a lateral decubitus position and the head raised by padding until precisely parallel to the X-ray table top. The head must be facing directly forward and must not move during the procedure. A straight 22-gauge spinal needle is usually used. It may be difficult to detect spinal fluid with a smaller needle. The needle is carefully passed up to but not beyond the lateral margin of the bony spinal canal. Differing tissue resistance (i.e., adipose tissue, muscle, and fascia) is felt by the operator during needle passage. The needle passes safely posterior to the internal carotid artery. Rarely, a tortuous vertebral artery or an anomalous position of a posterior inferior cerebellar artery may be directly in the path of the needle. Puncture of either artery could result in a fatal outcome since neither artery is accessible for direct pressure to control bleeding.[15] Large epidural veins are present at the C1–C2 level, and puncture of a vein occurs frequently. It serves as a landmark for the dura. Careful further advancement of the needle up to 2 mm will reach the dura. The needle should be sharp since it can displace the dura medially before entering the subarachnoid space.[16] A very controlled needle jab will pierce the dura. When the needle passes through the dura, it is very near the spinal cord lateral margin. The needle stylet is removed. Clear spinal fluid will appear in the hub of the needle spontaneously or with gentle aspiration. Occasionally, careful needle rotation will result in cerebral spinal fluid (CSF) flow, but the needle should not be advanced further because of risk of spinal cord injury. If contrast medium is to be injected, a preliminary small contrast injection is done carefully. If the contrast persists at the needle tip, it could be in the spinal cord. No more contrast is injected, and the procedure is terminated. Only free flow of the contrast medium test injection in the spinal fluid will allow further injection of contrast medium for CT myelogram.

MRI T2 myelogram effect may sometimes obviate the need for a myelogram by lateral C1–C2 puncture. Intravenous injection of contrast medium combined with MRI T2 myelogram with coronal, sagittal, and axial images can be very useful diagnostically in the case of spinal cord compression by neoplasm. The upper, lower, and peripheral tumor margins are delineated in the contrast enhancing tumor.

Cisternal Puncture

An MRI scan of the brain and upper cervical spine is suggested to exclude cerebellar tonsillar herniation before attempting the puncture. A cisterna magna puncture is very seldom necessary. It was previously done when lumbar puncture was not possible but was later supplanted by lateral C1–C2 puncture. The procedure is done with the patient in the sitting position, with the head slightly flexed on the neck. Hair is shaved from the occipital protuberance to the mid cervical level. An aseptic technique is used. The skin and deeper tissues down to the lower margin of the occipital bone (i.e., the opisthion) are infiltrated with 1% lidocaine local anesthetic solution. A 22-gauge straight spinal needle is inserted in the occipital midline below the external occipital protuberance and angled upward slightly. The needle tip is "walked" off the edge of the occipital bone and slowly advanced with gentle needle aspiration until clear spinal fluid is obtained. Samples of spinal fluid for diagnostic laboratory study are carefully obtained, or contrast medium is slowly injected for myelogram. Cisternal puncture was safely done with CT guidance in a patient with a previous MRA brain scan that demonstrated a posterior inferior cerebellar artery centrally in the cistern a magna, directly in the potential needle path.[17] CTA or MRA brain scan prior to lateral C1–C2 or cisternal puncture could possibly show aberrant position of a vertebral artery or posterior inferior cerebellar artery in the potential needle path and thereby avoid puncture of the artery (Figure 16.1).

SPINAL BIOPSY AND ASPIRATION/DRAINAGE PROCEDURES

The trainee should have a preliminary detailed knowledge of the skeletal, neural, and vascular anatomy of the spine before beginning spine SBT and interventional

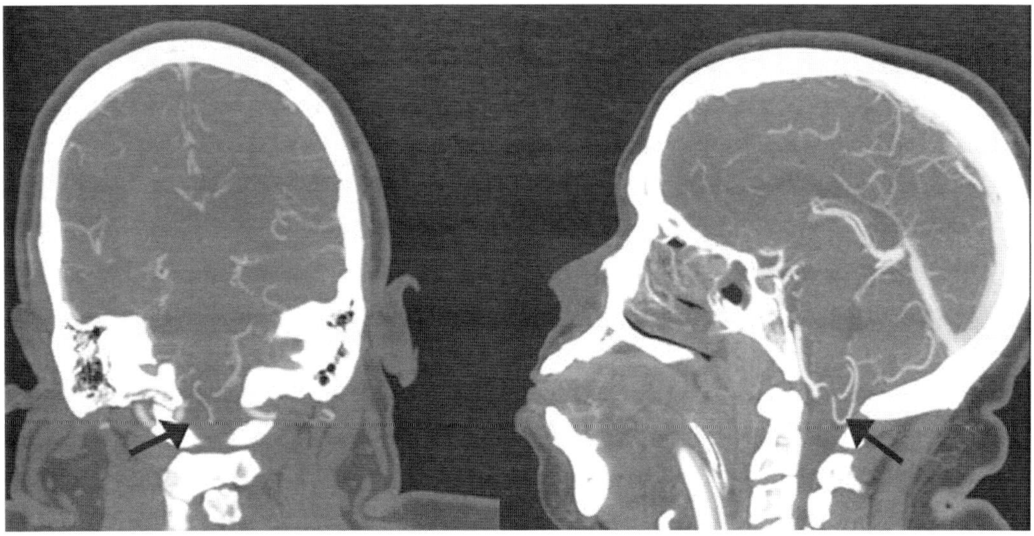

FIGURE 16.1 Computed tomography angiography (CTA). Posterior inferior cerebellar artery (*arrows*) extending below the foramen magnum centrally with risk of needle injury of the artery on cisternal puncture.

procedures. The anatomy along the projected track for biopsy should be clearly defined down to and beyond the biopsy target site.[18] The types and designs of needles and all other equipment to be used, components of a biopsy kit, and the technical skill of needle guidance to the target site are demonstrated to and studied by the trainee before the simulated procedure. Aseptic technique, including surgical scrub, sterile gown, cap, mask, and gloves, is reviewed with the trainee. Each trainee should use a full aseptic technique at least once in a simulated procedure. Prior to a patient procedure, the chart, medical history, laboratory studies, and diagnostic radiologic studies are reviewed. The procedure request is reviewed for appropriateness. All of these requisite points can be included in an SBT procedure. The C-arm fluoroscopy unit or CT scan techniques to be used in the simulated study and the expected radiation dose to the simulated patient are reviewed with the trainee.

Simulation-based training of spinal procedures is done in the simulation anatomical laboratory using a fresh, unembalmed cadaver, which provides the operator with a haptic sense of different tissue layers. Alternatively, an animal spine, such as a pig torso can be used. The simulation procedure is demonstrated and performed precisely as it would be in a patient.

Paraspinal Biopsy

The resident should have a complete preprocedure checklist noting all steps required for the procedure. Before the simulated procedure begins, a discussion is held with the trainee on the need for moderate sedation or deep, monitored sedation provided by anesthesiologist. Post-procedure recovery and patient follow-up are discussed. A decision is made on the possible required presence of a cytologist or pathologist for the procedure. Both anesthesia and pathology presence, if necessary, must be scheduled in advance of a real-life procedure. Bacteriology specimen containers and tubes for cultures are displayed and reviewed with the resident. The absolute requirement to obtain laboratory follow-up and review of histopathology, cytology, and bacteriological reports on the specimens obtained is discussed as an important progressive learning method. A sterile aseptic technique is planned and discussed with the resident. The skin entry site, needle angulation, and the anatomy along the needle track are discussed with the resident before the procedure is begun. Paraspinal biopsy-aspiration procedures are usually required for infection or neoplasm. The subarachnoid space, nerve roots, dorsal root ganglia, and spinal nerves must be avoided during needle passage.

A common approach for lumbar disc biopsy is the oblique dorsal transmuscular approach. A sample of the adjacent vertebral endplates should be obtained, in addition to disk specimens.[19] Spot radiograph or CT scan section documentation of the biopsy site is necessary. Under supervision, the resident performs the SBT paraspinal biopsy on the cadaver. Multiple needle passes to the target site are encouraged for each trainee. Once the skill is acquired by the trainee, individual practice is recommended.

SUGGESTED SIMULATION-BASED PROCEDURES FOR SPINAL BIOPSIES

Several types of spinal biopsies are amenable to SBT. They include:

- Oblique parasagittal intervertebral disc biopsy
- Oblique disc aspiration and disc and endplate biopsy
- Paraspinal periosteum/muscle biopsy
- Transpedicular lumbar vertebral body bone biopsy
- Transpedicular thoracic vertebral bone biopsy

The thoracic and cervical spine anatomy is more complex and compact, rendering needle placement and biopsy of bone or paraspinal tissues more hazardous than for the lumbar spine. Needle penetration control is carefully practiced with all techniques to avoid injury to tissues outside the target area.

Pigtail catheter drainage of paraspinal muscular or subperiosteal abscess is demonstrated, and the drainage kit components are reviewed with the resident. For suspected infection, aspirated laboratory specimens should be submitted from at least three areas of the lesion. Tissue samples are obtained for histopathological study since necrotic tumor may resemble abscess on some imaging studies. Tissue samples are also obtained from the lesion periphery.

Vertebral Bone Biopsy

Biopsy is by transpedicular or oblique lateral direct vertebral body biopsy. Careful needle control is necessary to prevent injury to adjacent tissues. C-arm radiographic spot film or CT axial images should be obtained to document the biopsy site.[20]

Percutaneous Vertebroplasty

Percutaneous vertebroplasty is an interventional procedure consisting of the injection of bone cement—polymethylmethacrylate (PMMA) into the vertebral body bone marrow through a bone needle by transpedicular or oblique vertebral body approach. The procedure was developed in France, in 1984, for the treatment of aggressive vertebral hemangiomas. Use of the procedure increased to include osteoporotic painful vertebral fractures and vertebral compression from trauma, metastatic neoplasm, and lymphoma. The procedure is indicated in the treatment of vertebral disease with severe, incapacitating pain that is unresponsive to conservative treatment.[18,21] The procedure is performed with biplane fluoroscopy or with C-arm fluoroscopic equipment with high-quality image resolution. Thoracic and lumbar vertebroplasty are performed with the patient in prone position, using a transpedicular or oblique vertebral body approach. Cervical vertebroplasty is performed with the patient in supine position, through an anterolateral vertebral body approach (Figure 16.2).

Preprocedural vertebral and adjacent soft tissue anatomy must be thoroughly reviewed at some time before the procedure. A CT scan of the procedure region is reviewed. Vertebral anatomic variations and pedicle shape, size, and angle relative to the vertebral body are studied. These anatomic characteristics will influence the decision to perform a transpedicular or oblique vertebral body approach, the needle size, needle entry site, and needle approach angle. Patients referred for vertebroplasty are often 60 years of age or older, with age-related osteoporosis and vertebral degenerative changes (i.e., hypertrophic bone and osteophyte formations, vertebral body deformities, scoliosis, previous vertebral compression fractures, and zygapophyseal joint degenerative arthritic changes). In these patients, the morphology, size, and orientation of the pedicles may be difficult to assess even with high-quality fluoroscopic equipment. Complete study of the patient's chart, examination of the patient, review of radiologic studies, and planning of the procedure may require as much or even more time than the actual patient procedure.

Needle Positioning and Simulation

Simulation in vertebroplasty has been done with whole-animal or torso (e.g., pig), isolated spine specimen, physical constructed models, and cadaver.[22] The use of a fresh, unembalmed cadaver allows the trainee to experience the feel of needle placement in passage through lumbar muscle and fascia and the distinctive bone resistance. Once the needle enters the bone, very limited opportunity is available to modify its direction. Vertebroplasty is best practiced first in lumbar vertebrae, which are larger and have larger pedicles than do thoracic and cervical vertebrae. The trainee's spatial and depth perception

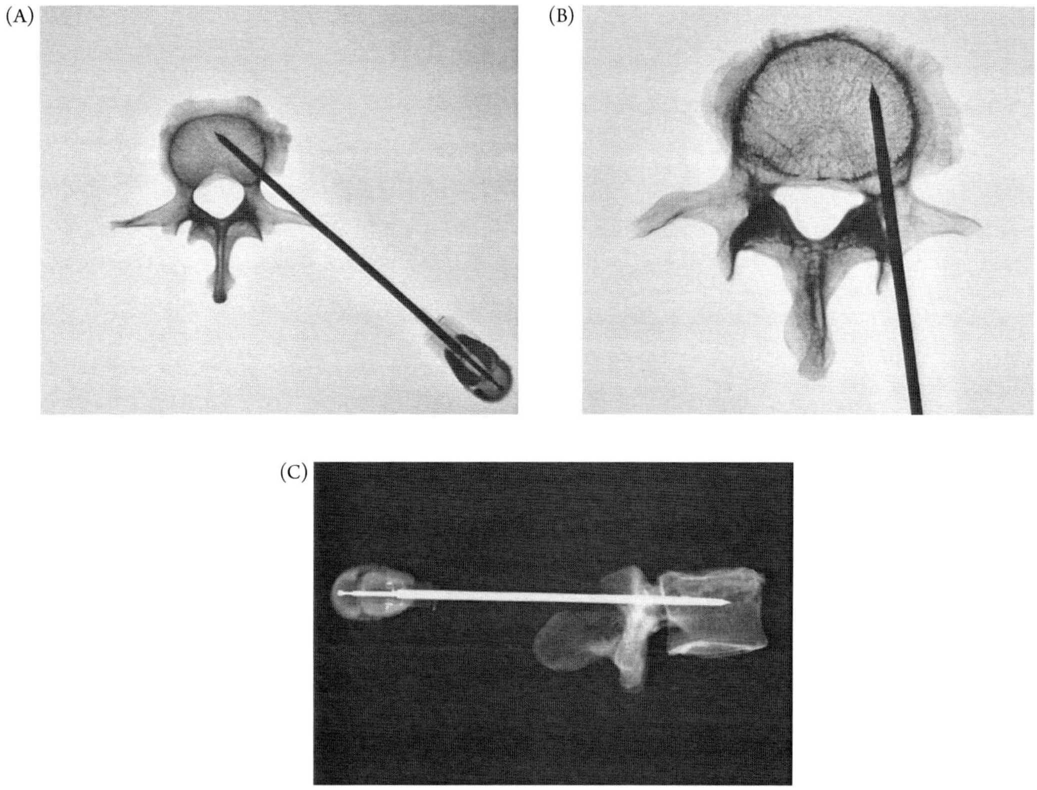

FIGURE 16.2 Vertebral body biopsy. (A) Oblique approach. (B and C) Transpedicular approach

is developed by repeated observation of anatomical spine specimens, spine models, and radiographic images. Pedicle alignment with the vertebral body should allow direction of the bone needle into the central vertebral bone marrow without risk of perforation of the medial or lateral cortex of the pedicle or the vertebral body cortex. Biplane and oblique imaging may be necessary to ensure correct direct needle passage through the pedicle into the desired bone marrow position.

Transpedicular Needle Placement

Patient preparation, positioning, sedation, and analgesia or anesthesia, and other procedure details precede the needle placement. With the patient in prone position, true anteroposterior (AP) and lateral baseline images are obtained. The superior and anterior vertebral endplates should be in the same plane. In the AP view, the spinous process should be in the midline, equidistant between the two pedicles. Occasionally, the spinous process may be angled slightly to one side, and this fact is considered in positioning the patient. In the lateral radiographic view, the vertebral posterior wall and pedicles should be aligned. The bilateral pedicle angles relative to the vertebral body are noted. The C-arm fluoroscopic unit arm is moved cephalad parallel to the pedicles, so that the pedicles in the AP view are projected in the middle to upper third of the vertebral body. The C-arm is then rotated obliquely to project the spinous process near the opposite pedicle. Correction is made for any spinous process intrinsic deformity. The pedicle medial border must be distinct and clear. Excessive C-arm rotation can reduce clarity of the pedicle medial margin and should be corrected. Clear, high-quality radiologic images are necessary for safely performing the procedure. The operator must take adequate time to fully assess the needle approach. The skin entry site is then marked over the pedicle in the superolateral quadrant adjacent to the center of the pedicle. The skin and superficial tissues and tissues down to the periosteum are infiltrated with 1% lidocaine local anesthetic solution. A skin incision is made to allow the entrance of a 13- or 11-gauge bone biopsy needle. The needle is advanced to the pedicle, and the needle tip is anchored in the cortical bone. Rotating the needle bevel may help to anchor the needle in cortical bone in the case of roughened or sloping bone margins. When the needle is in proper position, it is advanced with gentle bone hammer taps. AP and lateral fluoroscopy is used to frequently check the needle position as it is advanced. The needle must not break through the medial wall of the pedicle. The needle is advanced more rapidly when the tip is beyond the posterior vertebral margin. The final needle tip position is at the junction of the anterior and middle thirds of the vertebral marrow cavity. A second bone biopsy needle is often then placed in the opposite pedicle, with needle tip position in the vertebral bone marrow similar to the first needle.

Injection of PMMA Cement

Bone cement is a high-viscosity fluid resulting from mixing the copolymer powder PMMA with a monomer solvent, methylmethacrylate. Mixing and handling of the cement is difficult and requires practice in vitro by all operators, novice or experienced, before use in a vertebroplasty procedure. The cement vendor provides detailed product instructions. With mixing, an exothermic polymerization reaction begins, and the fluid viscosity thickens. Depending on the chemical characteristics of a particular mixture and extrinsic factors such as room temperature, the viscosity of the cement in 3–7 minutes will be too viscous to inject through the needle. The polymerization time for the cement used must be known, so that the PMMA will flow well through the needle and can be safely injected into the bone marrow. Manual cement injection can be done using 1 cc syringes filled to one-half to two-thirds capacity. The total volume injected through each transpedicular needle varies from 3 to 9 cc. This requires multiple syringes, with cement optimally prepared for each. Injection by mechanical or hydraulic injector is used with a larger capacity syringe.

The commonest complication of vertebroplasty is cement leak outside of the vertebral body through cortical bone defects or intravenous leak to epidural and paravertebral veins. A PMMA pulmonary embolism is a rare but known complication.[23] Cement injection is made under fluoroscopic control. The injection is stopped if cement leak into veins is noted. Intradural cement leak and post-vertebroplasty epidural hemorrhage are rare severe complications.[24,25]

Vertebroplasty is ideal for SBT. The trainee can learn all aspects of this technically difficult procedure before attempting the procedure in a patient.

INTERVENTIONAL NEURORADIOLOGY SIMULATION-BASED PROCEDURES

Computer software developments in endovascular simulation devices allow a variety of realistic appearing interventional procedures to be performed and recorded. Common carotid artery, cervical internal carotid artery stent placement. and intracranial arterial microstent procedures are possible with simulated guide catheter, micro guidewire and microcatheters. Aneurysm coiling simulation is possible. Custom clinical scenarios for SBT can be created using advanced software techniques, and simulation of clot removal devices in acute stroke treatment is possible. A review of an individual patient's actual imaging studies and subsequent procedure simulation is possible for planning purposes before the actual patient procedure is done.

CONCLUSION

Simulation-based training in neuroradiology is needed, necessary, and is now possible. SBT is particularly necessary in resident training, and even for review by qualified radiologists in high-risk interventional procedures and newly developed procedures. Verification of the validity of the metrics provided by computer-assisted high-fidelity simulation devices is necessary before consideration can be given for the use of such devices for accreditation of procedural skills. A standard methodology was described in this chapter for SBT in selected neuroradiology interventional procedures from which some metrics can be obtained over a period of time for the assessment of trainee development of knowledge and technical procedural skills. The combined experience of many teaching centers can assist in determining the durable, persisting benefits of SBT to medical education and interventional procedure safety for patients.

SIMULATION VIDEOS

Cerebral vascular and spine diagnostic and interventional simulation videos can be accessed at http://www.medschool.lsuhsc.edu/radiology/

REFERENCES

1. Desser TS. Simulation-based training: the next revolution in radiology education? *J Am Coll Radiol.* 2007;4:816–824.

2. Dutta S, Krummel TM. Simulation: a new frontier in surgical education. *Adv Surg.* 2006;40: 249–263.

3. Gould DA, Kessel DO, Healey AE, et al. Simulators in catheter-based interventional radiology: training or computer games? *Clin Radiol.* 2006;61:556–561.

4. Kohn JT, Corrigan JM, Donaldson MS, eds. *To Err Is Human: Building a Safer Healthcare System.* Washington, DC: Institute of Medicine/National Academy Press,1999.

5. Chamberlain D, Smith A, Woollard M, et al. Trials of teaching methods in basic life support:comparison of simulated CPR performance after first training and at 6 months, with a note on the value of re-training. *Resuscitation.* 2002;53: 179–187.

6. Gould DA, Reekers JA. Editorial. The role of simulation in training endovascular interventions. *Eur J Vasc Endovasc Surg.* 2008;35:633–636.

7. Gould DA, Reekers MD, Kessel, et al. Simulation devices in interventional radiology: validation pending. *J Vasc Interv Radiol.* 2009;20:S324-S325.

8. Gould DA, Patel A, Becker G, et al. SIR/ RSNA/CIRSE joint medical simulation task force strategic plan executive summary. *J Vasc Interv Radiol.* 2009;20:S284–S286.

9. Patel A, Glaiberman C, Gould DA. Procedural simulation. *Anesthesiol Clin.* 2007;25:349–359.

10. Gould DA. Invited Commentary. Training on simulators: limitations and relevance. *Eur J Vasc Endovasc Surg.* 2007;33:533–535.

11. Tubbs RJ, Murphy B, Mainiero MB, et al. High-fidelity medical simulation as an assessment tool for radiology residents' acute contrast reaction management skills. *J Am Coll Radiol.* 2009;6:582–587.

12. Mendiratta-Lala M, Williams T, de Quadros N, et al. The use of a simulation center to improve resident proficiency in performing ultrasound-guided procedures. *Acad Radiol.* 2010;17:535–540.

13. Aggarwal R, Black SA, Hance JR, et al. Virtual reality simulation training can improve inexperienced surgeons' endovascular skills. *Eur J Vasc Endovasc Surg.* 2006;31:588–593.

14. Glaiberman CB, Jacobs B, Street M, et al. Simulation in training: one-year experience using an efficiency index to assess interventional radiology fellow training status. *J Vasc Interv Radiol.* 2008;19:1366–1371.

15. Robertson HJ, Smith RD. Cervical myelography: survey of modes of practice and major complications. *Radiology.* 1990;174:79–83.

16. Orrison WW, Eldevik OP, Sackett JF. Lateral C1-2 puncture for cervical myelography. III. Historical, anatomic, and technical considerations. *Radiology.* 1983;146:401–408.

17. Pomerantz SR, Buchbinder B, Hirsch JA. Suboccipital puncture of the cisterna magna. CT guidance with intravenous enhancement to circumvent anomalous course of posterior cerebellar artery (PICA). American Society of Spine Radiology. Blog archive. Accessed August 25, 2009.

18. Fenton DS, Czervionke LF. *Image Guided Spine Intervention.* New York: Saunders (Elsevier)/Mayo Foundation; 2003.

19. Lis E, Bilsky MH, Pisinski L, et al. Percutaneous CT-guided biopsy of osseous lesion of the spine in patients with known or suspected malignancy. *AJNR Am J Neuroradiol.* 2004;25:1583–1588.

20. Pierot L, Boulin A. Percutaneous biopsy of the thoracic and lumbar spine: transpedicular approach under fluoroscopic guidance. *AJNR Am J Neuroradiol.* 1999;20:23–25.

21. Jensen M. Position statement on percutaneous vertebral augmentation: a consensus statement developed by the American Society of Interventional and Therapeutic Neuroradiology, Society of Interventional Radiology, American Association of Neurological Surgeons, and American Society of Spine Radiology. *J Vasc Interv Radiol.* 2009;20:S326-S331.

22. Abdala N, Abdala R, Da Costa J, et al. Manikin-type training simulator model for transpedicular puncture in percutaneous vertebroplasty. *Radiol Bras.* 2007;40:231–234

23. Kim Y, Lee JW, Park KW, et al. Pulmonary cement embolism after percutaneous vertebroplasty in osteoporotic vertebral compression fractures: incidence, characteristics, and risk factors. *Radiology.* 2009;251:250–259.

24. Chen Y, Tan TS, Chen WH, et al. Intradural cement leakage: a devastatingly rare complication of vertebroplasty. *Spine.* 2006;31:E379-E382.

25. Birkenmaier C, Seitz S, Wegener B, et al. Acute paraplegia after vertebroplasty caused by epidural hemorrhage. *JBJS.* 2007;89:1827–1831.

17

Simulation in Spinal Pain Management

ALAN D. KAYE, VALERIY KOZMENKO, AND BRAD J. HYMEL

MEDICAL SIMULATION-BASED training (SBT) is extensively used in academia and patient care today. Originally, anesthesiology was the principal field of medicine in which simulation was used, and the effectiveness of using simulation as a teaching tool resulted in an increased interest among other medical specialties in this unique interactive method of teaching and learning. In 2003, the Louisiana State University Health Sciences Center in New Orleans (LSUHSC-NO) pioneered a required SBT course for undergraduate medical student education.[1] In 2010, our institution developed an innovative method of teaching basic principles of pain medicine using a hybrid mixed-reality simulation.

Treatment modalities for pain in modern practice may be categorized into pharmacotherapy (most commonly used), psychological support, physical rehabilitation, and interventional procedures, including nerve root and spine facet joint injections. Effective SBT should provide education and experience in all aspects of pain management, and a multidisciplinary approach is recommended to investigate all possible options for optimal pain management.

At present, no simulator exists that will allow SBT in all aspects of chronic pain patient care. Management of a patient with chronic pain typically includes taking the patient's history, performing a thorough physical and neurological examination, and obtaining appropriate imaging and laboratory studies. The ramifications of chronic pain are multiple and include impaired patient activities of daily living, difficulty with ambulation, and depression. Chronic pain places significant strain on the health care economy.[2] Pain may also be related to complications of patient deconditioning, compensatory gait abnormalities, accidents, polypharmacy, and cognitive decline. Studies have shown that the prevalence of persistent pain increases with age.[3] Specifically, increases in joint pain and neuralgias are particularly common as one ages.[4] Complicating the problem, a majority of persons have significant pain problems and are undertreated.

It is clear that the treatment of pain begins with a detailed assessment of the origin of the pain, how the pain can be ameliorated, and the management modalities that are most effective for a particular patient. Such assessment is rarely simple, and current SBT is lacking in this aspect. Clinical manifestations of persistent pain are often complex and multifactorial in most populations. In addition, the perception of pain may differ among age groups and even in different cultures. Issues of physical accessibility to treatment, cost of drugs, the presence of coexisting illness, the use of concomitant medication, and the ability to understand the complaints of the patient are among factors that contribute to the complexity of pain management. The preliminary comprehensive pain assessment has multiple components, including a thorough medical history and physical examination with a review of systems, pertinent laboratory tests, imaging studies, and other diagnostic tests, all of which are eminently suitable for a training simulation model. Noting the temporal relationships of causative events and medical interventions can assist in pain diagnosis and sometimes in prognosis. In particular, the intensity, characteristics, frequency, location, and duration of the pain should be sought. Those factors that relieve or exacerbate the pain help to reveal the nature and origin of the pain. Subsequently, the medication history should be reviewed, including the use of over-the-counter herbal supplementation. A list of all adverse drug effects is obtained. The physical examination should focus on the neuromuscular system, with attention paid to impairments, weakness, hyper- or hypoalgesia, hyperpathia, allodynia, and focal or more generalized numbness and tingling. There may be pain trigger points, bony deformities, or local inflammation at sites that may suggest certain pathologies. With certainty, SBT has and will have the capacity to elucidate many of the features of pain assessment in the education of our health care trainees, including medical students, residents, and fellows.

Simulation-Based Techniques for Taking a Patient History

Multiple studies show that avatar-based simulations are highly effective in teaching decision-making and interpersonal communication skills in medicine, the military, business, negotiation, and other areas.[5–9] At LSUHSC-NO, an innovative avatar-based method of simulation for patient clinical history assessment has been developed and successfully utilized. The method is directly applicable to teaching the acquisition of history taking skills in patients with chronic pain. The software has a user-friendly interface with a three-dimensional (3-D) animated virtual patient that can answer the trainees' questions directly.

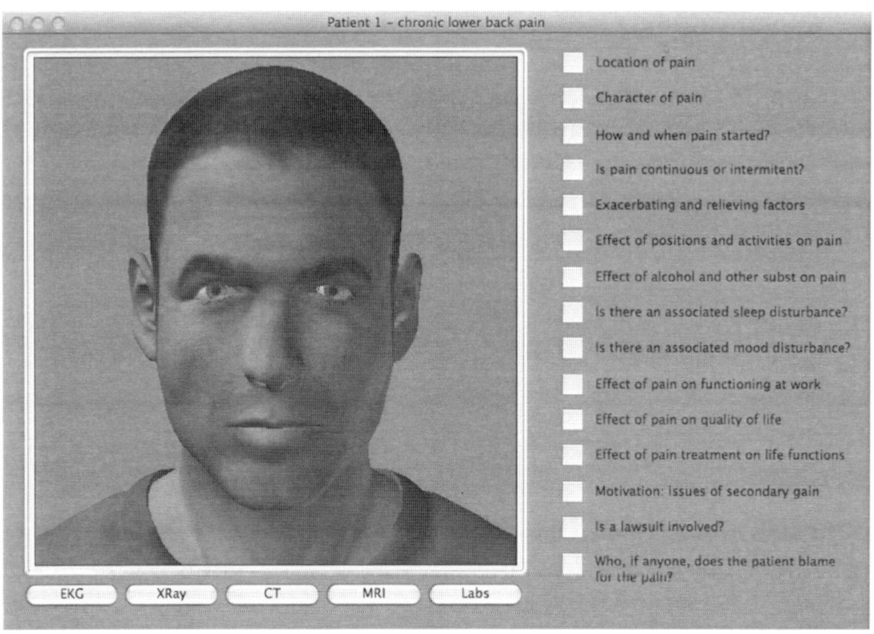

FIGURE 17.1 The Louisiana State University Health Sciences Center in New Orleans (LSUHSC-NO) proprietary avatar-based simulation software. Software and screenshot courtesy of Valeriy Kozmenko, MD.

Interacting with the virtual patient allows the trainees to take a detailed and/or focused history of the simulated patient and to begin the process of making topical diagnoses based on the results of the interview. The 3-D animation software allows the instructor to create male or female avatars of different ages and race. The LSUHSC-NO proprietary software avatar can be compiled for use on Apple Macintosh, Windows, or Linux computer systems.

Each simulation case is supplied with a library of the appropriate imaging studies, such as computed tomography (CT), magnetic resonance imaging (MRI), X-ray images, and laboratory data. The imaging studies and laboratory data are used in combination with the patient history and subjective complaints to select an appropriate method of treatment.

SIMULATION-BASED TECHNIQUES FOR PERFORMING INVASIVE PROCEDURES

Interventional pain modalities may help to determine the underlying cause of pain and assist in arriving at a precise diagnosis. Interventional procedures often alleviate the need for strong medication use, thereby sparing the patient from unwanted side effects associated with large analgesic drug doses. Specifically, focal nerve blocks are some of the most commonly used interventional procedures employed by pain physicians, and they assist not only with the diagnosis but also the prognosis, preemptive analgesia, and even definitive therapy.

At LSUHSC-NO, simulation-based techniques have been incorporated into technical skills training related to interventional pain procedures. After taking a simulated history and obtaining appropriate imaging and laboratory studies, the pain procedure trainees perform an injection of a steroid with or without local anesthetic into the simulated site of inflammation and/or into the epidural space. Each procedure is monitored by a pain procedure trained staff physician. Pre- and post-simulated procedure written and/or oral tests are given to assess trainee ability and progress in performance of the procedure.

Epidural injections can be done with the use of a part-task simulator or a cadaver. For example, the epidural injection simulator (EIS), a part-task trainer manufactured by Nasco, can be used for learning and practicing epidural puncture procedures. This simulator consists of a realistic torso connected to a portable electronic device. The simulator provides realistic feedback to the trainee to simulate the needle passing through different tissues. The torso has realistic bony structures, such as vertebrae and iliac crests. A loss of resistance is noted by the trainee when the needle enters the simulated epidural space with the use of a 16- or 18-gauge needle. The portable electronic device connected to the torso tracks the position of the tip of the needle and provides real-time feedback as the needle advances through the tissues. Depending on the learning objectives of the simulation-based scenario, epidural injection can be performed with or without the use of the visual feedback from the computer device (Figure 17.2).

The EIS can simulate different tissue densities based on such coexisting simulated medical conditions as pregnancy or obesity. Advantages of the EIS include low maintenance, affordable cost, high portability, standardized experience for trainees, immediate visual feedback during simulated procedures, and absent risk of patient infection. Its use, however, is limited only to performing epidural punctures.

In addition to the EIS, other part-task trainers can be used to teach technical skills related to invasive spinal procedures for pain management. For example, The Lumbar Puncture Simulator II, manufactured by Kyoto Kagaku, Ltd. (Figure 17.3) can be used by medical student and resident trainees alike to teach technical skills related to lumbar puncture.

Cadavers can also be used for SBT in invasive spinal procedures. For example, the Center for Advanced Practice at LSUHSC-NO is equipped with state-of-the-art cadaveric theaters capable of running 32 minimally invasive stations concurrently.

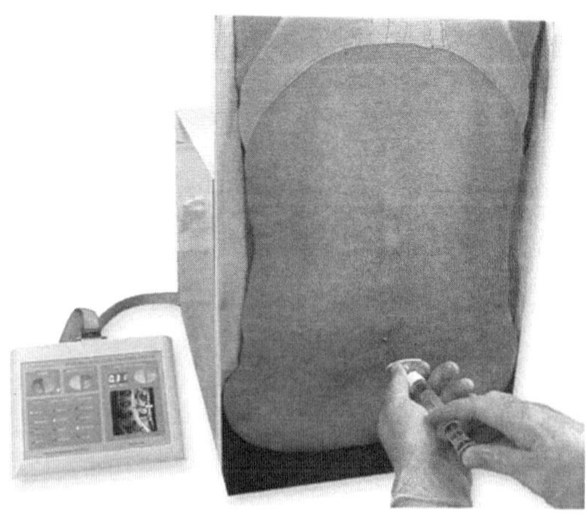

FIGURE 17.2 Nasco Epidural Injection Simulator. Reproduced with permission from Nasco (www.enasco.com).

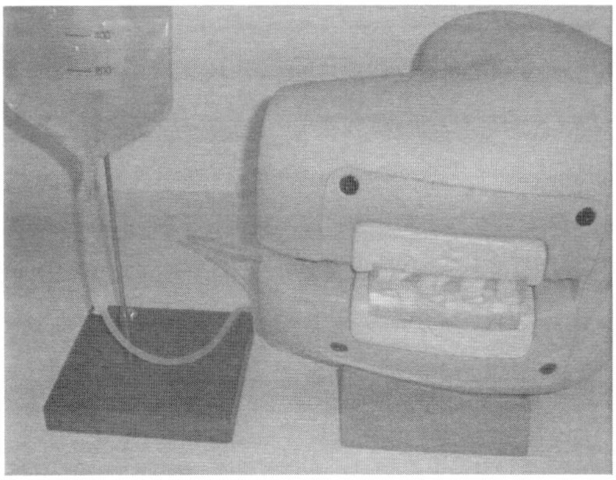

FIGURE 17.3 Lumbar Puncture Simulator II produced by Kyoto Kagaku, Ltd. Reproduced with permission from Kyoto Kagaku, Ltd. (www.kyotokagaku.com).

This setup provides an excellent opportunity to perform and practice complex pain interventional procedures, as compared with the limited use of low-back part-task devices for simple needle placement. Cadaver use allows trainee performance of cervical, thoracic, and lumbar spine needle placement for epidural injection, sacroiliac joint injection, facet joint injection, and selective nerve root block (SNRB). Combining the LSUHSC-NO proprietary avatar-based simulation virtual patient interaction with human cadaver spine interventional procedures provides the trainee with precise anatomical correlation and a SBT experience closely approximating a real patient procedure. The LSUHSC-NO software can be used to provide trainees with feedback on the effectiveness of selective nerve root blocks.

Pain management specialists often hail from the ranks of anesthesiologists, neurosurgeons, and neuroradiologists. The invasive procedures performed by these pain management specialists are a mainstay in the diagnosis and treatment of both acute and chronic pain. They range from direct percutaneous injections with short-acting local anesthetic solution to neurosurgical procedures using CT guidance. Cadaver SBT has become standard in training for such complex spinal nerve and spinal cord interventional procedures (Figure 17.5).

Simulation-based cadaver workshops are held regularly throughout the world, and are routine in interventional pain training programs. It should be noted that actual patient procedures are usually performed in a dedicated room with nursing staff and monitoring equipment. Imaging equipment, often C-arm fluoroscopy, CT, or occasionally MRI, is used to guide the interventions with a high level of accuracy. Ultrasound localization and guidance is often utilized due to its ease of portability and increasing popularity in regional anesthesia. Some patients require sedation, but most procedures can be performed with minimal

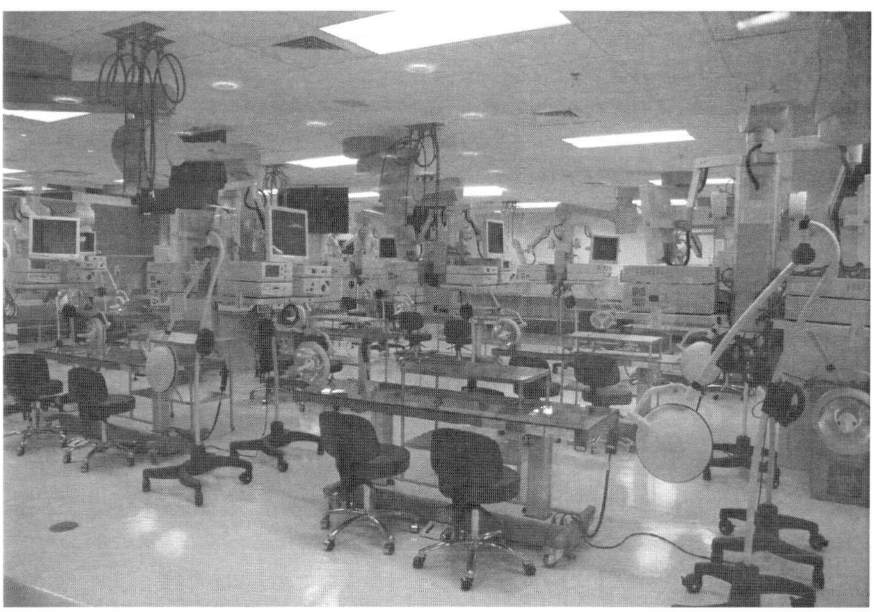

FIGURE 17.4 Louisiana State University Health Sciences Center in New Orleans (LSUHSC-NO), Center of Advanced Practice cadaveric laboratory. Photo courtesy of Valeriy Kozmenko, MD.

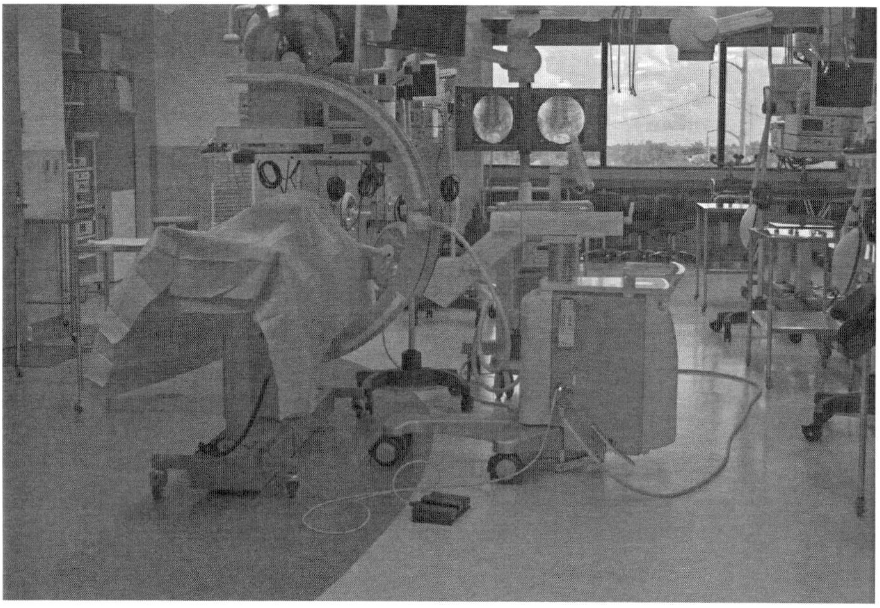

FIGURE 17.5 Louisiana State University Health Sciences Center in New Orleans (LSUHSC-NO) Center for Advanced Practice cadaveric laboratory. Photo courtesy of Valeriy Kozmenko, MD.

Table 17.1 Accuracy, specificity, and sensitivity of diagnostic examinations for back pain

DIAGNOSTIC TEST	ACCURACY	SENSITIVITY	SPECIFICITY
Clinical examination	46%–76%	0.8	0.82
Radiography	34%	–	–
Myelography	72%–91%	0.67–0.95	0.76–0.96
CT/MRI	70%–100%	0.80–0.96	0.68–0.95
Electromyography	78%	0.66–0.72	-

Reprinted with permission from Cosgrove MA, Towns DK, Fanciullo F, Kaye AD. Interventional Pain Management. In: Vadivelu N, Urman R, Hines R, eds. *Essentials of Pain Management*, Chapter 13. New York: Springer Science+Business Media; 2011:250–312. Modified from Rubin DI. Epidemiology and risk factors for spine pain. *Neurol Clin.* 2007;25:353–371.

parenteral medications (patient participation during some procedures is advantageous).

Multiple regional procedures or "blocks" done by anesthesiologists for pre- and postoperative pain are also utilized in acute and chronic pain management. An invaluable resource for a wide variety of these body regional procedures is the New York Society of Regional Anesthesia's website at www.nysora.com.

Interventional Procedures Commonly Employed for Spine Pain Management

Back pain is one of the most common causes for patients seeking medical attention. An estimated two-thirds of adults will experience low back pain at least once in their lifetime.[10] The etiology of back pain is often unclear, given that similar complaints and symptoms may result from various pathologic conditions, and imaging studies do not always specifically correlate, thus making accurate diagnosis and treatment difficult. Occupational injuries, compensation, and secondary gain issues confound the situation as well. A thorough history, physical examination, and the development of a cohesive and consistent treatment plan incorporating diagnostic procedures and therapeutic interventions provide the most effective care (Table 17.1).

Back pain can be divided into two categories—axial and radicular—but patients commonly have components of both. Axial back pain often originates in the spinal facet joints but can be secondary to pathology related to the intervertebral disk. Radicular pain usually results from nerve root irritation that may be the end result of many different processes. There are different approaches to the diagnosis and treatment of axial and radicular back pain through interventional procedures, but significant overlap exists. Patient responses to the procedures are sometimes difficult to predict, and evidence-based outcomes are difficult to interpret.[11–13]

A selected number of commonly performed invasive procedures in spinal pain management are now available. These procedures can be integrated into a SBT program in which trainees practice procedures on part-task trainers and/or cadavers until satisfying predetermined proficiency criteria established by instructors. Actual patient spine pain management procedures performed by trainees require preliminary full knowledge of the procedure and its risks by the trainee (as briefly outlined in the following procedure descriptions), direct supervision by a staff physician qualified and experienced in spine pain management procedures, and a comprehensive assessment of the trainee performance of the procedure. This assessment is addressed near the end of this chapter.

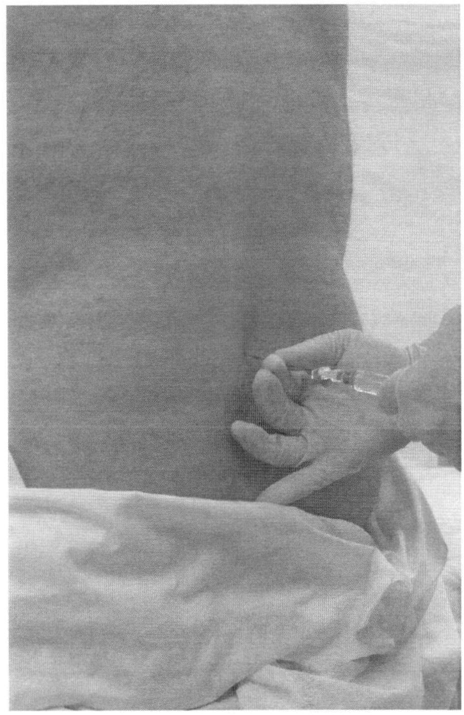

FIGURE 17.6 Patient epidural injection of local anesthetic and corticosteroid. Photo courtesy of Valeriy Kozmenko, MD.

EPIDURAL STEROID INJECTIONS: INTERLAMINAR AND TRANSFORAMINAL

Epidural steroid injection (ESI) is the most commonly performed injection for back pain. It may be performed in all segments of the spine, but is most commonly done in the lumbar and cervical regions. Our usual approach is through the interlaminar window, but this is not always possible. Previous surgical removal of bone and ligament, hardware implantation, and postsurgical scarring can make the interlaminar approach both difficult and risky. Transforaminal, caudal, or sacral approaches may be necessary due to anatomic alterations or pathologic changes in the spine. Clinical practice data has shown that cervical interlaminar ESI injection is safer than cervical transforaminal injection. Lumbar interlaminar ESI and lumbar transforaminal injection are equally safe and efficacious.[14–16]

Interlaminar Epidural Steroid Injection

The interlaminar ESI is usually performed with the patient in either prone or upright position, with X-ray fluoroscopic guidance (Figures 17.6 and 17.7).

The targeted level is identified by counting the lumbar or cervical vertebrae from a known level, such as T1 (first rib-bearing vertebra), T12 (last rib-bearing vertebra), the skull base, or sacrum. Anatomic variants, such as a sacralized L5 or a lumbarized S1 vertebra, may be present, and counting both up and down the spine is recommended. After skin preparation and regional draping utilizing standard sterile technique, the skin is anesthetized and a Tuohy epidural needle (18- or 20-gauge) is advanced through the skin and interspinous ligament until the ligamentum flavum is engaged. The loss of resistance technique with limited saline or air injection is used to identify and access the epidural space. In the cervical spine, the hanging drop technique may also be used. The needle tip location is confirmed with a lateral radiographic film and also by injection of radiopaque contrast medium, which shows a characteristic pattern (Figure 17.8).

The specific steroid dose is then injected, followed by a small amount of preservative-free sterile saline or local anesthetic solution. The addition

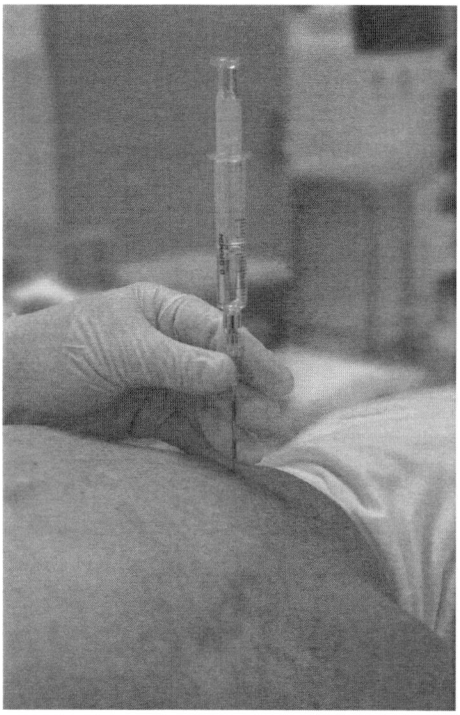

FIGURE 17.7 Interlaminar steroid injection in the cervical spine of a fresh cadaver specimen. Photo courtesy of Valeriy Kozmenko, MD.

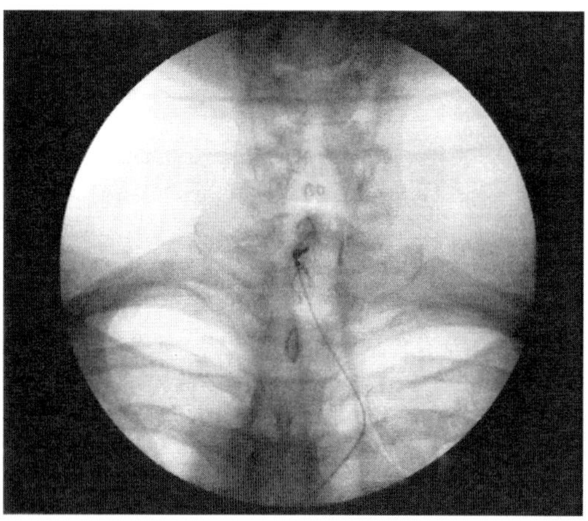

FIGURE 17.8 Cervical interlaminar epidural injection at C7-T1 interspace with spread of contrast outlining fat globules in the epidural space. Reprinted with permission from Cosgrove MA, Towns DK, Fanciullo F, Kaye AD. Interventional Pain Management, Chapter 13, p. 250–312. In: Vadivelu N, Urman R, Hines R, eds. *Essentials of Pain Management,* Chapter 13. New York: Springer Science+Business Media; 2011:250–312.

of local anesthetic provides some immediate pain relief, but increases the risk of post-injection muscular weakness. Careful monitoring is necessary after the procedure for detection of prolonged weakness or potential intrathecal injection. Injections are targeted at or below the corresponding level of the symptoms and the pathology shown on imaging studies. Severe spinal canal stenosis or disk herniation would suggest injection below the level due to the increased risk of arachnoid puncture (wet tap) or neurologic injury. The effects of the steroid injection usually occur within 24–48 hours and reach a maximum potential benefit by 7–10 days. The injection may be repeated monthly up to three times per year without significant systemic cumulative steroid side effects. Diabetic patients may experience some elevation of blood glucose levels from 2 days up to several weeks.

Transforaminal Epidural Steroid Injection

Transforaminal steroid injections target the nerve root laterally as it exits the neural foramen between two vertebral segments. Depending on modes of practice, they are performed for the same indications as interlaminar injections or after failure of a preceding interlaminar injection. Transforaminal injections are also utilized in patients whose anatomy does not allow for safe performance of the interlaminar approach (Figure 17.9).

A 22-gauge spinal needle is used to approach the nerve root in the foramen. An X-ray fluoroscopic view with 22 degrees lateral oblique rotation shows the characteristic "Scotty dog," appearance of the vertebral body, articular and transverse processes, and pedicle. The needle is advanced toward the "neck" or the 6 o'clock position just beneath the transverse process. This area above the nerve root is considered safer with regard to risk for intravascular injection and contact with the nerve root itself. This approach is also used for diagnostic nerve root blocks utilized in preoperative planning (Figure 17.10).

A preliminary needle aspiration and injection of a minimal amount of iodinated contrast medium will help to prevent inadvertent intravenous steroid injection, which can result in spinal cord infarction. Intraneural injection can be reduced by following the present American Society of Interventional Pain Physicians guidelines, which require a patient to be communicative so that initiation of an intraneural injection will be met with vocalization of discomfort

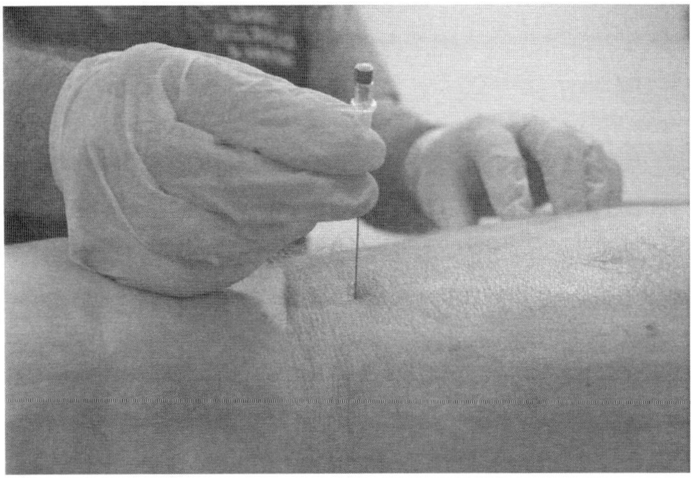

FIGURE 17.9 Lumbar transforaminal injection of steroid performed on a fresh cadaver specimen. Photo courtesy of Valeriy Kozmenko, MD.

from the patient, leading to immediate cessation of injection at that anatomical point. The use of contrast medium injection to assess for any vascular runoff and to verify contrast spread along the nerve root up to the epidural space is an absolute necessity. It should be noted that the risk of intra-arterial injection is higher when performing transforaminal injections in the cervical spine (Figure 17.11).

Cervical epidural injection with the use of a lateral radiographic view can reduce the risk of inadvertent improper location of injection and mitigate the risk of catastrophic spinal cord infarction.

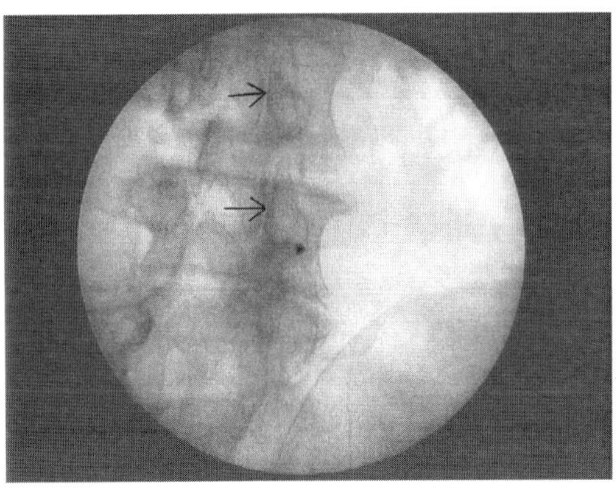

FIGURE 17.10 Arrows point to the left L2-L3 and L3-L4 facet joints. From this angle, a transforaminal or nerve root injection for L4 would be made at the black dot mark. Reprinted with permission from Cosgrove MA, Towns DK, Fanciullo F, Kaye AD. Interventional Pain Management. In: Vadivelu N, Urman R, Hines R, eds. *Essentials of Pain Management,* Chapter 13. New York: Springer Science+Business Media; 2011:250–312.

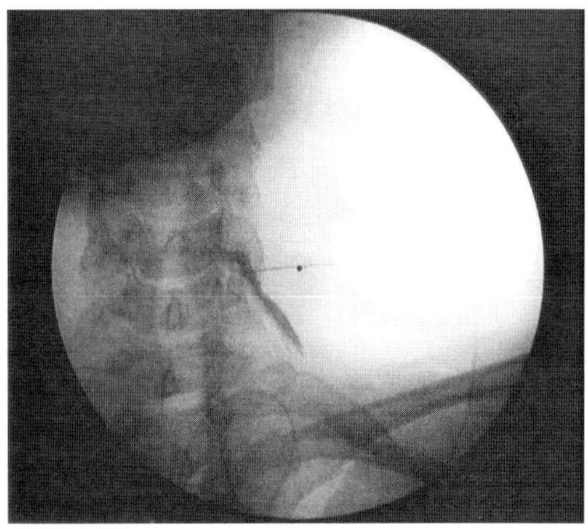

FIGURE 17.11 Cervical transforaminal epidural injection at C7-T1 level with spread of contrast medium along the nerve sheath to the epidural space. Reprinted with permission from Cosgrove MA, Towns DK, Fanciullo F, Kaye AD. Interventional Pain Management. In: Vadivelu N, Urman R, Hines R, eds. *Essentials of Pain Management,* Chapter 13. New York: Springer Science+Business Media; 2011:250–312.

FACET JOINT INJECTIONS

The zygapophyseal or facet joints are synovial joints located between adjacent vertebrae posteriorly, and these may be a site for axial back pain. The joints function in alignment of the spine and allow for forward flexion and extension and smaller amounts of lateral flexion, extension, and rotation. Abnormalities in their structure and alignment may cause substantial pain, which follows a characteristic referral pattern. After failure of conservative pain control measures, injections are targeted into the joint itself or to the sensory innervation of the joint. Facet injections are performed with the patient in the prone position, with a spinal needle using fluoroscopic guidance. The needle is directed into the joint space, which can contain only 1–2 mL of fluid. Diagnostic injections include local anesthetic solution alone, whereas a mixture of local anesthetic and steroid solution provides longer relief. Each articular facet receives sensory innervations from the dorsal nerve root above and below it. These nerves, known as the *medial branches*, may be anesthetized with local anesthetic diagnostically as well. This block can establish the specific contribution of the injected facet joint to the patients overall back pain, and also may indicate potential treatment success with radiofrequency neurolysis. The medial nerve block procedure is performed with X-ray fluoroscopic guidance, with the patient in the prone position. A spinal needle is directed to the lamina, where the medial branches come off the nerve roots at levels above and adjacent to each symptomatic joint level (Figure 17.12).

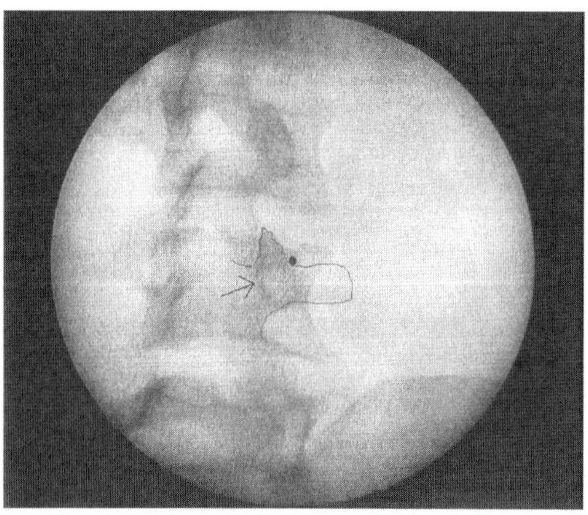

FIGURE 17.12 The arrow indicates the left pedicle of vertebra L4 and the dot indicates the location for needle placement for facet joint medial nerve branch block in the lumbar region. Reprinted with permission from Cosgrove MA, Towns DK, Fanciullo F, Kaye AD. Interventional Pain Management. In: Vadivelu N, Urman R, Hines R, eds. *Essentials of Pain Management*, Chapter 13. New York: Springer Science+Business Media; 2011:250–312.

A small amount of long-acting local anesthetic, usually less than 0.5 cc, is injected to anesthetize each medial branch. Pre- and post-injection patient verbalized pain scores and level of function are compared to establish the treatment efficacy. The patient also tracks the pain over the ensuing hours during previously painful positions and activities.

For a *lumbar facet block technique*, the lumbar spine is visualized in a 22-degree oblique angle with X-ray fluoroscopy. Thoracic facet joint disease is much less common but may be approached in a similar fashion. Patient participation during needle manipulation aids needle placement. Sedation can be used but is discouraged or minimized since it may alter the patient's subjective relief of symptoms.

PARAVERTEBRAL NERVE ROOT BLOCKADE

Using an aseptic technique and minimal local anesthetic solution injection, a 22- or 25-gauge spinal needle is inserted through the skin of the back and the adjacent muscle (Figure 17.13).

The puncture point is determined by an oblique radiographic view of the intervertebral foramen of interest. The needle is inserted with intermittent fluoroscopic visualization until reaching the bone. Correct needle placement is confirmed by posteroanterior and lateral radiographic views. Minimal injection of contrast medium confirms correct needle placement at the nerve sheath, and local anesthetic or a mixture of a long-acting local anesthetic and corticosteroid is injected.

EVALUATION OF TEACHING AND LEARNING IN SPINE PAIN MANAGEMENT SIMULATION

Assessment of educational activities is a complex process. In his book, *The Adult Learner*, Malcolm Knowles, a well-known scholar in adult education states, "Here is the area of greatest controversy and weakest technology in all education, especially in adult education and training." In the same book, Hilgard and Bower add, "It has been found enormously difficult to apply laboratory-derived principles of learning to improvement of efficiency in tasks with clear and relatively simple objectives. We may infer that it will be even more difficult to apply laboratory-derived principles of learning to the improvement of efficient learning in tasks with more complex objectives."[17] Further, these statements reflect not

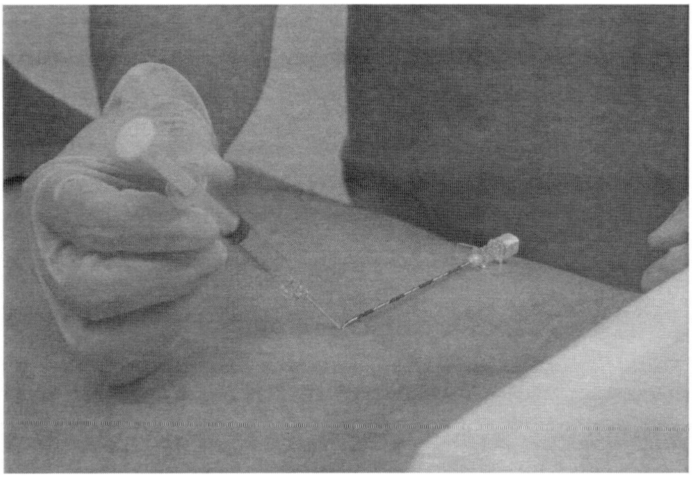

FIGURE 17.13 Paravertebral nerve root blockade. Photo courtesy of Valeriy Kozmenko, MD.

only challenges in evaluating training; they reflect challenges regarding the entire evaluation process, which is critical to improve teaching and learning.

A useful model for such an evaluation process regarding training effectiveness was developed by Don Kirkpatrick and consists of four levels of evaluation:

- *Level 1—Reaction evaluation*: Collecting the learners' opinions regarding the course and their positive or negative reactions to it. A post-activity survey regarding course content and structure would be an example.
- *Level 2—Learning evaluation*: Collecting data about knowledge, skills, and attitudes acquired during the session. Pre- and post-activity multiple-choice examinations regarding knowledge taught in the course would be an example.
- *Level 3—Behavior evaluation*: Collecting data about actual changes in trainees' behavior after the training. Unannounced direct observation of participants in the clinical environment would be an example.
- *Level 4—Results evaluation:* Collecting data on how the training course affected the entire organization. A review of the number of sentinel events, complications, or mishaps would be an example.[18]

As we have noted, simulation of chronic pain clinically encountered is a multifaceted and complex process. The assessment of the effectiveness of the SBT and patient procedure education in chronic spine pain management requires in-depth trainee cognitive, behavioral, and procedural skills evaluation. Since each method of evaluation has some advantages and disadvantages, a combination of several assessment tools is usually needed. At LSUHSC-NO, a trainee self-reflective assessment survey combined with a multiple-choice examination administered before and directly after the training and direct skilled supervisory observation with or without video recording has provided an effective method of measuring the trainees' abilities and progress. Detailed records of these educational experiences over an indefinite period of time are an invaluable asset in assessing the utility of simulation-based techniques and related patient training techniques in achieving successful patient outcomes with minimal complication rates.

CONCLUSION

Advances in the development of computer screen-based and mannequin-based simulators in combination with key principles of adult teaching and learning make simulation an invaluable tool in acquiring knowledge, communication, and procedural skills in spinal chronic pain management.

REFERENCES

1. Kozmenko V, Kaye A, Hilton C, Theory and Practice of Developing an Effective Simulation-Based Curriculum. In: Kyle RR, Murray WB, eds. *Clinical Simulation: Operations, Engineering and Management.* New York: Elsevier Academic Press; 2007:147.

2. Manchikanti L, Boswell MV, Singh V, et al. Comprehensive review of epidemiology, scope, and impact of spinal pain. *Pain Physician.* 2009;12:E35-E70.

3. Crook J, Rideout E, Browne G. The prevalence of pain complaints in a general population. *Pain.* 1984;18:299–314.

4. Badley EM, Tennant A. Changing profile of joint disorders with age: findings from a postal survey of the population of Calderdale, West Yorkshire, United Kingdom. *Ann Rheum Dis.* 1992;51:366–371.

5. Guyot P, Drogoul A, Honiden S. Power and Negotiation: Lessons from Agent-Based Participatory Simulations. *Proceedings of the Fifth International Joint Conference on Autonomous Agents and Multiagent Systems* (AAMAS-06), 2006:27–33.

6. Idaho Bioterrorism Awareness and Preparedness Program—Methodologies. Accessed June 25, 2010, at http://www.isu.edu/irh/IBAPP/methodologies.shtml

7. Serious Games Improving Training and Performance Metrics. *Serious Games Market.* Accessed December 15, 2011, at http://seriousgamesmarket.blogspot.com/2010/07/serious-games-improving-training-and.html

8. Radcliff BJ. Why Soft-Skills Simulation Makes a Hard Case For Sales Training. Accessed December 3, 2011, at www.competenet.com

9. Alexiou A. The virtual radiopharmacy laboratory: a 3-D simulation for distance learning. *J Educ Multimedia Hypermedia.* 2004;13: 307–322.

10. Rubin DI. Epidemiology and risk factors for spine pain. *Neurol Clin.* 2007;25:353–371.

11. Neumann N, Raj PP. Facet Syndromes and Blocks . In Raj PP, Abrams BM, Benzon HT, et al, eds. *Practical Management of Pain,* 3rd edition, Chapter 52. St.Louis, Mosby; 2000:745–752.

12. Cohen, SP, Raja SN. Pathogenesis, diagnosis, and treatment of lumbar zygapophysial (facet) joint pain. *Anesthesiology.* 2007;106:591–614.

13. Maugars Y. Assessment of the efficacy of sacroiliac corticosteroid injections in spondylarthropathies: a double-blind study. *Br J Rheumatol.* 1996;35:767–770.

14. Bogduk N, Dreyfuss P. *International Spine Intervention Society Practice Guidelines for Spinal Diagnostic and Treatment Procedures.* San Francisco: International Spine Intervention Society; 2004.

15. Anderson EF. Epidural and intrathecal narcotics for pain relief. *S D J Med.* 1984;37:7–12.

16. Magora F. Observations on extradural morphine analgesia in various pain conditions. *Br J Anaesth.* 1980;52:247–252.

17. Knowels MS, Holton EF, Swanson RA. *The Adult Learner: The Definitive Classic in Adult Education and Human Resource Development.* New York: Elsevier; 2005:542.

18. Kirkpatrick DI. *Evaluating Training Programs: The Four Levels,* 2nd edition. San Francisco: Berrett-Koehler; 1998.

18

Cervical Transforaminal Epidural Steroid Injections and Simulation–Based Training

CHARLES N. APRILL

SIMULATION-BASED TRAINING (SBT) can be very effective in progressively improving technical and cognitive skills in interventional diagnostic and therapeutic procedures, before their application in actual clinical practice.[1,2] In particular, SBT is especially well suited for practicing and perfecting key skills related to clinical procedures with high inherent risks of severe complications. Cervical transforaminal epidural steroid injection (TFEI) is one such procedure. Although it can be efficacious in the treatment of cervical radicular pain, this procedure must be performed carefully and precisely, with complete knowledge of cervical spine neural foraminal regional anatomy. No allowable margin of error exists for the correct needle placement in the neural foramen. In fact, improper needle placement for epidural steroid injection (ESI) may result in known severe complications, including quadriplegia and death.

Simulation-based training, in the form of a preliminary detailed, comprehensive didactic lecture, a pre-test (e.g., a multiple-choice written test), simulation-based deliberate practice, a post-practice test, and trainee interview, has been shown to result in progressive trainee procedural skills improvement[1,2] The distributed practice (i.e., practice repeated during several sessions spaced over a period of time) of simulation-based exercises with pre- and post- intervention tests over a period of time results in the best procedural skills improvement in trainees.[1] Trainee self-assessment and interview with mentors after completion of SBT adds further to trainee comprehension of the procedure.

One model of SBT for cervical TFEI begins with the anatomical study of cervical spine dried skeletal bone to provide the trainee with a clear understanding of the neural foraminal bone margins. A fresh, unembalmed cadaver is used for TFEI procedure practice. The procedure is demonstrated stepwise by a skilled, highly experienced staff physician preceptor. The trainee then performs the cervical TFEI repeatedly, with the skilled preceptor supervising and grading each procedure on a multipoint scale log. Subsequent practice TFEI sessions are graded, and scores are compared with all previous SBT practice sessions. Trainee skill in the SBT for cervical TFE needle placement is required to be up to the expert level. During SBT, the preceptor frequently emphasizes the use of C-arm fluoroscopy in needle placement, contrast medium limited volume injection through the needle, and the routine taking of radiographic spot films of needle position and contrast medium injection. The subsequent participation of the trainee in actual patient TFEI is carefully and constantly monitored, and the trainee is assisted by a skilled, experienced physician proctor.

Given its particular importance in TFEI, the remaining portion of this chapter focuses on the key technical and therapeutic aspects of the procedure. Such background knowledge can be given as a pre-SBT didactic lecture, or as an expert lecture or text-based reading assignment with the administration of a pre-test. Following this, faculty-tutored SBT can commence using a cadaveric model.

HISTORY OF TRANSFORAMINAL EPIDURAL STEROID INJECTION

The term "epidural" denotes a space within the spinal canal but is also applied to a variety of injection procedures. They may be classified as to region of interest: cervical, thoracic, or lumbar, and route of administration: caudal, interlaminar, or transforaminal. Each procedure involves directing a needle to a specific target using an imaging modality to guide and document final needle position. This chapter limits discussion to fluoroscopic guidance for cervical transforaminal injections. These procedures require injection of a contrast material to demonstrate the dispersal pattern of the injectates and documentation of that pattern with radiographic spot films. Finally, a report detailing the procedure, including the specific technique used, details of injected solutions (contrast medium, local anesthetic, and corticosteroids), and recording the initial post-treatment outcome is prepared for the permanent record.

Interest in the lumbar transforaminal approach emerged in the last quarter of the 20th century, in an attempt to deliver more target-specific injections.[3–5] The cervical literature is sparse by comparison to that of the lumbar spine; cervical transforaminal injection was first reported in 1988.[6] A descriptive outcome study by Bush and Hillier employing this approach followed in 1996.[7] The transforaminal approach was adopted to deliver therapeutic agents to more specific targets influenced by observations that lumbar transforaminal injections appeared to be effective in treating lumbar radicular pain.[8,9]

In 2009, Levin published the results of an extensive Medline/PubMed search and searches of large review articles on the major interventional spine topics.[10] This review was performed to find all prospective, double-blind, randomized, placebo-controlled trials in the English language interventional spine literature. The author concluded that "Fluoroscopically guided lumbosacral transforaminal epidural corticosteroid injections are effective in the treatment of acute/subacute lumbosacral radicular pain, and in preventing future surgeries." No firm conclusions were drawn about cervical epidural steroid injections (CESI).[11]

RELEVANT ANATOMY

The spinal epidural space is a continuous potential space in the vertebral spinal canal extending from the foramen magnum to the sacral hiatus, interposed between the dural sac and the osseoligamentous wall of the vertebral spinal canal. The epidural space is bounded posteriorly by the lamina and ligamentum flavum. The anterior boundary is formed by the posterior intervertebral disc margin and the posterior longitudinal ligament. The lateral boundary of the epidural space is fenestrated by paired nerve root canals or foramina at each segment. The vertebral pedicles are interposed between the successive intervertebral foramina and nerve root canals.

The dural sac almost fills the vertebral spinal canal and extends downward from the foramen magnum, terminating in the sacral canal. At each vertebral segment, paired dural nerve root sleeves extend toward the root canals. The cervical dural root sleeves are short and nearly horizontal in orientation, traversing the center of their respective neural foramina. The dural root sleeve contains the dorsal and ventral rootlets of the segmental nerve. The dorsal ganglia lie generally in the mid-zone of the root canals, between the pedicles of adjacent vertebrae. The dura and arachnoid membranes form a "water-tight" seal at the proximal end of the ganglion. Cerebrospinal fluid fills the root sleeve but does not extend beyond the ganglion. Occasionally, ectasia of a dural root sleeve will occur, resulting in extension of the subarachnoid space beyond usual boundaries. The nerve root sleeves usually communicate freely with the subarachnoid space.[12] A plexus of valveless veins occupies the spinal canal anterior epidural space.[13] Paired anterior internal epidural veins run the length of the vertebral canal. There are numerous interconnecting veins crossing the floor of the canal, the anterior internal vertebral venous plexus (AIVV).[14] These veins communicate freely with the basivertebral veins, at the center of the posterior wall of each vertebral body and the anterior internal vertebral venous plexus. Several radicular veins traverse each nerve root canal. They lie predominantly in the ventral root canal and connect the epidural venous plexus with descending cervical veins.

Segmental arteries traverse the cervical nerve root canals.[15] They course primarily in the anterior root canals along the anterior aspect of the segmental dural root sleeve. Some arterial branches perfuse the dorsal ganglia and segmental neural elements and, as such, are radicular arteries. Other branches penetrate the dura, running along the segmental rootlets and anastomosing with the anterior spinal artery. They are, therefore, medullary arteries. Varying numbers of medullary arteries of differing sizes are found in the cervical region, contributing to the blood supply of the cervical spinal cord. The radicular and medullary arteries of the cervical spine arise primarily from the vertebral artery.[16,17] Some arise from the ascending cervical and posterior cervical arteries. Medullary arteries penetrate the dura and divide into anterior and posterior branches, eventually reaching the anterior and paired posterior spinal arteries. Cervical medullary arteries are variable in size and distribution. There are usually two or three arteries of moderate size in adults. They may be present at any segment and on either side.[18,19]

SPONDYLOGENIC PAIN

Spondylogenic pain is pain arising from a component of the spine or its supporting structures and is synonymous with other terms such as *nonspecific* or *idiopathic spinal pain*. The International Association for Study of Pain (ISAP) published a taxonomy, defining clinical terms used to describe pain, in an effort to standardize the use of terminology.[20] *Somatic pain* results from noxious stimulation of a musculoskeletal component of the body and arises as a result of stimulation of nociceptive nerve endings in bone, ligament, joint, muscle, or tendon. *Visceral pain* occurs with noxious stimulation of a body organ or its capsule. Both somatic and visceral derangements cause pain in the location of the source structure, but the pain is often vague and ill-defined.

Referred pain is pain perceived in areas adjacent to or remote from the source of pain. *Convergence* is the physiological basis for referred pain. Sensory neurons from different peripheral sites converge on common neurons in the spinal cord and thalamus that relay to higher centers in the brain. Without additional sensory input, the brain may not be able to determine the specific site of the initial input. Referred pain is a misperception of the origin of the signal that reaches the brain. Somatic cervical spinal pain syndromes may be expressed topographically as neck pain. Local pain is often accompanied by somatic referred pain, perceived in the shoulder girdle, upper extremity, and, occasionally, the chest wall.

Radicular pain occurs when there is irritation or injury of a spinal nerve or its roots. Simple compression of a normal nerve or nerve root does not provoke pain. Pressure on a spinal nerve or its roots may produce a conduction block of axons. Sensory axon conduction block results in loss of sensation or "numbness." Motor axon block results in weakness. Compression alone can result in radiculopathy, without radicular pain. Pressure on a previously injured or damaged nerve or root provokes pain. Local ischemia or inflammation can induce ectopic impulses in a dorsal root canal ganglion, resulting in radicular pain. Radicular pain is discretely localized; band-like in distribution; shooting, lancinating, or shocking in quality; and may have a cutaneous component.

PREPROCEDURE EVALUATION

A practitioner of spinal interventions is responsible for assessing the clinical condition and appropriateness and risks of a given procedure. The practitioner must attempt to understand the pain and associated disability. The patient is the primary source of that information. What is the primary complaint? Is this an acute or a chronic problem; a constant or recurring problem? Is local pain somatic or visceral? Is there a radicular or somatic referred component? One must localize the somatic component and the location of radiating pattern. The pain character and intensity are as important as the location. What are the mechanical aspects (i.e., what provokes and relieves the pain)? For example, a 35-year-old woman presents with recent onset of left posterior and lateral aching neck pain for no apparent reason. Constantly present, the aching varies from moderate to severe on occasion. There is diffuse aching of left posterior shoulder girdle muscles. She has recurring episodes of severe, "sharp, stabbing" left upper extremity pain, extending along the posterior arm, medial forearm, and into the left third finger. No arm weakness, frequent "tingling" of the whole upper extremity, and normal strength and reflexes are noted. Prolonged sitting, particularly at a console or working at a desk aggravates the neck pain. Neck extension and left-side bend induces a painful "shocking" sensation in the left arm. Although intermittent, the arm pain is the dominant complaint. She has axial somatic neck pain, with somatic referred pain to the left shoulder girdle and left upper extremity radicular pain, without radiculopathy.

Self-rating of pain, employing a specific method such as a visual analog scale (VAS), is essential. What is the intensity rating at the time of assessment? Range of intensity is determined by noting the pain rating at its best and worst. Patients can express their pain on pain drawings, which should be correlated with the description of symptoms. These instruments are very useful in assessing the immediate response to an intervention.

Simple psyche screening questionnaires to assess anxiety, depression, self-perception of disability, and somatization are useful in assessing pain behavior. What has been the response to any previous interventions or procedures? Finally, what medications, at what doses have been used to treat, and what has been the response? Psychological factors contribute to pain and influence the outcome of interventions. There is no simple screening tool; therefore, one must know his or her patient and remember that "history repeats itself." The medical history includes a review of all allergies and idiosyncratic reactions, any current illness or infection, and chronic conditions such as cardiovascular disease, diabetes, seizures, and respiratory and renal disorders. All impact how procedures will be performed. The history of all surgical procedures and their outcomes should be explored. A complete list of current medications is mandatory. A general review of systems should include information about sleeping pattern. Social habits, such as tobacco and alcohol use or abuse, are important. The patient's work and/or avocations may pertain to complaints and should be explored. A family history may contribute to recognition of an underlying hereditary disorder.

The physical examination on the first patient encounter is general but focuses on primary and secondary complaints. Developmental status, and any deformities or postural aberrations should be recorded. The level of distress during interview and examination, the patient's willingness and ability to cooperate with interview/examination, and the patient's demeanor and orientation should be observed and recorded along with routine vital signs. Examination may include assessment of gait and both sitting and standing postures. Passive or active movements of the cervical spine through the range of motion are observed. Palpation of regional musculature and bony prominences helps to localize somatic pain. Injections into the spinal neuraxis require a basic neurologic examination prior to the procedure. On a case-by-case basis, examination of core and extremity strength, weakness, range of motion, and reflexes contribute to formulating a diagnostic hypothesis.

Spine imaging plays a definite role in the evaluation of spine pain complaints, both in demonstrating relevant pathology and in aiding in planning a safe and efficient approach for procedures. Modern imaging modalities provide excellent depictions of spine anatomy. However, many lesions evident in the maturing spine are clinically insignificant,[21] and imaging studies often demonstrate irrelevant pathology. Computed tomography (CT) or magnetic resonance imaging (MRI) may demonstrate a left cervical C3–C4 disc protrusion in a patient complaining of right arm pain and altered sensation radiating to the right forearm, thumb, and index finger. It cannot be overstated that a significant incidence of pathology is seen in asymptomatic subjects.[22] Scans should be reviewed overall, but with particular attention paid to areas that might be related to the patient's underlying complaints, as gleaned from the interview and examination. Not all abnormalities need to be targeted, but rather those most likely to be associated with the expressed symptoms and physical findings.

TFEI INDICATIONS, CONTRAINDICATIONS, PREDICTORS

The preprocedure evaluation should provide a basis for a hypothesis as to the nature of the underlying spinal disorder. Cervical transforaminal epidural injections are indicated when a patient expresses constant or frequently recurring episodes of radicular pain. Additionally, they are indicated in patients with somatic spinal pain associated with mixed somatic referred and radicular pain to one or both extremities or the chest wall.

Absolute medical contraindications include a bleeding diathesis, systemic infection or local infection in the procedure field, pregnancy, and inability or unwillingness to cooperate and participate in the procedure. Absolute psychiatric contraindications include active psychosis, and homicidal and suicidal ideation. Studies have shown a relationship between physical and sexual abuse and various types of pain. Relative medical contraindications include significant competing disease (i.e., uncontrolled hypertension, diabetes, congestive heart failure, and anticoagulation therapy). Relative psychiatric contraindications include personality disorders, bipolar disorder, severe depression, lack of social support, and drug dependence/abuse. Correlation of failed spinal surgery with childhood trauma has revealed definite pain procedure risk factors. These include physical, psychological, and/or sexual abuse; emotional neglect; abandonment; chemical dependency; and/or loss of a primary caregiver.[23–25] There is risk of a major depressive disorder in patients with chronic pain. Pure psychogenic pain is rare and used pejoratively. Almost all chronic pain can be altered by psychological adjustments. Without these issues being addressed, successful diagnosis and treatment is unlikely.

Negative predictors for procedure successful outcome include an external locus of control, "just fix me" attitude, unstable relationships, poor vocational adjustment, neurocognitive deficits, inability or unwillingness to participate in active rehabilitation, unreasonable expectation of procedures, ongoing litigation, symptoms inconsistent with pathology, high level of fear avoidance, inability to actively exercise, and a catastrophizing cognitive style. Positive predictors for procedure successful outcome include a history of adherence to treatment regimen; positive support system; compliance, currently and historically; and appropriate expectations.

MINOR COMPLICATIONS

Vasovagal Response

Vasovagal responses during pain interventional procedures are not rare. About 1 in 14 patients undergoing cervical interlaminar epidural injection will experience a vagal response. Gender incidence varies, and women are at greater risk than men. Vasovagal response is five times more common in cervical than in lumbar procedures. Usually a minor complication, such events at times may be quite severe. Vigilant screening is necessary to discover previous episodes; suspect "fainters." Pretreat the patient with atropine when suspicious, and recognize the early signs (i.e., "I feel sick," nausea, perspiration, and slowing of pulse rate).

Contrast Material

Allergic reactions to modern contrast media are extremely rare, and some reactions may be related to preservatives, such as methylparaben. Wang et al[26] reviewed 84,928 intravenous nonionic contrast injections noting "allergic" reactions in 545 (0.6%). Seventy-seven percent of the reactions were "mild," primarily urticaria, and successfully treated with diphenhydramine. Twenty-one percent had moderate reactions with respiratory symptoms, facial edema, or both. Corticosteroid administration, either intravenously or by inhaler, was effective in controlling these reactions. Only 2% of the total number of reactions (0.0012% overall) were severe. Of this group, eight were in women and three were in men. Three were unresponsive, and cardiorespiratory arrest occurred in one. There were no deaths and no long-term sequelae in 10 of the 11 patients with severe reactions.

Contrast medium is used to document where the injectate is spreading and to determine where it is not spreading. Modern nonionic contrast agents are safe for transforaminal injections. Unintentional vascular or even subarachnoid spread of contrast medium will cause no problems. In those very rare instances of documented history of severe allergic reaction to nonionic contrast medium, gadolinium may be used in limited volume as a substitute radiographic contrast agent.[27]

Diabetics taking Metformin are at risk for contrast medium–induced nephropathy (CIN) if exposed to nonionic or ionic contrast media during radiographic procedures. Solomon found no change in renal function in those subjects who had normal renal function prior to testing. Some patients with normal renal function, however, exhibited increases of serum creatinine with high contrast loads.[28] This should not be a problem with epidural injections as the contrast doses employed are very limited and much lower than the volumes delivered in intravascular and other radiologic procedures. Total contrast doses in excess of 100 cc are common for enhanced CT scans or angiograms. Nonetheless, diabetic patients with renal impairment should temporarily discontinue Metformin for 48 hours after the contrast procedure, with the prior approval of their primary physician.

Local Anesthetic Reactions

The local anesthetics employed in the epidural injections are lidocaine and bupivacaine. These amides are primarily metabolized in the liver and excreted in the urine. Their allergic potential is very, very low. Ester-based local anesthetics (i.e., procaine hydrochloride) have a higher incidence of allergic reaction. A large survey attests to the overall safety of the amides as spinal anesthetics.[29] For epidural injections, lidocaine may be employed in concentrations of 0.5% to 4.0% and bupivacaine at 0.25% to 0.75%. The percentage concentration of the anesthetic is reduced with increasing volume delivered. Although central nervous system and/or cardiovascular system toxicity can occur following the epidural, intravenous, or subarachnoid injection of local anesthetics, the toxic dose levels are far greater than for the drug concentration employed in epidural injections: 40 cc of 1.0% lidocaine (400 mg) delivered to the epidural space of test subjects resulted in average peak plasma concentrations safely below neurotoxic levels.[30] One author recommended the maximum epidural dose of lidocaine be 500 mg and 225 mg for bupivacaine.[31]

Acute cardiac complications, such as decreased cardiac output, can occur from intravascular injection of lidocaine or bupivacaine. One study has shown that normal cardiac function is maintained in subjects with lidocaine plasma levels of 4 to 8 mcg/mL. Plasma levels this high require doses of over 400 mg of lidocaine.[32] In human volunteers, slow intravenous injection of bupivacaine to produce plasma concentrations equivalent to those achieved during epidural injections did not cause significant cardiovascular change.[33] Between 0.75 and 2.0 cc of higher concentrations of bupivacaine for transforaminal injections are not toxic in the epidural space, nor are these doses toxic if technical misadventure results in delivery to the vascular system or subarachnoid space. Because of the longer half-life of bupivacaine, this anesthetic should be avoided in cervical injections. Inadvertently misplaced cervical injection into the subarachnoid or subdural space results in prolonged anesthetic effects, specifically affecting respiratory function.

Steroid Preparation Reactions

The steroid preparations most frequently employed in ESI are methylprednisolone acetate, triamcinolone acetonide, betamethasone sodium phosphate and acetate, and dexamethasone sodium phosphate. All corticosteroids have systemic effects when injected into the epidural space. Side effects may include fever, myalgia, malaise, fluid and electrolyte imbalance, hypertension, hyperglycemia, myopathy, ulcers, immunosuppression, behavioral changes, allergic reaction, and pituitary-adrenal suppression. Abrupt steroid withdrawal after prolonged oral use may precipitate acute adrenal insufficiency. Most of these side effects are clearly associated with the systemic absorption of corticosteroid and subsequent transient adrenal hypercortical effect, and could account for many of the "minor" complications associated with epidural injections.

The cardiovascular system is affected directly and indirectly by ESI. Direct effects are due to steroid receptors on heart and smooth muscle. Indirectly, steroids increase sodium uptake and vascular tone, raising blood pressure. Judicious steroid use is prudent in patients with cardiac disease, hypertension, and congestive cardiac failure. Dose and frequency of administration must be carefully monitored in this group. Remember that patients may be receiving "steroid shots" from other physicians for unrelated problems.

Epidural steroid injection related endocrine system alterations include decreased adrenocorticotropic hormone (ACTH), thyroid-stimulating hormone (TSH), follicle-stimulating hormone (FSH), and testosterone. Epidural steroid injections can suppress adrenal function for weeks,[34] and these changes are largely dose related. Bizarre responses do occur rarely: a 24-year-old man underwent a second cervical ESI of 60 mg of methylprednisolone for ongoing severe arm pain, and a cushingoid appearance developed 1 month later and persisted for 12 months.[35]

Does injection of corticosteroids increase the risk of infection? Infections do occur in patients following ESI.[36] Postoperative infections are increased in hip replacement patients who received preoperative steroid injections.[37] No studies have been done on outcomes of spine surgery after ESI, but suppression of the immune system suggests there is inherent risk, especially in the first 4 weeks following injection of steroid.

Epidural administration of glucocorticoids results in potent suppression of insulin action, and this should be taken into account when patients with diabetes receive ESIs.[38] Statistically significant elevations in blood glucose levels occur in diabetic subjects. This effect peaks on the day of the injection and lasts approximately 2 days.[39]

The musculoskeletal system suffers from some bone mineral density loss, muscle weakness and wasting, and predisposition to avascular necrosis of bone with long-term oral steroid use. Although systemic corticosteroids may be associated with loss of bone mineral density, a prospective study of 204 patients followed for 1 year after standard doses of epidural steroids revealed no change in bone mineral density.[40] The currently used steroids contain preservatives, and Bernat felt that seizures following intrathecal cortisone acetate were due to the 0.9% benzyl alcohol.[41] Benzyl alcohol is common in depot steroids and is neurotoxic.[41] Hodgson et al[29] reported that there was no concrete evidence of neurotoxicity of intrathecal steroids, but did not recommend purposeful delivery of these agents into the subarachnoid space.

MAJOR COMPLICATIONS

Directing a needle deep into the tissues in and about the spine approaches sensitive spaces and structures of the neural axis, thus risking a spectrum of possible major complications.

Infection

Infection following epidural injection is a serious issue. It has been described as a rare complication,[42] but the possibility of procedure-related infection must be a concern for the injectionist. Analysis of the American Society of Anesthesiologists (ASA) Closed Claims database from 1970 to 1999 revealed that infection was the third most common complication of chronic pain procedures, accounting for 13% of all complications.[9] Any penetration of the skin surface by the needle, which is then placed in deep spaces in and about the spine, has the potential of introducing organisms that may cause subsequent infection.[43] Standard aseptic preparations and draping of the local injection site and strict aseptic technique will minimize this complication. Diabetics and immunocompromised patients are a subgroup that should be recognized prior to procedures. Antibiotic prophylaxis should be considered for immunocompromised patients undergoing transforaminal injection. Antibiotics should not be mixed with the nonionic contrast medium during any epidural injection. Accidental delivery of antibiotics into the subarachnoid space is to be avoided.

Bleeding, Hematoma

Many veins lie in the needle path or near the end point targets of transforaminal epidural injections. Furman et al reported the incidence of fluoroscopically confirmed "vascular uptake" occurring during cervical transforaminal injections.[44] Observing blood at the needle hub reliably predicts intravascular penetration with 97% specificity, but this finding has low sensitivity (45% overall). The absence of blood in the needle hub despite aspiration is not reliable. The incidence of vascular uptake with cervical TFE is almost 20%. Kim et al have recently reported a much higher rate of vascular uptake for cervical transforaminal injections, over 50%.[45] Although neither author specified, most of the vascular uptake seemed to be venous, and no complications occurred. Venous uptake during epidural injections is common and innocuous, as long as it is recognized and needle adjustment is made before injecting physiologic solutions.

The incidence of epidural hematoma is approximated to be less than 1 in 150,000 for epidural interlaminar injections.[46] There are rare anecdotal reports of hematoma following cervical transforaminal injections, but no clinically significant hematoma has been reported.

The potential for bleeding and hematoma formation is increased in patients with a coagulopathy or liver disease, or in patients taking anticoagulant medications. It is crucial that the injectionist be familiar with the patient's coagulation status and with common anticoagulant and antiplatelet medications.[47] Anticoagulant therapy should not be interrupted until there is full understanding of the reason for the therapy. Interruption of anticoagulant therapy is usually best left to the physician managing and prescribing the patient's anticoagulation. Epidural steroid injections are elective procedures, and interrupting anticoagulant therapy may increase the risk of serious complications such as stroke, myocardial infarction, or pulmonary embolus.

The following guidelines for performing spinal procedures in anticoagulated patients are based on the second American Society of Regional Anesthesia and Pain Medicine (ASRA) Consensus Conference on Neuraxial Anesthesia and Anticoagulation in 2003.[46] Warfarin therapy should be discontinued 4–5 days before spinal procedures, and the international normalized ratio (INR) should be within normal range at the time of the procedure. Thienopyridine derivatives (e.g., clopidogrel, ticlopidine) should be suspended 7 days and 14 days, respectively, prior to spinal procedures to allow for recovery of primary and secondary platelet aggregation and platelet–fibrinogen binding.

Low-molecular-weight heparin should be held for at least 12 hours before the procedure in thrombosis prophylactic dosing and at least 24 hours in therapeutic dosing. Aspirin and nonsteroidal anti-inflammatory drugs have not been found to have any contraindications for spinal procedures.

Dural Puncture

Transforaminal injections place the dural root sleeves at risk. Dural puncture is reportedly rare when the procedure is performed by expert interventionalists.[48] Minor complications, including headache secondary to dural puncture, occurred in less than 0.5% in over 4,300 procedures. Failure to recognize subarachnoid spread results in injection of anesthetic and steroid into the subarachnoid or subdural space, and delivery of anesthetics in sufficient quantity and concentration into these spaces may produce significant spinal block that may impair respiration. These misadventures are avoided by selection of appropriate target; proper needle size; good visualization; a cooperative, comfortable, but minimally sedated patient; and precise technique.

Brain and Spinal Cord Infarct

Arterial filling during transforaminal injections has been rarely reported. Only two cases of cervical medullary artery filling during transforaminal injection have been reported.[49–51] In both instances medullary artery filling was recognized during real-time fluoroscopy. Transforaminal injections are hazardous because of important arterial structures in the target field. Delivery of a particulate steroid into an artery may result in embolization of particles, larger than capillaries, with subsequent ischemia and/or infarction of the perfused tissue. Unpublished, anecdotal reports of catastrophic neurological complications associated with epidural injections were circulating during the last decade; Brouwers et al[52] reported the first such occurrence in 2001. Central cervical spinal cord infarction occurred in conjunction with a fluoroscopically guided C6 transforaminal injection. This was likely the result of embolization of the anterior spinal artery watershed by way of a cervical medullary artery.[19]

Since the first report in 2001, an alarming number of case reports of catastrophic neurological complications have appeared in the literature. In a mail-in survey, Scanlon et al[53] collected 287 responses from physician members of the American Pain Society. There were 78 major neurologic complications associated with cervical TFE. All procedures involved injection of particulate steroid preparations, and vertebrobasilar arterial distribution brain and/or cervical spinal cord infarctions occurred. There are more events than case reports; many are encountered in the context of medicolegal proceedings.

Clearly, the following preventive measures are needed if cervical TFEI injection is to be done safely:

- Recognition of intra-arterial injection when it occurs is critical. Careful real-time fluoroscopy, in the frontal plane, during slow injection of an adequate volume of nonionic contrast medium to opacify vessels is mandated. Visualization of vessels can be enhanced by digital subtraction angiography (DSA).
- Injection of a small test dose of concentrated local anesthetic solution before injecting steroids, especially with particulate steroid varieties, to test for onset of neurological signs, may allow recognition of unexpected flow in the vertebral or medullary arteries.
- Currently, the presumed mechanism of spinal cord injury is an embolic shower of particles from the steroid preparation into the circulation of the anterior spinal artery.[55,56] A third safety measure is to avoid entirely the use of particulate steroids for all transforaminal epidural injections.

Dexamethasone sodium phosphate is a nonparticulate steroid. Derby et al[55] found the particle size in this preparation to be approximately 10 times smaller than red blood cells, and the particles do not appear to aggregate. They have lower density than the particles and aggregates of methylprednisolone acetate, triamcinolone acetonide, and betamethasone sodium phosphate/acetate, the most commonly used agents. In a comparison study, Dreyfuss et al[57] reported that dexamethasone was slightly less effective than triamcinolone, but the difference was not statistically significant. There have been no reported infarcts when dexamethasone has been used for transforaminal injections. Two animal studies have demonstrated severe neurologic injury to the animals when particulate steroid preparations were injected into the carotid[58] and vertebral[59] arteries, but there was no evident injury to those animals receiving intra-arterial injections of the nonparticulate preparation, dexamethasone. A theoretically safer nonparticulate agent appears to be a valid alternative to the particulate agents that have been used to date.

EPIDURAL INJECTION TECHNIQUES

Equipment

FLUOROSCOPY

Image guidance is mandatory for cervical TFE. This chapter focuses on X-ray fluoroscopic guidance only. The procedure demands precise needle placement for selective administration of medications. The X-ray fluoroscopic instrument of choice is the C-arm, which can be moved in any plane to provide optimal imaging for direct needle insertion and to verify, and document, the final needle position and contrast spread. Digital subtraction imaging (DSI), although not at present the standard of care, can provide significant useful information when used correctly. The C-arm fluoroscope is used to align the skin entry point with the target. A needle can then be advanced parallel to the beam. A historical record of all procedures must be archived either with hard or digital images, and images must document both the needle in safe position prior to the injection of contrast medium and the contrast dispersal pattern. Injection must include real-time viewing of the slow injection of contrast material in the coronal plane. The report should include statements as to the presence or absence of vascular uptake (either venous and/or arterial), and spread in the nerve root canal, central spinal canal, or subarachnoid space.

Miscellaneous Supplies

Aseptic technique demands the use of sterile gloves. Although the effectiveness of masks, caps, and gowns in the control of infection with regard to minimally invasive spinal injections has never been demonstrated, some have advocated their use.

Transforaminal epidural injections are best accomplished with 25- or 22-gauge needles. In almost all cases, a 3.5-inch needle length suffices. Although some have advocated the use of blunt needles to prevent unintentional arterial injection, no evidence exists as to the validity of this claim, as has been addressed in detail.[3] In addition, blunt needles require an introducer needle to puncture the skin, are difficult to control, and, in at least one small study, have been shown not to decrease the incidence of vascular puncture.

To limit needle movement during the attachment of multiple syringes once optimal needle position is obtained, a small-bore low-volume extension tube is attached. This also allows the physician to stay out of the fluoroscopy beam during the injection of contrast medium using active fluoroscopy, as mandated for patient safety.

The use of nonionic, water-soluble contrast media is mandated. Injection of contrast medium validates that the needle is in correct position, and that the subsequent active injectate will cover the targeted anatomical structure. The dispersal pattern ensures that the needle tip has not unintentionally strayed into a dangerous position (i.e., intrathecal or intra-arterial).

Transforaminal epidural injections employ local anesthetic in concentrations high enough to cause sensory nerve block. This provides reliable negative information: if the patient has minimal or no relief of primary pain, and there is significant numbness in the specific dermatome of the targeted nerve, one can make the assumption that the pain is not associated with that specific level. This might be helpful in ruling out this level as associated with the pain generator. If a patient presents with right upper extremity radicular pain, and there is correlating pathology by imaging, the complete relief of the index pain following TFE implicates that pathology as the pain source.

Patient Monitoring

Monitoring devices such as pulse oximetry, noninvasive blood pressure, and electrocardiogram (ECG), must at the least be available, and their use is required if any sedation is contemplated. An ongoing conversation with the patient is always an appropriate and accurate monitor of the patient's comfort, level of consciousness, and cardiac and respiratory status pre-, peri-, and post-procedure.

Intravenous Access

Intravenous access is recommended before transforaminal injections. Complications requiring the use of intravenous medications, such as allergic reactions and severe vasovagal reactions, are rare but do occur.

Sedation

Transforaminal injections should be minimally painful. If sedation is utilized, intravenous access is obviously required, except when only mild oral medications are utilized. Minimal, light sedation may have a place in the markedly anxious patient.

At all times during the course of the procedure, the patient must be able to converse with the attending physician. Sedation can never take the place of technical competence.

Preparation and Drapes

When aseptic precautions are utilized, infection following epidural administration of corticosteroids is quite rare. The skin at and around the point of needle insertion is prepared using iodine-based solution (e.g., povidone-iodine) or chlorhexidine, with or without alcohol, followed by sterile towels to cordon off the area. In following the sterility initiated in the "prep and drape," sterile technique is mandated throughout the procedure.

CERVICAL TRANSFORAMINAL STEROID INJECTION PROCEDURE

The patient is placed in the supine oblique position, with a pillow under the head for support. The C-arm is maneuvered to obtain an oblique view, with caudal tilt of the image intensifier, so that the chosen foramen is seen at its widest diameter in respect to both cephalo-caudal and ventral-dorsal dimensions. This is the so-called *foraminal view* (Figure 18.1).

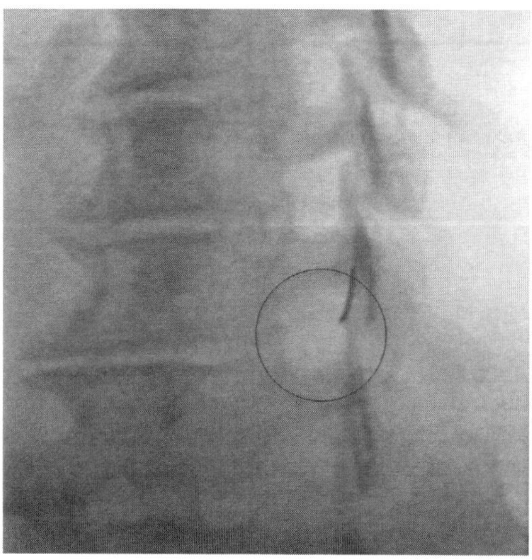

FIGURE 18.1 Left anterior oblique position, optimal for viewing the left C6-C7 nerve root canal (*circle*). Procedure needle is directed to the posterior root canal, against the superior articular process (SAP) of C7.

In this position, the X-ray beam is focused parallel to the foramen and nerve. An essential understanding of the shape of the foramen is paramount to the safe performance of this procedure. In this foraminal view, the actual foramen is not the aperture it appears. In actuality, it is shaped like a funnel, with the central part hyperlucent, while the actual outer edge is ill-defined and indistinct, in that it lies over the posterior and anterior bony elements. The target is the superior articular process (SAP), the posterior wall of the root canal. The procedure needle is inserted and directed to contact the bone of the SAP at the posterior margin of the nerve root canal. The actual distance between the skin and SAP is rarely greater than 1 inch; the needle is advanced quickly under active fluoroscopy and is positioned in a few seconds. Although some radiation exposure to the needle guiding hand is inevitable, using pulsed, low-dose fluoroscopic modes results in an overall low radiation dose. This technique is analogous to that utilized for cervical discography and stellate ganglion blocks. Once the SAP is contacted by the needle, the depth must be determined. Frontal fluoroscopy demonstrates the medial-lateral position. The needle should project over the middle third of the SAP. The needle can then be advanced toward the uncinate line to lie in the medial third of the root canal. Vascular structures are less prevalent in this area. Radiographic images documenting precontrast needle position are then archived (Figures 18.2 and 18.3).

Using active fluoroscopy in the anteroposterior position, contrast material is injected slowly. The contrast medium volume should be sufficient to clearly visualize spread of the solution, and flow should be seen in the nerve root canal with spread around the dorsal ganglion. There may be distal flow along the anterior ramus and/or spread into the lateral regional epidural space. If foraminal stenosis is present, minimal contrast may be seen entering the spinal canal. Transient local pressure and paresthesias often accompany the injection. If significant venous uptake occurs, the needle is repositioned slightly, either medially toward the uncinate process or laterally. A repeat contrast injection is made after any repositioning of the needle.

If vascular flow into the spinal canal occurs, a medullary artery may have been cannulated, and the procedure should be terminated. If there is upward vascular flow lateral to the uncinate processes, the vertebral artery has been injected and the procedure is terminated. If there is any hint of a question in the

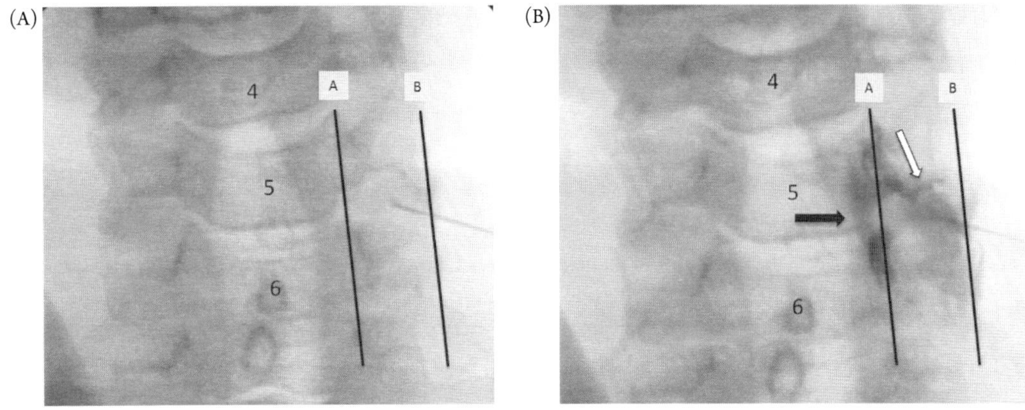

FIGURE 18.2 (A) Frontal (anterior/posterior) view of mid cervical spine. The needle is projected over the mid zone of the left C5-C6 nerve root canal. Medial vertical line A, through uncinate processes, represents the lateral limit of the central canal. The lateral-most line B, at the lateral margin of the articular processes, represents the lateral limit of the C5-C6 nerve root canal. (B) Same view after injection of 0.75 cc of contrast medium. Spot film demonstrates spread of solutions into the lateral epidural space (*black arrow*) and left C5-C6 nerve root canal (*white arrow*).

operator's mind about the safety of the injection, the procedure should be terminated immediately. Once a safe contrast pattern has been documented, frontal and anterior oblique images are obtained to document the procedure for the medical record.

A test dose of local anesthetic solution (e.g., 0.5 cc of lidocaine 4%) may be used as a final precaution. Following the injection, the patient is quietly observed for 2 minutes. The patient is questioned as to feeling sensation in the upper and lower extremities and asked to slowly wiggle fingers and toes. Karasek et al[54] reported transient quadriparesis following a test dose of local anesthetic; this was felt to be the result of transient spinal cord "anesthesia" due to injection into a medullary artery. The procedure was aborted, and the patient recovered completely in less than a half hour. The absence of any sensory or motor change after 2 minutes is a good indication that there has been no spread into a medullary artery.

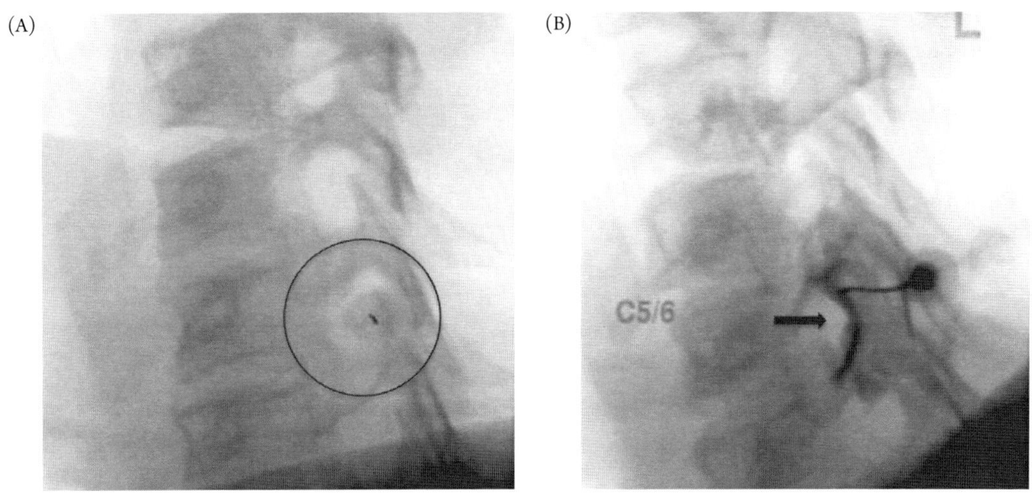

FIGURE 18.3 (A) Left anterior oblique view of mid cervical spine. Circle surrounds left C5-C6 root canal. Procedure needle is projected over the posterior root canal. (B) Same view after injection of 0.75 cc of contrast material. Spot film demonstrates spread of solutions in the posterior root canal, behind the left C6 dorsal ganglion (*black arrow*).

A nonparticulate corticosteroid can then be slowly injected. The steroid volume should be small (e.g., 1.0 cc of dexamethasone, 10 mg or equivalent is sufficient). The steroid solution should not be mixed with the local anesthetic solution.

Post-Procedure Care

Following the injection, the patient is taken to a recovery area for observation, where physiologic monitoring is continued until discharge. Recovery room personnel should be trained to recognize any emergent situations that may present. Complications require diagnosis and treatment in a timely and appropriate manner. Although rarely needed, immediate access to oxygen, airway supplies, and emergency medications must be available. In that sensory and/or motor deficit is often noted when local anesthetics are utilized, accurate neurologic assessment is of particular importance.

Prior to discharge, the patient is evaluated for degree of pain relief from the initial, preprocedure level. Assessment by the physician, or other trained personnel, must include those provocative movements that initiate an increase in the index pain. Sensory change in the selected target dermatome should be noted. This post-procedure evaluation must be included in a specific, detailed, accurate procedure note dictated following any medical intervention.

On discharge, written instructions should be provided to the patient. These instructions should detail information about a follow-up appointment, care of the injected area, and on contacting medical help if the patient believes that a complication due to the procedure is occurring.

CONCLUSION

Corticosteroids placed within the epidural space are rationally used for treatment of radicular type pain thought to be of an inflammatory origin. Common sense dictates that an injection specifically and precisely targeting the pain generator with a concentrated active component will have more benefit when compared to a dilute preparation placed in an area distant from the pathology. This is borne out in the literature, where precise, selective, transforaminal epidural placements of corticosteroids have evidenced long-term benefit.

Evaluation of the patient following each injection and further treatment, based on some evidence of past benefit and a rational expectation of future pain relief, are the essence of evidence-guided medicine.

Today, for patients with radicular pain, transforaminal injection of corticosteroid should be considered prior to any surgical intervention. As with all medical interventions, there is a risk–benefit ratio that must be considered. Transforaminal injections can involve significant morbidity and even mortality. As pointed out early in this chapter, SBT can be a useful addition to traditional methods for initial training in this important technique. With prudence, vigilance, and meticulous technique, the risks are minimized.

REFERENCES

1. Monsky WL, Levine D, Mehta TS, et al. Using a sonographic simulator to assess residents before overnight call. *AJR*. 2002;178:35–39.

2. Sica GT, Barron DM, Blum R, et al. Computerized realistic simulation: a teaching module for crisis management in radiology. *AJR*. 1999;172:301–304.

3. Krempen JF, Smith BS. Nerve-root injection: a method for evaluating the etiology of sciatica. *J Bone Joint Surg Am*. 1974;56:1435–1444.

4. Tajima T, Furukawa K, Kuramochi E. Selective lumbosacral radiculography and block. *Spine*. 1980;5:68–77.

5. Stanley D, McLaren MI, Euinton HA, et al. A prospective study of nerve root infiltration in the diagnosis of sciatica. A comparison with radiculography, computed tomography, and operative findings. *Spine*. 1990;15:540–543.

6. Morvan G, Mempoint D, Bard M, et al. Direct intra-foraminal injection of corticosteroids in the treatment of cervico-brachial pain. In: Baird M, Laredo J, eds. *Interventional Radiology in Bone and Joint*. New York: Springer Verlag; 1988:25.

7. Bush K, Hillier S. Outcome of cervical radiculopathy treated with periradicular/epidural corticosteroid injections: a prospective study with independent clinical review. *Eur Spine J*. 1996;5:319–325.

8. Vallee JN, Feydy A, Carlier RY, et al. Chronic cervical radiculopathy: lateral-approach periradicular corticosteroid injection. *Radiology*. 2001;218:886–892.

9. Slipman CW, Lipetz JS, Jackson HB, et al. Therapeutic selective nerve root block in the nonsurgical treatment of atraumatic cervical spondylotic radicular pain: a retrospective analysis with independent clinical review. *Arch Phys Med Rehabil*. 2000;81:741–746.

10. Levin JH. Prospective, double-blind, randomized placebo-controlled trials in interventional

spine: what the highest quality literature tells us. *Spine J.* 2009;9:690–703.

11. Fitzgibbon DR, Posner KL, Domino KB, et al. Chronic pain management: American Society of Anesthesiologists Closed Claims Project. *Anesthesiology.* 2004;100:98–105.

12. Tarlov IM. Spinal perineurial and meningeal cysts. *J Neurol Neurosurg Psychiatry.* 1970;33: 833–843.

13. Crock HV, Yoshizawa H, Kame SK. Observations on the venous drainage of the human vertebral body. *J Bone Joint Surg Br.* 1973;55:528–533.

14. Gershater R, St Louis EL. Lumbar epidural venography. Review of 1,200 cases. *Radiology.* 1979;131:409–421.

15. Dommisse GT. *The Arteries and Veins of the Human Spinal Cord from Birth.* New York: Churchill Livingstone; 1975.

16. Turnbull IM, Brieg A, Hassler O. Blood supply of cervical spinal cord in man. A microangiographic cadaver study. *J Neurosurg.* 1966;24:951–965.

17. Launay M, Chiras J, Bories J. Angiography of the spinal cord: venous phase. Normal features. Pathological application. *J Neuroradiol.* 1979;6:287–315.

18. Dommisse GF. The arteries, arterioles, and capillaries of the spinal cord. Surgical guidelines in the prevention of postoperative paraplegia. *Ann R Coll Surg Engl.* 1980;62:369–376.

19. Huntoon MA. Anatomy of the cervical intervertebral foramina: vulnerable arteries and ischemic neurologic injuries after transforaminal epidural injections. *Pain.* 2005;117:104–111.

20. Merskey H, Boqduk N. *Classification of Chronic Pain. Descriptions of Chronic Pain Syndromes and Definition of Pain Terms.* 2nd edition. Seattle, WA: IASP Press; 1994.

21. Okada E, Matsumoto M, Ichihara D, et al. Aging of the cervical spine in healthy volunteers: a 10-year longitudinal magnetic resonance imaging study. *Spine.* 2009;34:706–712.

22. Ernst CW, Stadnik TW, Peeters E, et al. Prevalence of annular tears and disc herniations on MR images of the cervical spine in symptom free volunteers. *Eur J Radiol.* 2005;55:409–414.

23. Schofferman J, Anderson D, Hines R, et al. Childhood psychological trauma and chronic refractory low-back pain. *Clin J Pain.* 1993;9:260–265.

24. Nickel R, Egle UT, Hardt J. Are childhood adversities relevant in patients with chronic low back pain? *Eur J Pain.* 2002;6:221–228.

25. Linton SJ. A prospective study of the effects of sexual or physical abuse on back pain. *Pain.* 2002;96:47–51.

26. Wang CL, Cohan RH, Ellis JH, et al. Frequency, outcome, and appropriateness of treatment of nonionic iodinated contrast media reactions. *AJR Am J Roentgenol.* 2008;191:409–415.

27. Shetty SK, Nelson EN, Lawrimore TM, et al. Use of gadolinium chelate to confirm epidural needle placement in patients with an iodinated contrast reaction. *Skeletal Radiol.* 2007;36:301–307.

28. Parra D, Legreid AM, Beckey NP, et al. Metformin monitoring and change in serum creatinine levels in patients undergoing radiologic procedures involving administration of intravenous contrast media. *Pharmacotherapy.* 2004;24:987–993.

29. Hodgson PS, Neal JM, Pollock JE, et al. The neurotoxicity of drugs given intrathecally (spinal). *Anesth Analg.* 1999;88:797–809.

30. Braid DP, Scott DB. The systemic absorption of local analgesic drugs. *Br J Anaesth.* 1965;37:394–404.

31. Covino B. Clinical pharmacology of local anesthetic agents. In: Cousins M, Bridenbaugh P, eds. *Neural Blockade in Clinical Anesthesia and Management of Pain.* Philadelphia: JB Lippincott; 1988:111.

32. Jorfeldt L, Lofstrom B, Pernow B, et al. The effect of local anaesthetics on the central circulation and respiration in man and dog. *Acta Anaesthesiol Scand.* 1968;12:153–169.

33. Mather LE, Tucker GT, Murphy TM, et al. Cardiovascular and subjective central nervous system effects of long-acting local anaesthetics in man. *Anaesth Intensive Care.* 1979;7:215–221.

34. Tuel SM, Meythaler JM, Cross LL. Cushing's syndrome from epidural methylprednisolone. *Pain.* 1990;40:81–84.

35. Benzon HT. Epidural steroid injections for low back pain and lumbosacral radiculopathy. *Pain.* 1986;24:277–295.

36. Gaul C, Neundorfer B, Winterholler M. Iatrogenic (para-) spinal abscesses and meningitis following injection therapy for low back pain. *Pain.* 2005;116:407–410.

37. Kaspar J, Kaspar S, Orme C, et al. Intra-articular steroid hip injection for osteoarthritis: a survey of orthopedic surgeons in Ontario. *Can J Surg.* 2005;48:461–469.

38. Ward A, Watson J, Wood P, et al. Glucocorticoid epidural for sciatica: metabolic and endocrine sequelae. *Rheumatology.(Oxford).* 2002;41:68–71.

39. Gonzalez P, Laker SR, Sullivan W, et al. The effects of epidural betamethasone on blood glucose in patients with diabetes mellitus. *PMR.* 2009;1:340–345.

40. Manchikanti L, Pampati V, Beyer C, et al. The effect of neuraxial steroids on weight and bone mass density: a prospective evaluation. *Pain Physician.* 2000;3:357–366.

41. Bernat JL. Intraspinal steroid therapy. *Neurology.* 1981;31:168–171.

42. Windsor RE, Storm S, Sugar R. Prevention and management of complications resulting from common spinal injections. *Pain Physician.* 2003;6:473–483.

43. Kabbara A, Rosenberg SK, Untal C. Methicillin-resistant Staphylococcus aureus epidural abscess after transforaminal epidural steroid injection. *Pain Physician.* 2004;7:269–272.

44. Furman MB, Giovanniello MT, O'Brien EM. Incidence of intravascular penetration in transforaminal cervical epidural steroid injections. *Spine.* 2003;28:21–25.

45. Kim DW, Han KR, Kim C, et al. Intravascular flow patterns in transforaminal epidural injections: a comparative study of the cervical and lumbar vertebral segments. *Anesth Analg.* 2009;109: 233–239.

46. Horlocker TT, Wedel DJ, Benzon H, et al. Regional anesthesia in the anticoagulated patient: defining the risks (the second ASRA Consensus Conference on Neuraxial Anesthesia and Anticoagulation). *Reg Anesth Pain Med.* 2003;28:172–197.

47. Layton KF, Kallmes DF, Horlocker TT. Recommendations for anticoagulated patients undergoing image-guided spinal procedures. *AJNR Am J Neuroradiol.* 2006;27:468–470.

48. Derby R, Lee SH, Kim BJ, et al. Complications following cervical epidural steroid injections by expert interventionalists in 2003. *Pain Physician.* 2004;7: 445–449.

49. Baker R, Dreyfuss P, Mercer S, et al. Cervical transforaminal injection of corticosteroids into a radicular artery: a possible mechanism for spinal cord injury. *Pain.* 2003;103:211–215.

50. Rathmell JP, Aprill C, Bogduk N. Cervical transforaminal injection of steroids. *Anesthesiology.* 2004;100:1595–1600.

51. Bogduk N, Dreyfuss P, Baker R, et al. Complications of spinal diagnostic and treatment procedures. *Pain Med.* 2008;9:S11-S34.

52. Brouwers PJ, Kottink EJ, Simon MA et al. A cervical anterior spinal artery syndrome after diagnostic blockade of the right C6-nerve root. *Pain.* 2001;91:397–399.

53. Scanlon GC, Moeller-Bertram T, Romanowsky BS, et al. Cervical transforaminal epidural steroid injections. More dangerous than we think? *Spine.* 2007;32:1249–1256.

54. Karasek M, Bogduk N. Temporary neurologic deficit after cervical transforaminal injection of local anesthetic. *Pain Med.* 2008;9:227–234.

55. Derby R, Lee SH, Date ES, et al. Size and aggregation of corticosteroids used for epidural injections. *Pain Med.* 2008;9:227–234.

56. Tiso RL, Cutler T, Catania JA, et al. Adverse central nervous system sequelae after selective transforaminal block: the role of corticosteroids. *Spine J.* 2004;4:468–474.

57. Dreyfuss P, Baker R, Bogduk N. Comparative effectiveness of cervical transforaminal injections with particulate and nonparticulate corticosteroid preparations for cervical radicular pain. *Pain Med.* 2006;7:237–242.

58. Okubadejo GO, Talcott MR, Schmidt RE, et al. Perils of intravascular methylprednisolone injection into the vertebral artery. An animal study. *J Bone Joint Surg Am.* 2008;90:1932–1938.

59. Dawley JD, Moeller-Bertram T, Wallace MS, et al. Intra-arterial injection in the rat brain: evaluation of steroids used for transforaminal epidurals. *Spine (Phila Pa 1976).* 2009;34:1638–1643.

19

Simulation in Musculoskeletal Radiology

MICHAEL MARISTANY, STEPHANIE CASEY, AND LEONARD R. BOK

SIMULATION PROCEDURES AND DICTATIONS FOR MUSCULOSKELETAL JOINT INJECTIONS

SIMULATION IN medicine has come a long way since the introduction of Milton Bradley's "Operation Game" in 1965. At that time, the idea of physicians using simulation for training or practicing surgery would have been thought ridiculous; the "Operation Game" was merely child's play. Such thinking has clearly changed. In 2009, writing in the *Journal of Graduate Medical Education*, Richard Satava suggested that "medical education is undergoing a complete revolution."[1] He argued furthermore that "simulation is and will be pervasive."[1] Writing in *Radiology* in 2007, Becker stated that "medical simulation is as relevant to radiology as it is to other medical specialties."[2]

With sophisticated, computerized, mannequin simulation models becoming increasing available, a shift away from the "see one, do one, teach one" process for learning how to perform procedures has occurred. Patient safety is now paramount.[3] Complex integrated systems are now used in simulation-based education utilizing mannequins, computers, advanced machine control devices, and audio-video equipment. These systems allow for life-like simulations of everything from angiograms to laparoscopic surgeries. With improving accessibility to these technologies, trainees should soon be able to achieve proven, increased level of competence before performing procedures on patients. Simulation-based education, however, does not have to be complex. Simulation can be high-fidelity or low-fidelity. Simulation can be individually based or team/group based.

Simulation-Based Training in Arthrography

Simulation-based education is applicable in musculoskeletal radiology (MSK) for developing familiarity with a variety of procedures most commonly involving the joints. Joint pain is a common malady, particularly in our aging population. It often requires visualization of small structures and/or lesions for accurate diagnosis. These structures are often in close proximity to one another and may have suboptimal signal-to-noise ratios (SNR) for ease of detection, given the size of some joints, particularly the hip and shoulder. Arthrography helps overcome these obstacles and allows for better visualization of hyaline cartilage, fibrocartilage, ligaments, tendons, sequela of synovitis, intra-articular loose bodies, and other processes by producing improved spatial resolution through distention of the joint and other structures, and by producing improved contrast resolution through the introduction of a contrast agent. Arthrography is particularly necessary in evaluating the glenoidal labrum and articular cartilage in the hip, superior labrum anterior to posterior (SLAP) tears, and in postsurgical joints. Joint arthrography with radiographs is only used occasionally to ensure needle placement in the synovial joint space for specific injections. Computed tomography (CT) arthrography is useful for postoperative joint assessment, particularly when a metal plate or other device has been placed near the joint. Similarly, preoperative planning may be necessary with a CT arthrogram. Magnetic resonance imaging (MRI) arthrography provides superior soft tissue differentiation and is most useful in hip, shoulder, and knee joints. Specialized MRI coils may be necessary for small-joint optimal detail. Magnetic resonance imaging arthrography is particularly useful in sports medicine, where rapid decision-making, treatment, and joint mobilization are required. Other invasive procedures commonly performed in musculoskeletal radiology include biopsies of bone or muscle, spine epidural steroid injections, and spinal facet joint injections.

This chapter focuses primarily on joint injections. Because the tactile (i.e., haptic) elements in these procedures are extremely important for proficiency, simulation-based training (SBT) can be effective and efficient in providing practice. This haptic element is in addition to the visual guidance provided by the imaging modality of choice, such as fluoroscopy, CT, or ultrasonography (US). Fresh, unembalmed cadaver is a good substrate for simulation-based education in this area because its use provides tactile feedback to the trainee otherwise only available in a living patient. The student can learn the feel of puncturing the joint capsule or entering the epidural space prior to performing the procedure on a patient. Such SBT will help the student avoid the question "are you in yet?" Other radiology educators report utilizing cadavers in a similar manner to train novice or beginner residents.[4] They describe an introductory lecture and two subsequent 4-hour training sessions with a lightly embalmed cadaver brought to the fluoroscopic suite. The Louisiana State University Health Sciences Center in New Orleans (LSUHSC-NO) has a simulation center within the school of medicine that occupies two floors. On one floor, the Center for Advanced Practice (CAP), a demonstration laboratory is housed, containing space for unembalmed cadaveric SBT. This laboratory has operating room lighting and video capability.

The following is a description of a simulation study day in the laboratory. The table with specialized lighting and video equipment and operator was reserved and a portable C-arm X-ray fluoroscopic unit was brought to the site (Table 19.1). Lead aprons were provided for all personnel present. The fresh, unembalmed cadaver was utilized during the day by the musculoskeletal radiology, interventional radiology, breast radiology, neuroradiology, and spine pain interventional services.

Joint injections were conducted on the cadaver using fluoroscopic needle guidance. The individual joint procedures and the associated fluoroscopy were videotaped separately. The LSUHSC-NO musculoskeletal division, as a result of these joint studies, can provide trainees with both written and video material for guidance with SBT. The Accreditation Council for Graduate Medical Education (ACGME) criteria and guidelines for resident training provide the context for LSUHSC-NO's approach to simulation. Specifically, the department of radiology seeks to teach and achieve appropriate outcomes in all six ACGME competencies: patient care, medical knowledge, practice-based learning and improvement, interpersonal and communication skills, professionalism, and systems-based practice.[5] The Dreyfus Model of knowledge/skill acquisition[5–7]

Table 19.1 List of equipment and supplies for the day of cadaver simulation lab. Courtesy Stephanie Casey

Unembalmed cadaver: shoulder, elbow, wrist, hip, knee, ankle, and foot joints
Medical instruments and supplies
Fluoroscopy unit: C-arm portable X-ray unit with high resolution

is also utilized. The ACGME modification of the five-stage Dreyfus Model of knowledge acquisition includes five levels: novice, competent, proficient, expert, and master.[7]

The musculoskeletal SBT curriculum is at an early stage of development. It addresses patient care, medical knowledge, and interpersonal and communication skills (procedure reporting). The curriculum supplies tables and figures for each joint, as well as example dictations. This format focuses on the radiology novice- and beginner-level trainee. The goal is to advance the trainee skills and knowledge efficiently and effectively to the competent stage, at which the trainees will begin to perform procedures on patients under expert-level supervision. Patient safety, comfort, and dignity are enhanced by beginning training with simulated procedures. Novice and beginner trainees can benefit from the provided prepared printed materials in understanding MSK interventional procedures. Typical patient informed consent, complications, and adverse reactions are discussed with the trainees as part of the SBT curriculum.

Five typical joint injections have been videotaped on the unembalmed cadaver: the shoulder, elbow, wrist, hip, and knee joints. In addition to the videotape with skilled instructor explanation and guidance, written simulation materials are provided for SBT for each joint. A dictation example is included for each joint injection to assist the trainee in dictating the report of the simulated procedure.

Prior to the simulation procedure, the student should understand the anatomy of each joint. For each joint, the videos provide an introduction, and the printed material focuses the trainee's attention to the most pertinent structures involved in understanding and performing a procedure. For example, a trainee would find it helpful to note in his or her documentation for the hip joint injection that the femoral vein, artery, and nerve are near the needle track of the anterior approach for the hip arthrogram, and to understand why the needle direction along the lateral margin of the femoral head is necessary when performing the injection. The trainee may use the procedure description as a prompt during the procedure. After the procedure, the student may attempt first to reproduce the template without prompting and then after looking at the procedure description as a reminder.

Five videotaped and scripted simulated joint injection procedures have been developed. The shoulder arthrogram is presented here as an example. The same set of materials is available for the other joints to be studied.

Shoulder Arthrogram

The trainee watches the videotape and receives instruction from the musculoskeletal radiologist. The trainee is given printed materials, including the tables listing instruments and supplies for joint injection (Tables 19.1 and 19.2), indications for arthrography (Table19.3), which structures are better evaluated with arthrography rather than CT or MRI scan without intra-articular contrast (Table 19.4), the anatomic structures within or near the track of the needle approach (Table 19.5), and the advantages and disadvantages of the different approaches for shoulder join injection (Table 19.6). An illustration with anatomic landmarks and an X marking the target puncture site is provided. Frequent clinical indications for pre MRI scan shoulder arthrography include rotator cuff tear, glenoid labrum injury,synovitis, joint instability and intraarticular loose body (Figure 19.1).

Procedure for Shoulder Joint Arthrogram by Anterior Approach

The patient/cadaver is placed on the fluoroscopy table in the supine position. Real-time dynamic evaluation of the glenohumeral joint with fluoroscopic

Table 19.2 List of instruments and supplies used to perform joint injections. Courtesy Stephanie Casey

Metallic object/Kelly clamp
Ink marker
25-gauge local anesthesia needle
1% lidocaine without epinephrine
18-gauge needles, 1.5 inch to draw up lidocaine and medication
Sterile gloves
Adhesive bandage
Sterile 4×4 gauze pads
22-gauge, 3.5 inch spinal needle
Sterile connecting tubing
Nonionic contrast medium
Gadolinium contrast medium
Leur-lock syringe 10-mL, 12-mL

Table 19.3 Shoulder Table I: Arthrogram indications. Courtesy Micheal Maristany

Indications for shoulder arthrogram:
Instability of the joint
Muscle, ligament, and labral disease
Previous trauma
Impingement of bone on tendon, muscle, cartilage
Osteoarthritis
Surgical planning:
Computed tomography (CT) arthrogram useful pre- and postoperatively

Table 19.5 Shoulder Table III: Anatomic structures within or near the tract of approach. Courtesy Micheal Maristany

Anatomic structures within or near the needle track on joint approach:
1. Anterior approach:
Subscapularis, labrum, long head of the biceps tendon, subdeltoid/subacromial bursa, and subcoracoid bursa.
2. Posterior approach:
Teres minor, labrum

evaluation of the joint in internal and external rotation is performed.

The arm is abducted and externally rotated, and a weighted sandbag is placed in the patient/cadaver palm for passive stabilization.

The target site for the shoulder joint injection at the junction of the middle and inferior third of the anterior aspect of the glenohumeral joint is localized with a metallic object and marked with an ink marker. The skin overlying the shoulder joint is then prepped and draped following routine sterile technique. A 25-gauge local anesthetic needle is positioned over the target site.

For subcutaneous anesthesia, 8–10 mL 1% lidocaine is administered. A 22-guage spinal needle is then advanced toward the target site, into the glenohumeral joint. Intra-articular location of the needle is confirmed with 1 mL of nonionic contrast medium. This is followed with the injection of 12–15 mL of a dilute 1:200 gadolinium contrast mixture.

The simulation report by the resident notes that the patient tolerated the procedure well with no immediate complication or describes any complication that occurred during the simulation scenario.

Table 19.4 Shoulder Table II: Structures better evaluated with arthrogram. Courtesy Michael Maristany

Shoulder joint structures better evaluated with magnetic resonance imaging (MRI) arthrogram vs. noncontrast MRI labrum injury:
Articular cartilage
Rotator cuff musculotendinous injury
Depiction of the anatomy of the joint space
Possible communications to the subacromial/subdeltoid or subcoracoid bursa
Adhesive capsulitis
Intra-articular loose bodies

Discussion

The LSUHSC-NO approach attempts to create a program that fits the needs of novice and beginner trainees and addresses the haptic and the visual elements of procedures. This approach allows for introduction to the procedure and limited individual practice. It does not provide the opportunity for deliberate practice over long periods of time.[8] The use of a fresh or lightly embalmed cadaver has the advantage of realistic practice while optimizing patient safety. It does require preprocedural coordination, a strong support system in the anatomy department, and some cost for laboratory space, cadaver, C-arm fluoroscopy, and the necessary supplies. Available part-task training devices are not optimal for arthrography simulation, and it is possible that physical or computer-based simulators may be developed in the future that will reduce or eliminate the need for cadaver use in arthrographic SBT.

Formal physical and mental task analysis for arthrography has not yet been performed at LSUHSC-NO. Nevertheless, the curriculum and simulations are informed by fellowship-trained and experienced musculoskeletal radiologists as content experts.[9] The program continues to refine evaluation techniques to develop more critical and reproducible objective assessment.[1] Face validity is considered present in the cadaveric approach for SBT. The

Table 19.6 Shoulder Table IV: Advantages and disadvantages of different arthographic approaches to the shoulder joint. Courtesy Micheal Maristany

Anterior vs posterior shoulder joint needle approaches for arthrography:

1. Anterior approach:

   Advantages: Larger target, easier positioning for patients with poor mobility

   Disadvantages: Possible spurious injection of the subscapularis; if the rotator interval anterior approach is attempted, biceps tendon, subdeltoid/subacromial bursa and subcoracoid bursa spurious injection is possible.

2. Posterior approach:

   Advantages: There are fewer structures along the path of the injection site. Most shoulder pain and instability is anterior. Posterior approach is less likely to obscure pathology with the tract of the needle and lidocaine injection.

   Disadvantages: Positioning for the exam is less well tolerated and requires better mobility of the shoulder.

group participating at this institution is currently too small to attempt more rigorous validity studies.[10,11] It is important for a radiology department to be actively involved in simulation in the interests of continuous patient safety and the efficient, effective learning of trainees. The medical specialties of anesthesia and surgery have already developed advanced SBT; robust simulation programs are necessary in musculoskeletal radiology and will develop with the validation of simulation devices, methods, and metrics for trainee performance evaluation.

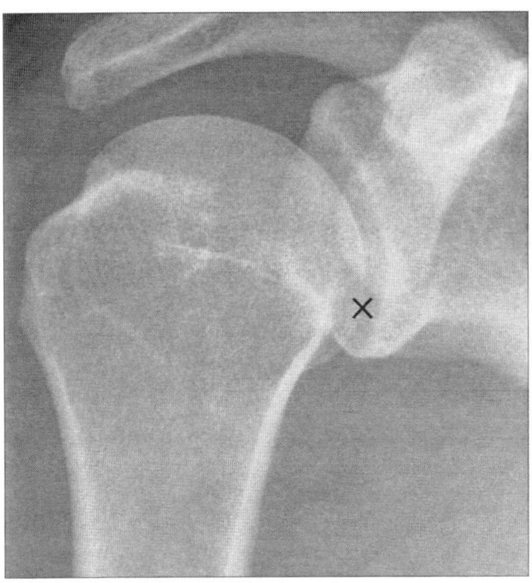

FIGURE 19.1 Glenohumeral joint injection anterior approach: target site for injection is at the junction of the middle and inferior third of the anterior aspect of the glenohumeral joint. Courtesy Stephanie Casey.

The LSUHSC-NO radiology simulation program elected to begin with MSK procedures using a relatively high-fidelity fresh cadaver simulation. There are, of course, other types of MSK simulations that can be created. For example, a computerized data bank of practice cases can be created at the institutional level. The cases can be presented as unknowns to be reported, with comparison and other studies available for correlation (i.e., high fidelity). Alternatively, they can be presented with questions to be answered and scored (i.e., intermediate fidelity). These approaches to simulation of image-based radiology procedures are utilized at the American College of Radiology (ACR) Learning Center and have been described in the medical literature for some time.[12,13] This approach, with the periodic oversight of a subject matter expert, may be quite useful in facilitating deliberate practice which, it has been argued, is the basis for expertise and mastery.[8]

CONCLUSION

The residents at LSUHSC-NO have reported simulation on fresh cadavers to be useful in increasing their confidence and understanding, as well as their skill at joint injection. Another center has reported a similar experience to that cited above.[4] Many other potential uses for SBT in musculoskeletal radiology exist, including computer-based simulation of cases. The literature will grow over the next several years as simulation in medical education becomes pervasive.

SIMULATION VIDEO

A video of a simulated shoulder arthrogram by posterior joint approach technique can be accessed at: http://www.medschool.lsuhsc.edu/radiology/

REFERENCES

1. Satava RM. The revolution in medical education—the role of simulation. *JGME.* 2009;1:172–175.
2. Becker, G. Simulation and the coming transformation of medical education and training. *Radiology.* 2007;245:7–9.
3. Stevens D. Finding safety in medical education. *Qual Saf Health Care.* 2002;11;109–110.
4. Dieudonne G, Mooney S, Bricker K, et al. A return to basics: a novel way to learn to perform musculoskeletal procedures. Paper presented at the 58th Annual Meeting of the Association of University Radiologists; March 23–26, 2010. San Diego, CA.
5. Batalden P, Leach D, Swing S, et al. General competencies accreditation in graduate medical education: an antidote to overspecification in the education of medical specialists. *Health Affairs.* 2002; 21:103–111. See also http://www.acgme.org
6. Dreyfus S, Dreyfus H. *A Five-Stage Model of the Mental Activities Involved in Directed Skill Acquisition.* University of California, Berkeley, Operations Research Center ORC-80-2; 1980;1–18.
7. Leach D. Changing education to improve patient care. *Qual Health Care.* 2001;10;ii54–ii58.
8. Ericsson KA, Krampe R Th, Tesch-Romer C. The role of deliberate practice in the acquisition of expert performance. *Psychol Rev.* 1993;100;363–406.
9. Johnson S, Healey A, Evans J, et al. Physical and cognitive task analysis in interventional radiology. *Clin Radiol.* 2006;61:97–103.
10. Gould D, Patel A, Becker G, et al. SIR/RSNA/CIRSE Joint Medical Simulation Task Force strategic plan executive summary. *J Vasc Interv Radiol.* 2007;18:953–955.
11. Dawson S. Procedural simulation: a primer. *Radiology.* 2006;241:7–25.
12. American College of Radiology. Education Center; Musculoskeletal MRI. Accessed June 29, 2011, at http://www.acr.org
13. Towbin A, Paterson, Chang P. Computer-based simulator for radiology: an educational tool. *Radiographics.* 2008;28:209–316.

20

Simulation in Vascular and Interventional Radiology

CHRISTOPHER VARGO, MALACHI G. SHEAHAN III, VERONICA CRISOSTOMO AYALA, HECTOR FERRAL, LEONARD R. BOK, AND THEA MORAN

ALTHOUGH SIMULATION in its current form is relatively new to radiology, many emerging viewpoints and trends related to it have already generated some controversy. The prospect of replacing traditional medical educational models with virtual reality (VR) and dramatically increasing the place of simulation in graduate medical education (GME) is now an actively discussed topic. Some postgraduate training programs, particularly anesthesia,[1] emergency medicine,[2,3] and surgery[4] already utilize simulation-based training (SBT) in one form or another. The requirement by the U.S. Food and Drug Administration (FDA) that simulation be part of the preparation for physicians to perform carotid angioplasty[5] is a strong indication that SBT is needed and can become part of the curriculum for GME in all aspects of interventional radiology (IR). Aspects of SBT in vascular and interventional radiology and in vascular surgery are presented in this chapter.

SIMULATION-BASED TRAINING IN INTERVENTIONAL RADIOLOGY

The goal of fellowship training in IR is to produce physicians who demonstrate competency in all aspects of minimally invasive vascular and nonvascular intervention.[6] Competency includes not only the technical skills required to perform a procedure safely but also the nontechnical skills inherent in day-to-day practice in the IR suite.[7] Such nontechnical skills include decision-making, communication, and teamwork.[7] Fellowship training in IR, as well as any GME in the United States, is primarily based on the master–apprentice educational model. In the apprenticeship model, fellows learn vascular and interventional procedures on patients under the supervision of an attending physician trained and experienced in the procedures.[8] Several scientific papers have discussed significant limitations of the master–apprentice model for medical postgraduate training. These include time-based (rather than proficiency-based) advancement of trainees, lack of uniformity in training criteria, decreased mentor clinical productivity while concentrating on apprentice training, increased procedure times for trainees, increased medicolegal costs, and most importantly, the potential for suboptimal results or injury to patients.[6–8]

In addition, the apprenticeship model is largely subjective, since it is predominantly based on the evaluations of mentors and sometimes lacks a structured educational basis.[8] According to Patel and Gould,[8] evaluations under these circumstances are susceptible to a host of errors and bias including *central tendency* (i.e., using the middle of the performance scale as an average), *recency error* (i.e., increased weight given to recent performance), *leniency error* (i.e., rating all trainees highly), *halo effect* (i.e., undue influence of a positive trait in a trainee), *harshness error* (i.e., rating all trainees strictly without justification), and *similarity error* (i.e., rating a trainee highly for traits similar to those of the evaluator).[8] Hospital credentialing in the realm of endovascular procedures has largely been based on the maintenance of a logbook from residency and fellowship delineating the number of various procedures performed.[9] Such a log may indicate involvement in a procedure, but it does not actually confirm proficiency.[9] Finally, trainee exposure to the appropriate number of endovascular procedures needed to achieve proficiency has grown increasingly difficult.

Continued technological developments in noninvasive imaging have largely eliminated the less complex diagnostic angiograms with which trainees could begin to master their catheter and guidewire skills.[6,10] In addition, increasing interest in endovascular procedures from other specialties in medicine has had a significant effect on the numbers of endovascular procedures performed in the IR suite. If adequate numbers of endovascular procedures cannot be maintained, IR fellowship training programs face increased risk for Residency Review Committee (RRC) citations, probation, or even loss of accreditation from the Accreditation Council for Graduate Medical Education (ACGME). The loss of basic endovascular procedures to noninvasive imaging, combined with the increasing division of caseload between multiple specialties, limits the trainee's ability to acquire the basic angiography skills "upon which more advanced interventional skills are based."[11] Without the availability of these basic procedures to hone essential technical skills, patients may be placed at risk as trainees attempt to acquire them in increasingly difficult endovascular procedures. These shortcomings of the master–apprenticeship training model have combined with the increasing emphasis on patient safety to shift the traditional educational paradigm and to bring endovascular simulation to the forefront.[8,12]

Dawson[13] has defined medical simulation as "the creation of an educational environment in which learning occurs through the use of a device, mannequin, or team, without the presence of an actual patient."[8,13] Four main categories of medical simulators have been used for endovascular training. They include synthetic/physical models, animal models, human cadavers, and VR machines.[7]

Synthetic or physical models are generally simple, inexpensive, reusable (to an extent), and portable.[7] An example is the use of mannequins for cardiopulmonary resuscitation training. Endovascular training has utilized various plastic models of the arterial system to allow trainees to practice vessel catheterization, balloon angioplasty, and stent placement, as well as to provide low-fidelity SBT of basic tasks.[7,14]

Animal models have a higher degree of face validity and can allow full procedural simulation.[7] Their use, however, is significantly limited by availability, high cost, species anatomic differences, lack of comparable pathology, and ethical debates.[7,15]

A human cadaver model connected to a mechanical pump has been used to simulate the arterial system for endovascular procedures. These simulations allow life-like replication of the arterial system with high fidelity and high face validity.[7,15] They also allow full procedural simulation and can be used repeatedly. If a stent or coils are deployed or embolic particle vessel occlusion is performed, that portion of the arterial system can no longer be used.[15] The main limitations of the cadaveric model includes high cost and subject availability.[7,15]

Virtual reality hybrid simulators are physical models attached to a computer interface that enables the trainee to navigate through the virtual environment with the use of instruments or catheters.[8] The benefits of VR simulators include the ability to capture specific data, the ability to record video/audio input, device reusability, minimal setup requirements, the potential for trainee assessment using computer-acquired metrics, and a high degree of realism.[7,8,16,17] Disadvantages include their cost, maintenance, and acceptability, as well as the present unavailability of true three-dimensional models in the VR format.[7]

In terms of endovascular simulation, several industry-created VR simulators are currently available. They include the CathLabVR Simulator (CAE Healthcare, Montreal, Canada), SimSuite® (Medical Simulation Corporation, Denver, Colorado), Vascular Intervention Simulation Trainer™ (VIST™) and Vascular Intervention Simulation Trainer—(VIST-C™) (Mentice, Gothenburg, Sweden), and the ANGIO Mentor™ (Simbionix, Cleveland, Ohio).[7] These devices not only allow trainees to manipulate guidewires and catheters in a "virtual patient" vascular system but provide some realistic haptic feedback that mimics the touch or "feel" of the procedure. These simulators offer various procedural modules. They include coronary angiography, coronary artery intervention, peripheral angiography, neurangiographic intervention, carotid artery intervention, renal angiography, renal artery intervention, iliac and superficial femoral artery intervention, and below-the-knee arterial intervention. Multiple case scenarios are available or can be constructed to present increasing levels of difficulty. Additional specific modules include abdominal aortic aneurysm (AAA) repair, aortic valve intervention, coronary sinus lead placement, electrophysiology (EP) ablation, cardiac transseptal puncture, foramen ovale closure, inferior vena cava filter placement, uterine artery embolization, and various peripheral embolization procedures, such as renal artery embolization, renal arteriovenous malformation/arteriovenous fistula embolization, selective arterial embolization for gastrointestinal bleeding, trauma embolization, and post AAA repair endoleak embolization.

Clinical simulation involving hemodynamic monitoring, complication management, and drug administration is also available. Various simulators are also able to provide post-procedure feedback with automated assessment of specific metrics (i.e., measures) of performance.[8] Now that these simulators have become available, the question becomes whether their use will translate into improved endovascular skills, reduced numbers of procedural errors, and improved patient care. Clinical simulators for laparoscopy, colonoscopy, and anesthesia have already been successfully validated.[9] To this end, the Society of Interventional Radiology (SIR), the Radiological Society of North America (RSNA), and the Cardiovascular and Interventional Radiological Society of Europe (CIRSE) have created a Joint Medical Simulation Task Force charged with "guiding the implementation of a robust infrastructure and process to support IR simulation development, assessment, validation, application, and dissemination."[6]

Multiple studies have been performed with various endovascular simulators in an attempt to confirm or refute their validity. These studies generally attempt to measure either trainee efficiency or procedural quality.[16] According to Duncan and Glaiberman,[16] efficiency in angiography can be measured by procedure time, amount of contrast medium injected, fluoroscopy time, supply use, and/or the number of catheter exchanges. Quality is usually measured by the computer-generated metrics provided by the simulators, based on such factors as stent diameter, residual stenosis, stent position, and vessel wall contact or scraping.[16] Glaiberman et al[18] studied IR fellows and staff during renal artery stenosis simulations on the Mentice VIST™ simulators. An "efficiency index" was created based on fluoroscopy time, procedure time, tools used, and the volume of contrast medium injected. The study reported a direct correlation between the experience and efficiency (i.e., efficiency index score) of the fellow or staff member being assessed, a finding that suggests construct validity.[18] Evidence of efficiency on a simulator or the successful participation in SBT of basic catheter techniques does not in itself ensure trainee proficiency in a procedural skill or his or her ability to perform a procedure in a quality manner.[7] For example, a study by Berry et al[19] compared experienced interventional radiologists to novices during a simulation of carotid artery stent placement. This study looked at the performance metrics provided by the Procedicus VIST™ simulator and concluded that, with the exception of performance time and fluoroscopic time used, construct validity of the other VIST™ metrics (i.e., contrast medium volume used, cine loops, tool/lesion ratio, lesion coverage, stent placement accuracy, and residual stenosis) was not confirmed. Ahmed et al[7] compared the results of 13 different studies involving simulator training and technical skills. A wide variability of results was found, with some studies suggesting construct validity and others unable to confirm this finding. It was concluded that "key questions about the exact role of the existing simulators in training programs remain and that they at this point will only function as an adjunct to... traditional teaching."[7] The SIR/RSNA/CIRSE task force recognizes the current deficiencies in evidence supporting the use of endovascular simulators.[10,11,20] The Task Force has noted that current simulator models are appropriate for gaining some aspects of endovascular experience, such as the correct sequence of procedural steps or the selection of appropriate tools,[10,11,20] but the ability of endovascular simulators to facilitate the acquisition of catheter manipulation skills is still unproved.[8]

TECHNICAL CONSIDERATIONS OF ENDOVASCULAR PROCEDURES

Given the strong movement toward the integration of simulation into training curricula, it is appropriate to review peripheral endovascular techniques and interventions. This wide spectrum of procedures will need to be included in a comprehensive curriculum, including vascular procedural simulation. The subsections below describe knowledge- and technical-based elements of some key peripheral endovascular techniques.

Diagnostic Catheter Angiography

Diagnostic angiography is the visualization and diagnostic evaluation of arterial vessels via direct catheterization and contrast medium injection.[21] Utilizing the Seldinger technique, a needle, flexible tip guidewire, and vascular sheath and/or catheter are passed into the lumen of an artery.[22] Manipulation of a catheter inserted through a 5- or 6-French vascular sheath can usually allow access into most arterial systems within the body. Arterial access is usually achieved via retrograde entry into the common femoral artery because it is large, superficial, and has the lowest risk of complications.[22] Additional sites of arterial access include brachial or radial access, or antegrade femoral access.[21,22]

Imaging of the arterial and/or venous systems usually occurs via digital subtraction angiography (DSA). During DSA, acquisition of a noncontrast image is first obtained and used to subtract the background from each subsequent contrast image.[23] The "subtracted" image reveals only the opacified blood vessels.[23] Due to high-image resolution, DSA is largely still considered the gold standard in arterial imaging. Diagnostic angiography, however, is an invasive procedure with complication risks (i.e., access site vascular injury, contrast media reactions, radiation exposure, contrast-induced nephropathy, stroke, peripheral embolization, and death).[21] The risk of potential complications from invasive DSA has led to the adoption of noninvasive imaging methods for routine vascular imaging. Computerized tomography angiography (CTA) and magnetic resonance angiography (MRA) have largely replaced catheter angiography for simple diagnostic vascular examinations. Several studies have shown MRA and CTA to be comparable to DSA in diagnostic image quality, especially within the aortoiliac, femoral, and popiteal arterial distributions.[24,25] Computed tomography angiography may be limited by vessel wall calcification (e.g., within the infrapopliteal arteries).[24,25]

Technique of Abdominal Aortography and Lower Extremity Angiography

Arterial access is usually achieved via retrograde entry into a common femoral artery via single-wall puncture with a micropuncture (i.e., 21-gauge) needle.[21,23] A 0.018-inch guidewire is passed through the needle, which is then replaced with a transition 4-French micropuncture catheter. The inner dilator of the micropuncture catheter is removed allowing passage of a 0.035-inch flexible tip guidewire with straight or J curved tip, which is then used to secure access into the aorta.[22,23] The micropuncture catheter is then removed and replaced with a 5-French vascular sheath that allows atraumatic catheter exchanges. A 5-French pigtail or Omniflush catheter is advanced over the wire, through the vascular sheath, into the abdominal aorta to the T12 vertebral body level. A biplane pressure-injected aortogram may then be obtained in slightly oblique anteroposterior (AP) and lateral projections.

The aortogram catheter is then withdrawn to a level just above the aortic bifurcation. A pelvic angiogram may then be performed.[21] Oblique imaging (i.e. 25–30 degrees) of the pelvis is indicated to allow visualization of the ipsilateral iliac artery bifurcation and contralateral femoral artery bifurcation.[21] A DSA of the right and left lower extremities is then performed utilizing a bolus chase technology. In the setting of critical limb ischemia and/or nonhealing wounds, selective catheterization of the popliteal artery is considered in order to allow optimal visualization of the infrapopliteal arteries.

Thoracic Aortography and Upper Extremity Angiography

After arterial access and sheath placement, a pigtail catheter is positioned in the ascending thoracic aorta 6–8 cm above the aortic valve, and a thoracic aortogram is obtained in the oblique 45-degree left anterior oblique (LAO) position. This allows optimal visualization of the brachiocephalic vessels. In the setting of trauma, an additional right anterior oblique (RAO) aortic arch arteriogram can be obtained in order to exclude occult injury. Selective catheterization of the subclavian arteries can be performed with a JB1, JB2, vertebral, or other catheter.[21,22] For older individuals with tortuosity of the thoracic aorta, or for those patients with a left common carotid artery origin from the innominate artery (i.e., bovine arch configuration), a Simmons or Vitek catheter may be needed.[21]

Angioplasty and Stenting of Aortoiliac Disease

Peripheral artery disease is estimated to affect as many as 12 million Americans.[26] Successful treatment requires lifestyle modification, medical management, and, when appropriate, endovascular intervention.[27] Surgical repair, including arterial bypass grafting or endarterectomy, has proven effective in providing long-term arterial patency with relief of symptoms. A significant perioperative mortality, however, has been reported.[28] As a result, endovascular treatment is often favored as the first line of treatment. The Trans Atlantic Inter Society Consensus (TASC) working group published standard guidelines for the surgical and endovascular treatment of arterial disease.[29,30] Current official recommendations include balloon angioplasty with or without stenting as initial therapy for TASC A- and TASC B-type lesions. These lesions include single-stenosis of less than 3 cm, single stenosis of 3–10 cm in length, two stenoses of less than 5 cm in length, or a single occlusion.[30,31] Since the development of the TASC guidelines, refinement of endovascular techniques, as well as the development of nitinol stents, has led to increasing utilization of endovascular treatment of extensive aortoiliac disease (i.e., TASC C and D lesions) that was originally reserved for surgical therapy. A meta-analysis performed by Jongkind et al[28] reported 4- and 5-year primary and secondary patency rates that ranged from 60% to 86% and 80% to 98%, respectively. According to this study, the primary patency rate of endovascular therapy was below that of surgical treatment, but secondary patency rates were comparable to operative repair.[27]

Angioplasty and Stenting of Femoral Popliteal Arterial Disease

Original TASC guidelines recommended angioplasty and, if needed, stenting for type A lesions with no specific recommendations for type B and C lesions.[32] Surgical bypass was the treatment of choice for TASC type D lesions.[33] The overall long-term primary patency rates of angioplasty and stenting have been disappointing in the treatment of superficial femoral and popliteal arteries.[34] Angioplasty has a reported 3-year primary patency rate of approximately 50%.[34] Patency rates of nitinol stents placed within the superficial femoral and popliteal arteries appear more promising, with 1- and 2-year patency rates between 76% and 97% and 60% and 84%, respectively.[34] In general, angioplasty and stenting compares favorably with surgical bypass for TASC A and B lesions within the femoral popliteal arterial distribution.[35] Patency rates for TASC C and D lesions are less encouraging, and they are not yet comparable to surgery. Decisions to treat TASC C and D lesions with endovascular therapy should be based on quality-of-life issues, patient preference, short-term healing goals, and increased surgical risk due to additional patient comorbidities.[35]

SIMULATION-BASED TRAINING IN VASCULAR SURGERY

Training in vascular surgery has undergone a dramatic paradigm shift over the past two decades. Advances in technology, devices, and techniques have thrust the specialty from a general surgery niche into an entirely new field, with its own independent certification and training programs. Currently, four different residency pathways are offered in vascular surgery, each with its own advocates.[36] An advocacy for less-invasive endovascular procedures has created a reduced volume of open surgical cases in the United States.[37] This situation is especially true with complex aortic cases, leading some to question how trainees will learn to perform these inherently difficult procedures.

Government emphasis on quality care, increased patient safety, and cost reduction has also placed a strain on residency programs. Continued resident duty hour restrictions[38] emphasize the need for more efficient surgical instruction. In this environment, simulation could be a valuable asset for training vascular surgeons. Simulators offer the ability to perform multiple procedures without facing the real-life challenges of anesthesia induction, operating room schedules, and copious paperwork. Additionally, simulation can allow repeated, deliberate practice of the same intervention without risk to a human patient. With proper integration, simulation may offer a more economic use of training time, perhaps the most valuable resource of a residency program.

SIMULATOR TYPES

Numerous low- and high-fidelity endovascular simulation devices exist for vascular surgical training, each with its own benefits and shortcomings. These devices can be broadly characterized into four categories: synthetic, cadaveric, animal, and VR.[7] Synthetic models range from low- to extremely high-fidelity. Blood vessel anatomy can be synthetically simulated using models as simple as a plastic tube or as complex as multimaterial sculptures (see Figure 20.1). Synthetic models can also be created for endovascular use. Systems of pressurized tubes can be used for simulated stent placement and catheter manipulation (see Figure 20.2).

Synthetic models can be inexpensive and are the most widely available tools for vascular simulation. Cadaveric models are excellent for SBT related to dissection, vascular exposure, and anastomosis creation. Fresh, thawed, unembalmed cadaver specimens have tissue handling properties (i.e., haptics) that are especially useful for mimicking live patients. Cadaver use in vascular surgery training is limited by availability and cost. Animal models can be used to simulate human procedures with extremely high fidelity. Their usefulness, however, is limited by the need for special handling facilities and staff, as well as by ethical and legal considerations. Virtual reality simulators can depict the vascular system with extremely high fidelity and allow for the performance of a variety of simulated interventional procedures (see Figure 20.3). These devices have the advantage of including standardized metric assessments. Virtual reality simulators allow learners to perform repeated, identical tasks until techniques are mastered (i.e., deliberate practice), possibly shortening the learning curve a trainee must usually experience in actual patient procedures. By downloading an actual patient's specific anatomy from radiologic studies such as CTAs or DSAs, these devices can be used for preoperative planning. This technique allows the surgeon to practice a real procedure in advance, helping him or her to select the operative approach and the device(s) for the actual intervention in advance. Virtual reality simulators are usually very costly and require dedicated staff to implement software updates and calibration.

THE USE OF SIMULATION IN TEACHING VASCULAR SURGERY

When considering SBT in vascular surgery, it is important to differentiate its use for *teaching* from its use for *testing*, realizing that it has helped to revolutionize both components of training. Other than some skill lab incorporation, guidelines from the ACGME with regard to SBT in vascular surgery remain less than clear. Additionally, at this time, none of the U.S. specialty boards accepts SBT experience as a proxy for patient case logs. Exposure to simulation varies among vascular fellowship training programs, with the high cost and maintenance of endovascular simulation devices precluding their use in some small training programs. One proposed lower-cost alternative is to set up regional centers where vascular surgery fellows can travel periodically for short training sessions.[39]

Evidence for simulator use in vascular training demonstrates that standardized simulation-based teaching methods may lead to more efficient trainee skill acquisition, particularly at the novice level.[40] As trainees advance, higher-fidelity models seem to offer more benefit.[41] Interestingly, training on endovascular

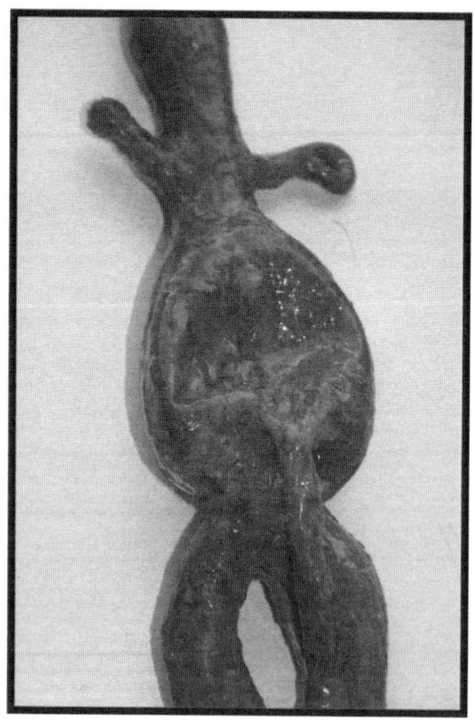

FIGURE 20.1 Synthetic simulation model of the abdominal aorta with aneurysm.

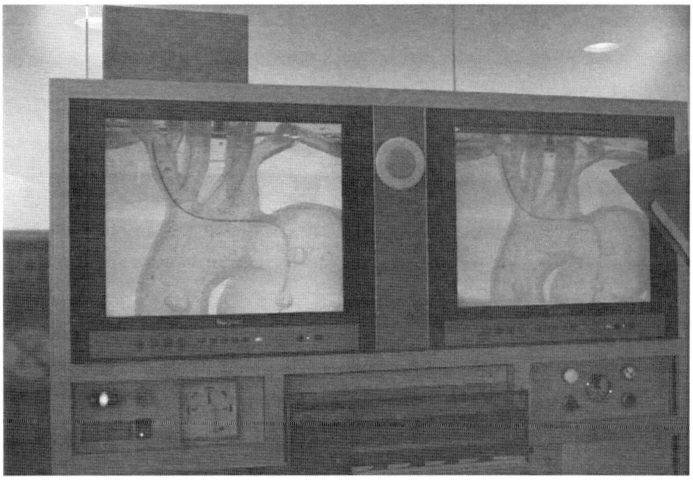

FIGURE 20.2 Systems of pressurized tubes for simulation.

simulators results in a subjective improvement in skills that may translate to applied skills in the operative theater.[42,43] Additionally, exposure to vascular simulation at the medical student level increases interest in vascular surgery as a specialty and helps to develop technical skills.[44] Although the effectiveness of simulation in vascular education needs continued validation, standardized simulation remains a part of most proposed vascular training strategies.[37,45–47]

THE USE OF SIMULATION IN TESTING IN VASCULAR SURGERY

Formal testing of surgical dexterity is not a modern concept. Fellowship in the Royal College of Surgeons of England required a technical skill examination through the early 1940s. In the United States, the American Board of Surgery conducted intraoperative assessments on prospective candidates through 1952. Both practices were halted due to logistical problems, such as time, cost, and standardization.[7]

In a prospective randomized trial, residents' scores on the multiple choice American Board of Surgery In-Training Exam (ABSITE) did not correlate with their technical ability, as measured by either skill testing or intraoperative assessment.[47] This fact supports the findings of a pilot study in technical skills assessment conducted as part of the European Board of Surgery Qualification in Vascular Surgery examination in 2002. European candidates performed a saphenofemoral junction ligation and a tibial artery anastomosis on open models. Additionally, dexterity was assessed with a knot-tying test. Internal consistency was demonstrated among the three technical exams, but the study found no correlation between technical ability and the candidates' scores on an oral knowledge examination. Also, no correlation existed between the individuals' operative experience, as reported by case logs and their technical performance.[7,48] Currently, the multiple choice Vascular Surgery In-Training Exam (VSITE) is the only standardized test given during vascular surgery residency, and no standardized method exists for surgical skill evaluation. In most programs, direct observation has been the only assessment tool utilized for the appraisal of

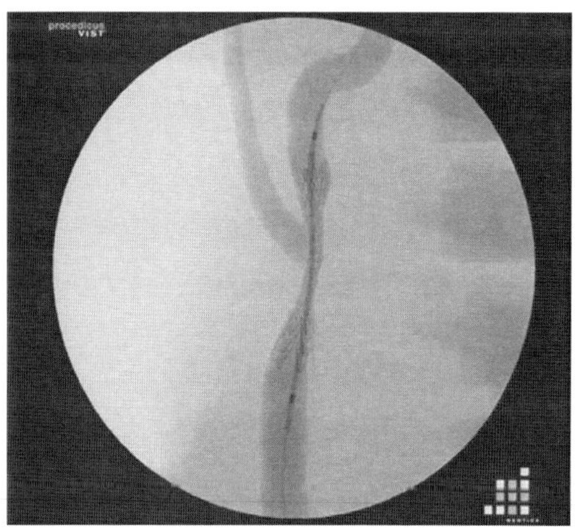

FIGURE 20.3 Virtual reality simulation of carotid artery stent procedure.

technical ability. Simulation-directed surgical skill testing offers a potential solution to these issues.

Some evidence exists supporting simulation as a valid means of skill testing in vascular surgery. Two studies have shown that performance of a carotid endarterectomy on a bench-top model can discriminate senior from junior trainees, but this ability to differentiate between trainee skills was lost when comparing individuals at more advanced levels of training.[49] The reason for this failure is more due to the fact that higher-level trainees have more likely mastered the technical skills related to carotid endarterectomy. Hence, their performances on a part-task trainer are similar. Furthermore, these bench models do not properly evaluate complex decision-making and crisis resolution In other words, technical competence on a bench model may not translate into an independent environment. Evaluating technical competence during a crisis situation, therefore, may help delineate between skill levels among advanced trainees. Simulated procedures in high-fidelity operating room theaters have been used successfully in this regard.[50]

Further research is also necessary to determine the ideal method for evaluating the trainees' performance on the simulator. The Imperial College Surgical Assessment Device uses electromagnetic sensors to track hand movements.[7] Economy of motion during simple tasks such as knot tying has been shown to correlate well with dexterity in complex procedures. No correlation between economy of motion and endovascular skill has yet been demonstrated. Virtual reality systems can often offer direct feedback metrics, such as procedure time, fluoroscopy time, handling errors, and contrast volume. Observer assessments can be performed with checklists, global assessments, or some hybrid method.[7]

SPECIAL CONSIDERATION: SIMULATION FOR CAROTID INTERVENTIONS

Perhaps more so than in any other vascular bed, simulation can play a vital role in instructing interventions in the cervical carotid artery circulation. Carotid stents were first approved by the FDA in 2004, for the prevention of stroke. Since carotid artery interventions provide a small absolute risk reduction for stroke, even a rare technical error can override a surgeon's margin of efficacy. Additionally, small missteps during a carotid stent placement can result in severe morbidity and even mortality. Clearly, carotid artery stent procedures must be assiduously learned prior to attempting independent performance. Only a few high-volume centers for carotid artery stent placement exist, however. Additionally, a paucity of experts is available to train novices. With this in mind, the FDA has mandated SBT experience prior to placing these new devices in patients.

Training on VR simulators has been shown to reduce fluoroscopy time, handling errors, and volume of contrast medium used in carotid interventions.[51] Improvement in technical performance has been demonstrated in both novice and experienced users[52,53] with the use of simulators. Of particular interest is the practice of SBT for individual case preparation or "mission rehearsal." Such pre-procedure preparation using simulation has demonstrated benefits in the preoperative selection of catheters, stents, and embolic protection devices, as well as the reduction of operative time and contrast medium volume.[54,55] Mission rehearsal can also be expanded to include the entire team of doctors, nurses, and technicians in a simulated operative suite.[56] One future benefit of simulation in carotid artery interventions will likely involve the initial training of novices. Prior to the performance of a carotid stent procedure in an actual patient, trainees can be instructed exclusively on a VR simulator until a predetermined benchmark of competency is demonstrated (i.e., proficiency-driven training). This model of skills acquisition will theoretically help reduce the morbidity associated with an interventionalist's learning curve as he or she becomes facile with carotid artery interventions.

Bench models for carotid endarterectomy have proved a valid tool for assessing basic skills, but advanced practitioners may require higher-fidelity instruction, such as occurs using a simulated operating room.[49,50] As simulation expands in training programs, a better understanding of its role will be evident in teaching and testing, complex decision-making, and crisis resolution.

THE FUTURE OF SIMULATION IN VASCULAR EDUCATION

In 2008, the Association of Program Directors in Vascular Surgery (APDVS) established an ad hoc simulation committee to address the need for standardization of simulation use in vascular training. The committee is currently working on a comprehensive curriculum for endovascular skills training, as well as on models for skills courses and standardized skill assessments. Obviously, the archetype is the work performed by the Fundamentals of Laparoscopic Surgery (FLS) committee formed by the Society of American

Gastrointestinal and Endoscopic Surgeons in the late 1990s.[57] Further studies are needed as consideration develops for integration of simulation into vascular surgery training. As further validation of these new training methods and assessment tools is provided, a more efficient and productive educational system will develop. At least one multicenter, randomized trial is currently under way to help determine the effect of a simulation-based curriculum on trainee performance. Eventually, evidence will need to accrue that SBT is successful in performing the ultimate goal: global improvement of patient outcomes.

PORCINE MODEL FOR THE TRANSJUGULAR INTRAHEPATIC PORTOSYSTEMIC SHUNT PROCEDURE

The transjugular intrahepatic portosystemic shunt (TIPS) is one of the most complex and technically difficult procedures performed in interventional radiology.[58–62] Teaching the technique for this procedure in the conventional fashion (i.e., in real time on a patient) is difficult. TIPS is performed in patients who suffer from chronic liver disease. The procedure in itself is technically difficult, and most patients with chronic portal hypertension have challenging and altered anatomy (i.e., a small hard liver, ascites, small hepatic veins, and small portal veins). If a trainee performing the procedure is inexperienced, it is not uncommon for the more experienced operator to take over the case when technical difficulties arise, thus, limiting the trainee's full "hands-on" learning experience. Simulation-based training is perfectly suited for training individuals in such circumstances, helping trainees gain experience in a difficult procedure prior to attempting it on patients. The porcine simulation model for TIPS has been successfully employed both for research[63,64] and for training purposes[65] prior to TIPS procedure performance in a patient. Its description in SBT follows.

Animal Preparation

The porcine model is an excellent simulation model for the TIPS procedure. Typically 35 to 45 kg Large White swine are employed since the hepatic vascular anatomy is very similar to human anatomy. The procedure is performed with the animal under general anesthesia. It is prepared by a veterinarian with expertise in swine anesthesia. The procedure must be conducted in compliance with the Guide for the Care and Use of Laboratory Animals and/or any other applicable local regulations. In addition, before beginning any training, approval of the model by the Institutional Animal Care and Use Committee (IACUC) is required.

After a 24-hour fast, the animal is premedicated by intramuscular injection of a combination of diazepam (0.1 mg/kg), ketamine (10 mg/kg), and atropine sulphate (0.04 mg/kg). Anesthesia is induced with intravenous propofol (2 mg/kg) through a venous access in an ear marginal vein, and it is maintained, after orotracheal intubation, with 10% desflurane in oxygen. Ketorolac (1 mg/kg) and tramadol (1.5 mg/kg) can be administered as intraoperative analgesics. The pig is secured on the operating table in the supine decubitus position with caudal extension of the forelimbs. Under sterile conditions, a surgical access to the jugular vein is obtained, and an introducer sheath of adequate size is placed.

Procedural Details

The tools for the procedure in a porcine model are the standard tools used in a TIPS procedure, including a portal vein access system (e.g., RUPS-100, Ring set, Haskal set, Cook, Inc. Bloomington, Indiana, or the Angiodynamics set, Angiodynamics, Queensbury, New York), angiographic catheters and guidewires, angioplasty balloons, and stents (e.g., Wallstent[R], Boston Scientific, Natick, Massachusetts, or VIATORR[R], W.L. Gore, Flagstaff, Arizona). The training should be conducted with the TIPS set that the trainee will eventually use in his or her clinical practice. This alignment allows the trainee to become familiar with equipment that he or she will be using and makes it easier for the trainee to focus on the actual procedure itself rather than the instruments during his or her first attempts on patients.

Once the animal has been anesthetized, prepared, and jugular access has been secured, the trainee is then guided through the steps of the procedure in the standard fashion. The proctor carefully monitors the trainee's movements and will be able to correct any wrong maneuvers by direct instruction, without having to "take over" the case.

Considerations

ACCESS TO THE MOST SUITABLE HEPATIC VEIN

The swine has very similar hepatic vein anatomy to humans. The most suitable hepatic vein is catheterized

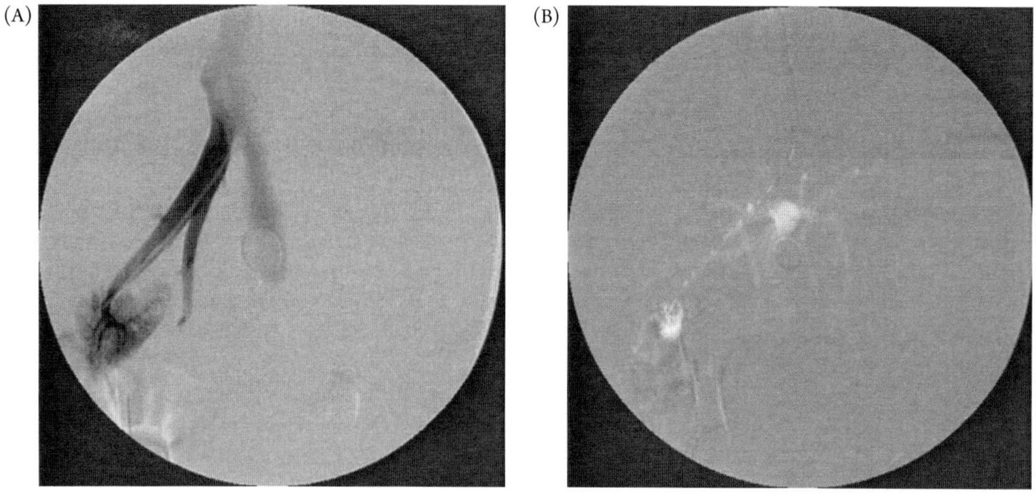

FIGURE 20.4 (A) Digital subtraction angiography (DSA) image of a hepatic venogram with iodinated contrast showing a widely patent right hepatic vein suitable to perform the transjugular intrahepatic portosystemic shunt (TIPS) procedure. (B) DSA image of a wedge hepatic venogram with CO_2 contrast with reflux of CO_2 into a patent portal vein.

by the trainee with the standard catheters and wires. At this stage, a free and wedge contrast venogram or a CO_2 venogram can be performed to ensure that the catheterized vein is the hepatic venous access of choice. (Figure 20.4 A,B). The swine model can also be used to teach the resident/fellow alternative portal vein localization techniques.

Once the optimal hepatic vein is secured and the location of the portal vein has been identified, then the TIPS equipment of choice is employed to perform the transhepatic puncture. The proctor can then guide the trainee in the use of the trocar needle and can point out the importance of needle direction to access the portal vein.

ACCESS INTO THE PORTAL VEIN

The trainee has the opportunity to try different maneuvers and techniques to advance the needle through the liver parenchyma to obtain access to the portal vein. This maneuver is probably the most difficult step of the procedure and, indeed, the most stressful to most operators (Figure 20.5 A,B).

Once the portal vein access is secured, then stent deployment and dilation is conducted (Figure 20.6 A–D). Again, training should involve the wires and stents that the trainee will eventually use in clinical practice. With these steps, a successful TIPS can be conducted in the swine model, as shown in the images.

TEACHING EXPERIENCE WITH THE SWINE MODEL

The swine simulation model for TIPS has been used for several years both in research[63,64] and training.[65] Experience has shown that the model is very useful, particularly for the novice trainee who has the "book" knowledge about the procedure but has not had the "hands-on" experience with it. In clinical practice, typically, the trainee assists in four to five procedures before he or she is allowed to take part as a primary operator. The advantage of using the swine model is that the trainee is allowed to be the primary operator from the beginning of the procedure, without the stress of having a live patient on the operating table. Several years of teaching physicians using this simulation model at international "hands-on" training courses in minimally invasive techniques has led one of the authors (Dr. Hector Ferral) to conclude that four to five swine procedures are needed by the novice trainee before he or she can be allowed to act as the operator in the unsupervised environment. If the trainee is in an environment where supervision is available, then one to two swine procedures may be sufficient to allow the trainee to become familiar with the steps of the procedure and to be able to function as a first operator under supervision by an experienced proctor.

The chief disadvantage of this animal model is that it is expensive and requires the availability of a

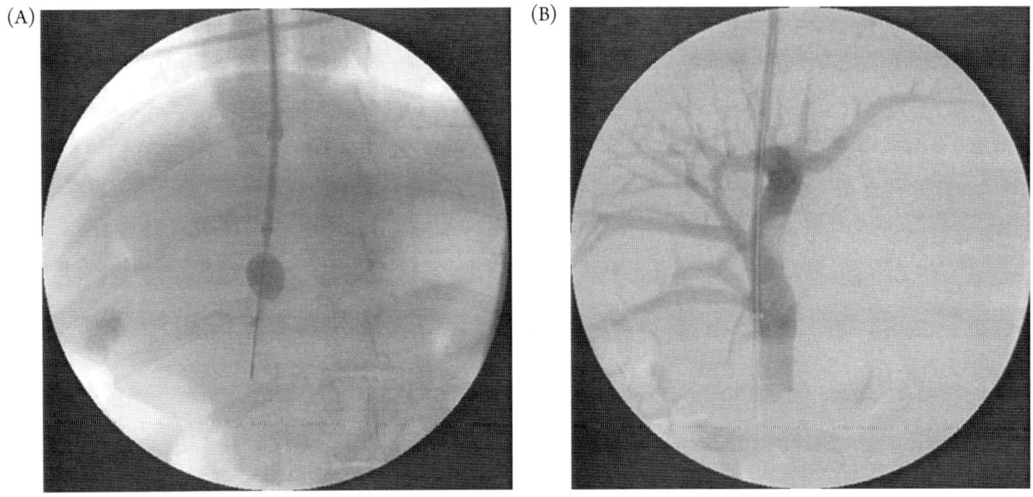

FIGURE 20.5 (A) Spot film demonstrates the access needle has been advanced through the liver parenchyma. (B) Digital subtraction portogram after successful entry into the portal venous system. The pig portal vein anatomy is very similar to the human portal vein.

fully staffed animal experimental laboratory. Additional disadvantages are moral objections by some groups and legal barriers in some jurisdictions. Based on early comparison of VR to porcine model training, it is possible that VR training may eventually successfully replace the porcine model for training purposes, yet its use for research purposes will likely persist.[65] A TIPS simulation, however, cannot be created and loaded onto a standard vascular simulator, which utilizes femoral artery access. TIPS simulation will require a device that provides simulated internal jugular vein access and VR TIPS procedure. In the meantime, until such a device becomes available and its validity for training proven, the porcine model certainly advances the interests of patient safety and efficient, effective training.

SIMULATION IN VENOUS ACCESS AND SOLID ORGAN PUNCTURE

Central and peripheral venous access are common procedures utilized by several subspecialities, including IR. Consequently, SBT in these techniques is an attractive teaching option and is taught in many simulation laboratories. Various peripheral venous simulators are available commercially for the practice of peripheral venous puncture. Central venous puncture part-task trainers, without or with ultrasound guidance capability, are also available. The most common SBT method utilized is via a vascular access mannequin, although other methods have been described.[66] For example, utilizing a specially prepared unembalmed cadaver with jell placed in the internal jugular vein is a potential but expensive method for jugular venous access SBT. Researchers have performed physical and cognitive task analysis for arterial and venous punctures.[67] Others authors have described methods to simulate ultrasound-guided procedures and needle puncture techniques.[68,69]

Solid organ puncture and other solid organ procedures may experience increased development of simulation devices over time. Researchers of Collaborators in Radiological Interventional Virtual Environments (CRaIVE) have performed physical and cognitive task analysis for both percutaneous transhepatic cholangiogram and nephrostomy.[70] A training system for endoscopic retrograde cholangiopancreatography (ERCP) exists, as well as novel approaches to training for percutaneous renal access using porcine kidneys or commercially available VR simulator (i.e., PERC Mentor™, Simbionix, Cleveland, Ohio).[71,72] Although these procedures are of particular interest to organ-based specialties, such as gastroenterology and urology, they have applications in IR as well. It is important, therefore, that IR be actively involved in the development, validation, and standardization of these simulation technologies and curricula. Simulation-based applications will become increasingly necessary for training in such procedures, given their increasing complexity and difficulty.

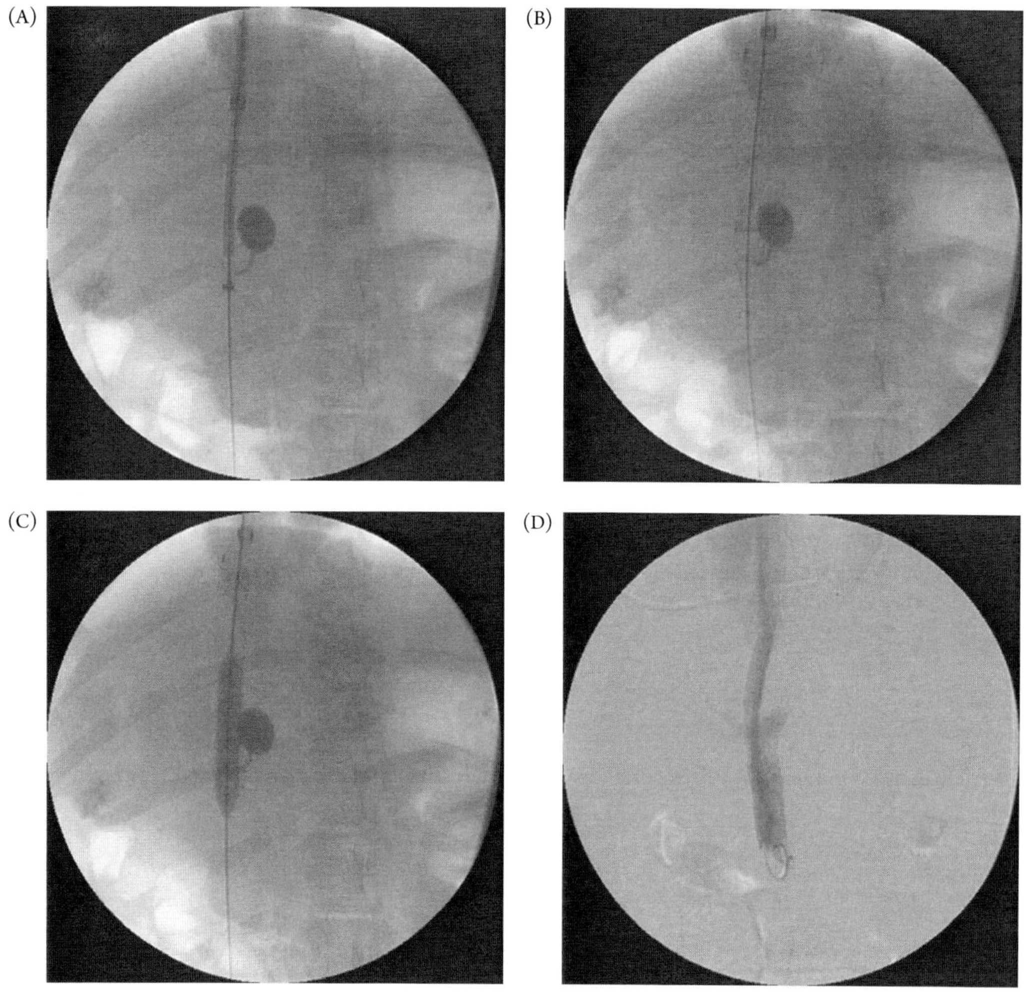

FIGURE 20.6 (A) Spot film during a pig transjugular intrahepatic portosystemic shunt (TIPS) shows the stent deployment step. A VIATORR stent (W.L. Gore, Flagstaff, Arizona) has been advanced into the portal vein and is still within the access sheath. (B) Spot film during a pig TIPS shows the stent deployment step. A VIATORR stent (W.L. Gore, Flagstaff, Arizona) has been successfully deployed within the portal vein through the transparenchymal tract. (C) The spot film demonstrates the stent dilation step. An angioplasty balloon has been employed to dilate the stent. (D) Digital subtraction portogram after completion of the procedure shows a widely patent TIPS.

CONCLUSION

Simulation in vascular and interventional radiology is an important topic with broad scope. It offers much promise for trainee development of skills in complex and sometimes hazardous procedures, without actual patient participation and risk.[73] Simulation devices are tools, not complete educational solutions. Validation of simulation technology and educational value must precede the regular curricular use of SBT for resident and fellow training in vascular and interventional radiology.

SIMULATION VIDEOS

Diagnostic and interventional vascular simulation videos may be accessed at: http://www.medschool.lsuhsc.edu/radiology/

REFERENCES

1. Gaba DM, Howard SK, Fish KJ, et al. Simulation-based training in anesthesia crisis resource management (ACRM): a decade of experience. *Simul Gaming.* 2001;32:175–193.

2. Ten Eyck RP. Simulation in emergency medicine training. *Pediatr Emerg Care.* 2011;27:333–341.

3. Okuda Y, Bond W, Bonfante G, et al. National growth in simulation training within emergency medicine residency programs, 2003–2008. *Acad Emerg Med.* 2008;15:1113–1116. [Epub August 20, 2008.]

4. Scott DJ, Dunnington GL. The new ACS/APDS skills curriculum: moving the learning curve out of the operating room. *J Gastrointest Surg.* 2008;12: 213–221.

5. Clair DG. Evolution of carotid stenting: regulatory issues. *Semin Vasc Surg.* 2008;12:64–68.

6. Gould D, Patel A, Becker G, et al. SIR/RSNA/ CIRSE Joint Medical Simulation Task Force strategic plan executive summary. *JVIR.* 2007;18:953–955.

7. Ahmed K, Keeling A, Fakhry M. Role of virtual reality simulation in teaching and assessing technical skills in endovascular intervention. *JVIR.* 2010;21: 55–66.

8. Patel A, Gould D. Simulators in interventional radiology training and evaluation: a paradigm shift is on the horizon. *JVIR.* 2006;17:S163-S173.

9. Gould DA. Interventional radiology simulation: prepare for a virtual revolution in training. *JVIR.* 2007;18:483–490.

10. Gould DA, Reekers JA. The role of simulation in training endovascular interventions. *Eur J. Vasc Endovasc Surg.* 2008;35:633–636.

11. Gould DA, Reekers JA, Kessel DO. Simulation devices in interventional radiology: validation pending. *JVIR.* 2006;17:215–216.

12. Patel AA, Glaiberman C, Gould DA. Procedural simulation. *Anesthesiology Clin.* 2007;25:349–359.

13. Dawson, S. Procedural simulation: a primer. *JVIR.* 2006;17:205–213.

14. Yamagami T, Osuga K, Yoshimatsu R, et al. Development of a portable training tool for simulating visceral angiographic procedures for beginners. *Cardiovasc Intervent Radiol.* 2009;32:412–416.

15.Garrett HE. A human cadaveric circulation model. *J. of Vasc Surg.* 2001;33:1128–1130.

16. Duncan JR, Glaiberman CB. Analysis of simulated angiographic procedures: part 1 - capture and presentation of audio and video recordings. *JVIR.* 2006;17:1979–1989.

17. Duncan JR, Kline B, Glaiberman CB. Analysis of simulated angiographic procedures. Part 2: extracting data from audio and video recordings. *JVIR.* 2007;18:535–544.

18. Glaiberman CB, Jacobs B, Street M. Simulation in training: one year experience using an efficiency index to assess interventional radiology fellow training status. *JVIR.* 2008;19:1366–1371.

19. Berry M, Reznick R, Lystig T, et al. The use of virtual reality for training in carotid artery stenting: a construct validation study. *Acta Radiol.* 2008;49: 801–805.

20. Gould DA, Kessel DO, Healey AE, et al. Simulators in catheter based interventional radiology: training or computer games? *Clin Radiol.* 2006;61:556–561. (Reprinted 2009).

21. Rajagopalan S, Mukherjee D, Mohler E. *Manual of Vascular Diseases.* Philadelphia: Lippincott Williams and Wilkins; 2005.

22. Valji K. *Vascular and Interventional Radiology,.* 2nd edition. Philadelphia: Elsevier; 2006.

23. Kessel D, Robertson I. *Interventional Radiology, A Survival Guide.* 2nd edition. Philadelphia: Elsevier; 2005.

24. Rieker O, Duber C, Neufang A, et al. CT angiography versus intraarterial digital subtraction angiography for assessment of aortoiliac occlusive disease. *AJR.* 1997;169:1133–1138.

25. Rieker O, Duber C, Schmiedt W, et al. Prospective comparison of CT angiography of the legs with intraarterial digital subtraction angiography. *AJR.* 1996;166:269–276.

26. Prince E, Murphy T, Dhangana R, et al. Evaluation and management of patients with peripheral artery disease by interventional radiologists: current practices. *JVIR.* 2008; 19:639–644.

27. Goel A, Findeiss L, Slim A. Medical management in peripheral arterial disease: a systematic approach to medical therapy. *JVIR.* 2010;21:603–605.

28. Jongkind V, Akkersdijk GJ, Yeung KK, et al. A systematic review of endovascular treatment of extensive aortoiliac occlusive disease. *J of Vasc Surg.* 2010;52:1376–1383.

29. Park KB, Do YS, Kim DI. The TASC classification system in iliac arterial stent placement: long term patency and clinical limitations. *JVIR.* 2007;18:193–201.

30. Dormandy JA, Rutherford RB. Management of peripheral arterial disease. TASC working group. Transatlantic inter-society consensus (TASC). *J Vasc Surg.* 2000;31:S1–S296.

31. Park KB, Do YS, Kim DI, et al. The transatlantic intersociety consensus classification system in iliac arterial stent placement: long term patency and clinical limitations. *JVIR.* 2007;18:193–201.

32. Hallett JW, Mills JL, Earnshaw JL, et al. *Comprehensive Endovascular Surgery.* Toronto: Mosby; 2004.

33. Ruef J, Hofmann M, Haase J. Endovascular interventions in iliac and infrainguinal occlusive artery disease. *J Interv Cardiol.* 2004;17:427–435.

34. Laird JR. Limitations of percutaneous transluminal angioplasty and stenting for the

treatment of disease of the superficial femoral and popliteal arteries. *J Endovasc Ther.* 2006;13 (Suppl 2): 1130–1140.

35. Surowiec SM, Davies MG, Eberly SW. Percutaneous angioplasty and stenting of the superficial femoral artery. *J of Vasc Surg.* 2005:41: 269–278.

36. Goldstone J, Wong V. New training paradigms and program requirements. *Semin Vasc Surg.* 2006;19:168–171.

37. Kwolek CJ, Crawford RS. Training the next generation of vascular specialists: current status and future prospects. *J Endovasc Ther.* 2009;16(Suppl I): 142–152.

38. Pastores SM, O'Connor MF, Kleinpell RM, et al. The Accreditation Council for Graduate Medical Education resident duty hour new standards: history, changes, and impact on staffing on intensive care units. *Crit Care Med.* 2011;39:2540–2549.

39. Dawson DL, Lee ES, Hedayati N, et al. Four-year experience with a regional program providing simulation-based endovascular training for vascular surgery fellows. *J Surg Educ.* 2009;66:330–335.

40. Bath J, Lawrence P, Chandra A, et al. Standardization is superior to traditional methods of teaching open vascular simulation. *J Vasc Surg.* 2011;53:229–234.

41. Sidhu RS, Park J, Brydges R, et al. Laboratory-based vascular anastomosis training: a randomized controlled trial evaluating the effects of bench model fidelity and level of training on skill acquisition. *J Vasc Surg.* 2007;45:343–349.

42. Dawson DL, Meyer J, Lee ES, et al. Training with simulation improves residents' endovascular procedure skills. *J Vasc Surg.* 2007;45:149–154.

43. Chaer RA, Derubertis BG, Lin SC, et al. Simulation improves resident performance in catheter-based intervention: results of a randomized, controlled study. *Ann Surg.* 2006;244:343–352.

44. Lee JT, Qiu M, Teshome M, et al. The utility of endovascular simulation to improve technical performance and stimulate continued interest of preclinical medical students in vascular surgery. *J Surg Educ.* 2009;66:367–373.

45. Woratyla SP, Rasmussen TE, O'Donnell SD, et al. Review of standards for competence in catheter-based endovascular procedures: a resource and strategy for the interventional vascular surgeon. *Vasc Endovasc Surg.* 2003; 37:39–46.

46. Bismuth J, Donovan MA, O'Malley MK, et al. Incorporating simulation in vascular surgery education. *J Vasc Surg.* 2010;52:1072–1080.

47. Scott DJ, Valentine RJ, Bergen PC, et al. Evaluating surgical competency with the American Board of Surgery In-Training Examination, skill testing, and intraoperative assessment. *Surgery.* 2000;128:613–619.

48. Pandey VA, Wolfe JHN, Liapis CD, et al. The examination assessment of technical competence in vascular surgery. *Br J Surg.* 2006;93:1132–1138.

49. Black SA, Harrison RH, Horrocks EJ, et al. Competence assessment of senior vascular trainees using a carotid endarterectomy bench model. *Br J Surg.* 2007;94:1226–1231.

50. Black SA, Nestel DF, Kneebone RL, et al. Assessment of surgical competence at carotid endarterectomy under local anaesthesia in a simulated operating theatre. *Br J Surg.* 2010;97:511–516.

51. Patel AD, Gallagher AG, Nicholson WJ, et al. Learning curves and reliability measures for virtual reality simulation in the performance of carotid angiography. *J Am Coll Cardiol.* 2006;47:1796–1802.

52. Calligaro KD, Toursarkissian B, Clagett GP, et al. Guidelines for hospital privileges in vascular and endovascular surgery: recommendations of the Society for Vascular Surgery. *J Vasc Surg.* 2008;47:1–5.

53. Rosenfield KM. Clinical competence statement on carotid stenting: training and credentialing for carotid stenting-multispecialty consensus recommendations. *J Vasc Surg.* 2005;41:160–168.

54. Hislop SJ, Hedrick JH, Singh MJ, et al. Simulation case rehearsals for carotid artery stenting. *Eur J Vasc Endovasc Surg.* 2009;38:750–754.

55. Roguin A, Beyar R. Real case virtual reality training prior to carotid artery stenting. *Catheter Cardiovasc Interv.* 2010;75:279–282.

56. Willaert W, Aggarwal R, Bicknell C, et al. Patient-specific simulation in carotid artery stenting. *J Vasc Surg.* 2010;52:1700–1705.

57. Peters JH, Fried GM, Swanstrom LL, et al. Development and validation of a comprehensive program of education and assessment of the basic fundamentals of laparoscopic surgery. *Surgery.* 2004;135:21–27.

58. Maynar M, Cabrera J, Pulido-Duque JM, et al. Transjugular intrahepatic portosystemic shunt: early experience with a flexible trocar/catheter system. *AJR Am J Roentgenol.* 1993;161:301–306.

59. Haskal ZJ, Rees CR, Ring EJ, et al. Society of interventional radiology technology assessment committee. Reporting standards for transjugular intrahepatic portosystemic shunts. *J Vasc Interv Radiol.* 2003;14:S419–S426.

60. Haskal ZJ, Martin L, Cardella JF, et al. Society of interventional radiology standards of practice committee. Quality improvement guidelines for transjugular intrahepatic portosystemic shunts. *J Vasc Interv Radiol.* 2003;14:S265–S270.

61. Haskal ZJ, Brennecke LH. Transjugular intrahepatic portosystemic shunts formed with

polyethylene terephthalate-covered stents: experimental evaluation in pigs. *Radiology.* 1999;213:853–859.

62. Haskal ZJ, Davis A, McAllister A, et al. PTFE-encapsulated endovascular stent-graft for transjugular intrahepatic portosystemic shunts: experimental evaluation. *Radiology.* 1997;205:682–688.

63. Teng GJ, Bettmann MA, Hoopes PJ, et al. Comparison of a new stent and Wallstent for transjugular intrahepatic portosystemic shunt in a porcine model. *World J Gastroenterol.* 2001;7:74–79.

64. Shi HJ, Cao AH, Chen J, et al. Transjugular intrahepatic portosystemic shunt with autologous endothelial progenitor cell seeded stent: a porcine model. *Acad Radiol.* 2010;17:358–367.

65. Berry M, Lystig T, Beard J, et al. Porcine transfer study: virtual reality simulator training compared with porcine training in endovascular novices. *Cardiovasc Interv Radiol.* 2007; 30:455–461.

66. Mahne A, Dravid V. Interventional radiology simulation lab: initial experience with US-guided right internal jugular central venous access catheter placement. Presented at the 59th Annual Meeting of the Association of University Radiologists, 2011. San Diego, CA.

67. Johnson SJ, Healey AE, Evans JC, et al. Physical and cognitive task analysis in interventional radiology. *J Clin Radiol.* 2006;61:97–103.

68. Mendiratta-Lala M, Williams T, de Quadros N, et al. The use of a simulation center to improve resident proficiency in performing ultrasound-guided procedures. *Acad Radiol.* 2010;17:535–540.

69. Magee D, Zhu Y, Ratnalingam R, et al. An augmented reality simulator for ultrasound guided needle placement training. *Med Bio Eng Comput.* 2007;45:957–967.

70. CRaIVE, collaborators in Radiological Interventional Virtual Environments. Accessed July 8, 2011, at http://hpv.csbangor.ac.uk/CRaIVE/projects.php

71. Frimberger E, von Delius S, Rosch T. A novel and practicable ERCP training system with simulated fluoroscopy. *Endoscope.* 2008;40:517–520.

72. Stern J, Zeltser, Pearle M. Percutaneous renal access simulators. *J Endourol.* 21;3:2007:270–273.

73. Satava R. Disruptive visions: surgical education. *Surg Endosc.* 2004;18:779–781.

21

Simulation in Cardiothoracic Radiology

MICHAEL L. STEIGNER, FRANCINE JACOBSON, AND FRANK J. RYBICKI

THE USE OF SIMULATION IN CARDIAC IMAGING

THE ORIGINS of simulation for use in training began in the field of cardiology with the development of "Harvey," a life-sized manikin developed by Dr. Michael S. Gordon, at the University of Miami. Harvey was capable of simulating 20 different conditions that were used to develop physical examination skills in medical students and house staff, as well as for continuing physician education.[1–2]

Cardiology patient simulators are still in use today. Ewy et al[3] demonstrated that fourth-year medical students trained with the use of a cardiology patient simulator scored significantly higher on multiple-choice examinations, skills tests on the simulator, and skills tests on live patients when compared with students trained on live patients only.

Cardiac imaging has rapidly advanced in recent years, yet training in imaging modalities has lagged behind. In a recent survey of diagnostic radiology chief residents from 112 Accreditation Council for Graduate Medical Education (ACGME)-certified diagnostic radiology residency programs, only 17% believed that they were being adequately trained for cardiac imaging, whereas 92% believed that cardiac imaging was important.[4] Currently, initial certification by the American Board of Radiology (ABR) includes "Cardiac" as a virtual section in the oral examination. Regardless of future changes in board structure, cardiac requirements will surely remain.[5] One obstacle in cardiac imaging training is a relative shortage of clinical staff with expertise in the subject. Also, dedicated cardiac rotations are scarce and can compete with other subspecialties for time within a training program.[6] Even with these shortcomings, simulation can be robustly used to enrich the overall educational experience for trainees. Computer-based simulation has been used to prepare radiology residents for on-call duties. Towbin et al[7] developed a picture archiving and communication systems (PACS)-based simulator, which used full digital imaging and communications in medicine (DICOM) datasets to simulate the clinical experience. Residents were able to review the simulation-based cases as they would in a routine clinical workflow, submit findings, and receive immediate feedback from the actual subspecialty dictated report. This setup allowed residents the ability to grade their own findings for accuracy. Towbin also suggested that simulation can be used for focused review by a diagnostic category (e.g., liver tumors), and the utility could be expanded for experienced radiologists approaching new imaging studies.

The current paradigm for cardiac computed tomography (CT) training primarily exists in continuing medical education (CME) training courses. The American College of Radiology (ACR) has established practice guidelines for the performance and interpretation of cardiac CT.[8] Training courses for radiologists are structured to meet ACR training requirements. The ACR recommends 50 mentored cases over the previous 36 months. These courses rely almost exclusively on computer-based simulation in the form of mentored case review. Previously acquired cardiac CT datasets are rendered anonymous and loaded onto three-dimensional (3-D) postprocessing workstations. Learners then work through the cases in a mentored review as a way to satisfy the training requirements. The data supporting the validity of this training method in cardiac CT are limited. Ripsweden et al[9] tested the learning curve effect of the interpretation of 100 consecutive cases aimed at diagnosing coronary artery disease in two radiologists and two radiographers, all without prior experience in interpreting cardiac CT. This study showed a learning curve effect with positive predictive value and a decrease in the interpretation time by half.

Brigham and Women's Hospital (BWH) has implemented a simulation-based program to teach radiology residents cardiac CT. The residents are given a structured training program during a dedicated week for cardiac CT training. Initially, the residents are tested on the first day of this rotation, with multiple-choice questions and practical examination of postprocessing and interpretation skills to serve as a baseline to measure the effectiveness of the training program. Residents are then directed to a collaborative intranet webpage (Microsoft Sharepoint 2007, Microsoft Corporation, Redmond, Washington) that describes the objectives of the rotation and lists the steps required to complete those objectives. First, the residents view cardiac CT online training videos freely available on the web, courtesy of the Society of Thoracic Radiology.[10] Next, the residents watch training videos on the use of the 3-D workstation (VitreaWeb Vital Images, Minnetonka, Minnesota). An extensive reading list is supplied, as recommended by ACR practice guideline for the performance and interpretation of cardiac CT. Each resident then independently works through a minimum of 50 cardiac CT cases using a Vital Images workstation. In addition, each resident is given hands-on training during the case review by a subspecialty-trained radiologist with experience in cardiac CT. During the week, the residents participate in the acquisition, reconstruction, postprocessing, interpretation, and reporting of live cases. Residents are also given hands-on training for image acquisition. At the completion of the rotation, each resident is tested with a multiple-choice examination, as well as a practical examination. The preliminary results of data collected suggest an ongoing improvement in individual confidence, diagnostic accuracy, and image postprocessing skills with decreased interpretation time.

The ACR has also described practice guidelines for the performance and interpretation of cardiac magnetic resonance imaging (MRI).[11] The recommended number of mentored cases to be reviewed by a radiology trainee is also 50. Although this is a logical training approach, to date, no objective data are available to support these training methods for cardiac MRI.

ECHOCARDIOGRAPHY

Echocardiography presents both technical challenges in image acquisition and cognitive challenges in conceptualizing 3-D relationships using two-dimensional (2-D) cardiac projections. Simulators have been developed as an aid in teaching both transthoracic and transesophageal approaches. Weidenbach et al[12] developed an augmented reality simulator that uses 3-D echo datasets registered with the heart model for spatial and temporal congruency. A dummy transducer with a 3-D tracking system is then used to simulate image acquisition. The 2-D image is displayed with the 3-D reference image to depict the virtual scan plane (Figure 21.1).

The simulator is used with an integrated training system to augment the trainee's experience. Weidenbach et al have expanded the training system to include congenital heart lesions and validated it for pediatric echocardiography.[13] Bose et al[14] have

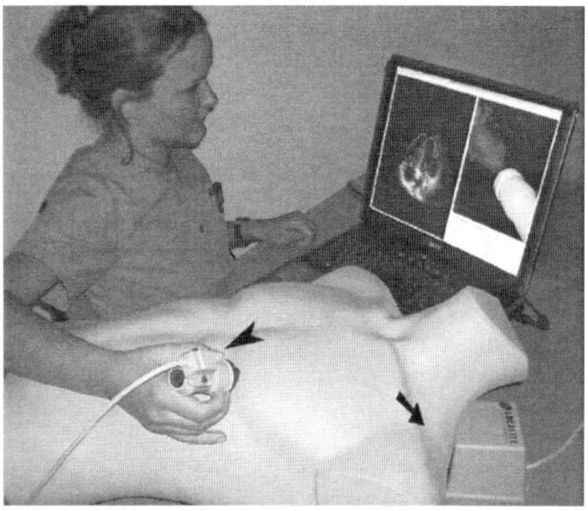

FIGURE 21.1 Echocardiography simulator as it was used in training course. The hollow dummy torso is only used to provide realistic setting: *arrow*, electromagnetic transmitter; *arrowhead*, sensor of tracking system. Reprinted from Weidenbach M, Razek V, Wild F, et al. Computer-based training in two-dimensional echocardiography using an echocardiography simulator. *J Am Soc Echocardiogr.* 2005;18:362–366, with permission of the publisher, Elsevier.

described another transesophageal echocardiography (TEE) simulator. Testing of this device with a group of anesthesia residents showed that those trained on it scored significantly better in the post-training test than did those who did not use the simulator.[15] Using Internet-based cardiac CT datasets, Kempny and Piórkowski[16] have developed a novel simulation technique for TEE called CT2TEE. Using a 3-D cardiac model constructed with volumetric CT data registered with respect to the position of the esophagus, virtual TEE projections are created (Figure 21.2). The simulator is freely available online.[17]

RESEARCH RELATED TO RADIATION EXPOSURE

The complex motion of the heart includes translation, rotation, and deformation. This fact, coupled with the respiratory excursions of the diaphragm, makes the heart the most complex organ routinely imaged. The imaging acquisition technology has been largely driven by the need for faster, higher-resolution images required for reliable, reproducible cardiac imaging.[18] With technological advances, scientists and imagers are charged with testing safe and efficient systems to be applied to human subjects. Hence, the use of simulation has become a mainstay for preclinical cardiac imaging research.

With a new climate of concern about radiation exposure,[19] CT vendors and investigators have responded with techniques and technologies to reduce patient exposure. Cardiac CT, once shunned because of high radiation doses, now is routinely performed at radiation levels competitive with, and even lower than, digital subtraction angiography. In 1999, in order to calibrate CT scanners, Stefan Ulzheimer and Willi Kalender[20] developed the first phantom in cooperation with Quality Assurance in Radiology and Medicine (QRM) (Möhrendorf, Germany, http://www.qrm.de). The phantom is

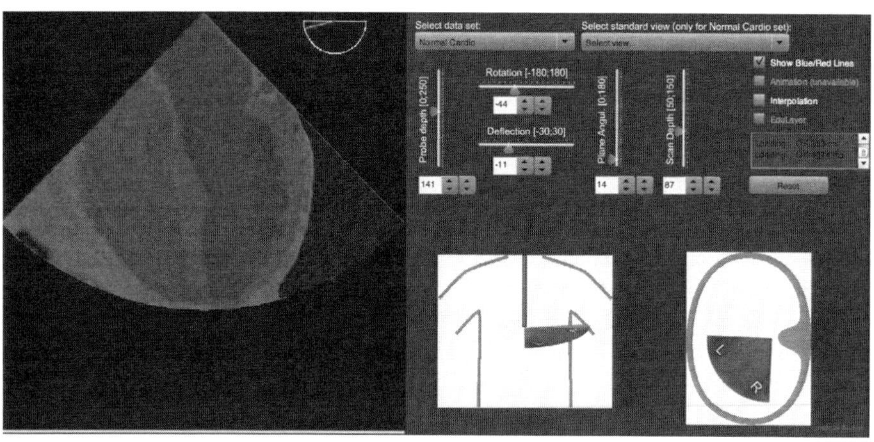

FIGURE 21.2 Internet-based simulator of transesophageal echocardiography using a three-dimensional cardiac model constructed with volumetric computed tomography data. The simulated image is a four-chamber view of the heart. The simulated imaging plane is demonstrated with the coronal and axial cartoons.

manufactured using materials that simulate the density and attenuation of the tissues of the thorax; thus, imaging has noise properties similar to human thoracic CT. Rings can be placed around the phantom to simulate varied attenuation from different sized patients. Spaces within the phantom are available for inserts. For example, a cardiac calibration insert can be placed in the center of the phantom, which contains multiple cylinders of calcification varying in size and density. McCollough et al[21] have used this phantom to develop a consensus standard for quantification of coronary artery calcium. This phantom has also been used to compare the dose performance of 64-channel single-source CT and 64-channel dual-source CT (DSCT).[22]

Physical phantoms have been developed to simulate cardiac anatomy and physiology. Toepker et al[23] developed a phantom to simulate low-attenuation stenoses in a coronary artery. Plastic vessel phantoms were created in four different sizes ranging from 2 to 4 mm. Each vessel phantom contained a fixed radiolucent concentric narrowing with an associated diameter stenosis of 50%, designed to simulate noncalcified coronary artery plaque. The phantoms were mounted on the robotic arm of a cardiac motion simulator that simulated a heart rate of 70 beats per minute. The phantom was then put into a water tank filled with saline that fitted inside the thorax phantom. Imaging with DSCT showed that the low-attenuation stenosis could be reproducibly measured, although DSCT may underestimate the degree of stenosis. The accuracy of measurements was also demonstrated to be independent of motion.

The reference standard for quantitative cardiac function is cardiac MRI (CMR). Limitations to its use include clinical contraindications, such as claustrophobia and patients with implanted devices. In addition, only a limited inventory of scanners equipped with appropriate gradients and trained imagers is currently available. Cardiac CT can robustly assess function, and improved temporal resolution makes CT competitive with MR studies, such as steady-state free precession, with best temporal resolution in the order of 80 milliseconds.[24] Spatial resolution is more complex as the MR scan can be intimately related to the field of view, which, in turn, determines spatial resolution. In general, however, MR spatial resolution is less than that of CT. This is one reason that CT approaches have entirely dominated clinical noninvasive coronary artery imaging. Cardiac MRI, however, has outstanding contrast resolution with a spectrum of inherent contrasts, as opposed to CT, in which the main source of contrast is intravenously injected contrast medium containing iodine. Groen et al[25] used an anthropomorphic moving heart phantom (Limbs & Things. Bristol, U.K.) to compare CMR, DSCT, and single-source MDCT in assessing left ventricular ejection fraction and cardiac output at a range of different heart rates (Figure 21.3).

Variable flow settings were created with a gas pump to simulate heart rates from 50 to 100 beats per minute. The end-diastolic volume (EDV) was determined by filling the phantom with water, and the end-systolic volume (ESV) was calculated from the stroke volume, which was determined using a gas flow analyzer. Cardiac output (CO) and ejection fraction (EF) were also calculated. The phantom was then scanned using 64-slice MDCT, DSCT, and 1.5 Tesla MR. The short axis images were then used to trace the endocardial borders. The functional parameters of EDV, ESV, CO, and EF were calculated. The results showed that DSCT deviated least from the reference parameters. Cardiac MR showed an underestimation of EF and CO. Groen et al[25] suggested that the structural overestimation of the EDV and ESV leading to underestimation of the EF and CO was due to the limited spatial resolution of CMR. Sixty-four-slice MDCT showed variable results, with large limits of agreement likely due to the decreased temporal resolution of single-source MDCT that typically has half the temporal resolution of DSCT.

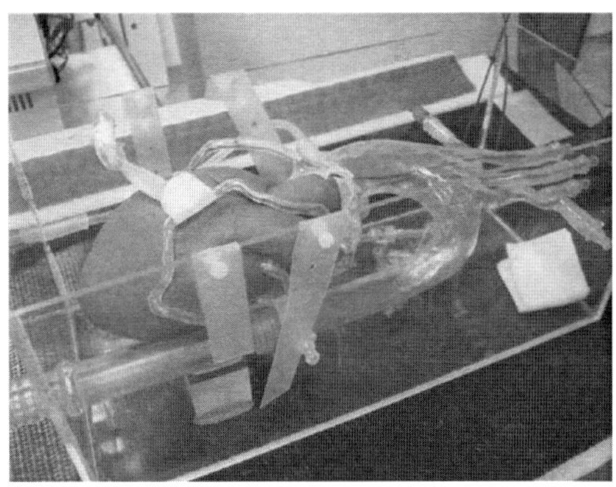

FIGURE 21.3 The moving anthropomorphic heart phantom. Reprinted from Groen JM, van der Vleuten PA, Greuter MJ, et al. Comparison of MRI, 64-slice MDCT and DSCT in assessing functional cardiac parameters of a moving heart phantom. *Eur Radiol.* 2009;19:577–583, with permission of the publisher, Springer Science+Business Media.

Horiguchi et al[26] used a cardiac phantom to study in-stent visibility obtained with prospective and retrospective ECG-gated 64-detector MDCT at 140 kV and 120kV. Multiple heart rates and stent types were studied. They used a commercially available prototype cardiac phantom constructed from a rubber balloon driven by a controller with an electrocardiograph (ECG) synchronizer (Figure 21.4).

Coronary artery cylinder models with artificial in-stent restenosis have been manufactured. Neointimal hyperplasia was simulated using acrylonitrile-butadiene-styrene resin material with an attenuation of 40 Hounsfield Units (HU), similar to an in-stent restenosis. Twelve different coronary stents were prepared, inserted into a coronary model, filled with dilute contrast material, attached to the balloon phantom, and surrounded by corn oil to simulate epicardial fat. Their results showed improved visibility of in-stent restenosis with 140 kV prospectively ECG-gated CTA compared to 120 kV retrospectively ECG-gated helical CTA with a theoretical radiation dose reduction of 34%–42%.

Computer-based simulation (CBS) has also been used to simulate cardiac anatomy and physiology. Computer-based simulation involves digital modeling of an anatomic and physiologic phantom, then generating imaging data using models of the imaging process. The main advantage of computer-generated phantoms is their verity. Segars et al[27] developed a computed-generated phantom using a hybrid model based on patient imaging data using more complex mathematical primitives to define the organs and structure. This four-dimensional (4-D) extended cardiac-torso phantom (XCAT) provides a high-resolution computer model of human anatomy and physiology that is reported to be suitable for CT and MRI. Anatomical patient variation, such as gender, can be applied to the model. Motion, the fourth dimension, is included in the phantom to simulate ECG-gated cardiac motion and respiratory motion (Figure 21.5).

The 4-D XCAT has generated 3-D and 4-D datasets from patient anatomies (e.g., an adult male and a 12-year-old boy). Iodinated contrast has been modeled, and global and regional cardiac wall motion abnormalities have been simulated (Figure 21.6).[28]

Tobon-Gomez et al[29] used the XCAT methodology to modify the cardiac phantom to include modeling of myocardial trabeculae and papillary muscles. They were able to generate CMR datasets using an MRI simulator developed by Kwan et al[30] Tobon-Gomez et al[29] tested the performance of the virtual datasets to clinical datasets. They showed a good match between the local appearance of the real and simulated images. The Segars team has continued to develop the model. The most recent advancement includes the ability

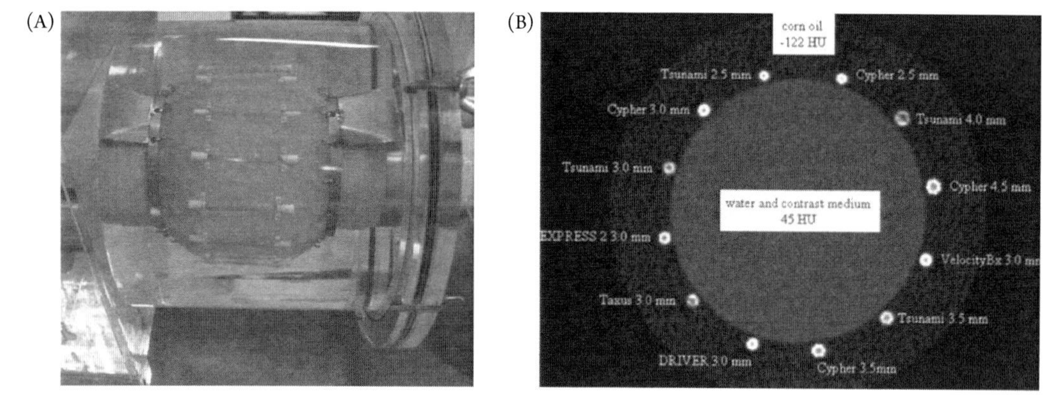

FIGURE 21.4 (A) Cardiac phantom and stented coronary artery models. Close-up view of balloon component of the cardiac phantom (Alpha 2, Fuyo Corp.). Balloon attached with the stented coronary artery models ($n = 12$) was surrounded by corn oil. (B) Transaxial computed tomography (CT) image of cardiac phantom. The balloon was filled with a mixture of water and contrast medium (45 HU at 120 kV) to simulate weakly enhanced myocardium (at arterial phase) and was submerged in corn oil (−122 HU at 120 kV), simulating epicardial and pericardial fat. Coronary artery models ($n = 12$) were attached to the balloon surface. Reprinted from Horiguchi J, Fujoka C, Kiguchi M, et al. Prospective ECG-triggered axial CT at 140-kV tube voltage improves coronary in-stent restenosis visibility at a lower radiation dose compared with conventional retrospective ECG-gated helical CT. *Eur Radiology*. 2009;19:2363–2372, with permission of the publisher, Springer Science+Business Media.

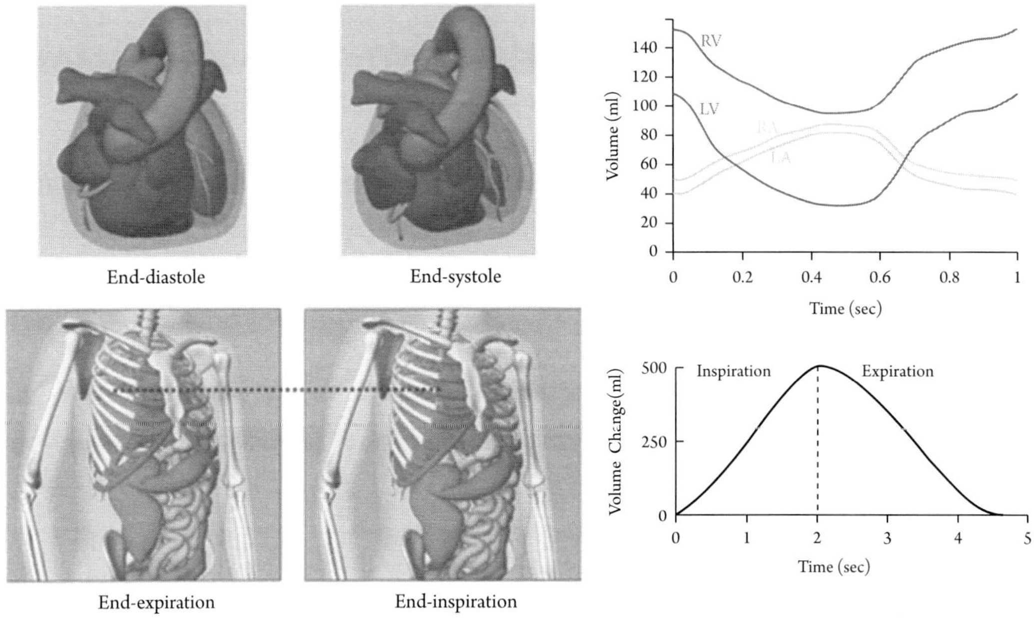

FIGURE 21.5 Cardiac and respiratory motions of the four-dimensional XCAT. Plots of the volume change in the cardiac chambers and lungs are shown to the right. Reprinted from Segars WP, Mahesh M, Beck TJ, et al. Realistic CT simulation using the 4D XCAT phantom. *Med Physics.* 2008; 35:3800–3808, with permission of the publisher, American Association of Physicists in Medicine.

to simulate post-infarct remodeling effects on left ventricular function (Figure 21.7).[31]

THE USE OF SIMULATION IN THORACIC IMAGING

Development of Hybrid Images for Nodule Detection

The detection of lung nodules as signal within anatomic noise has a long history in radiology. In part, this is due to the high radiographic contrast between soft tissue nodules and air, the primary substance in lung parenchyma. The detection of lung nodules has always been an important basic clinical skill for the radiologist. Detection, however, is not always simple. For example, projection radiography or summation shadow-gram of the chest are both areas in which even large nodules can be easily overlooked, particularly where the soft tissue structures of the mediastinum and abdomen are projected with the lung. Ribs can also cause difficulty in nodule detection. Furthermore, the superimposition of normal structures or extraneous chest wall nodules, tubing, etc. can result in visualization of nodular opacities that are spurious or artifactual.

Image perception researchers have used an alternative method to create simulated nodules by placing artificial nodules on normal image backgrounds. The simplest formulation uses a sphere of plausible density placed in a realistic location. Molded wax phantom nodules were taped onto the back of an anthropomorphic chest phantom for comparison of nodule detection from digital and conventional (analog) chest radiographs at the University of Alabama in Birmingham in a study reported in 1986.[32]

Although pathological diagnosis remains the gold standard for confirming whether a nodule is benign or malignant, removal of every detected lung nodule is both unrealistic and impracticable. Consequently, secondary "brass" standards have been developed to assess the malignant potential of detected nodules. Although no longer in common use, the Zerhouni Phantom[33] for the detection of calcification in a lung nodule to provide evidence for benign etiology, does give a rigorous approach to the use of simulation to assess the characteristics of pulmonary nodules. In this seminal work, the anthropomorphic CT phantom reproduced transverse sections of the thorax, duplicating the shape and CT density of the soft tissue and bony structures within each section. Peripheral rings of "fat equivalent" plastic were added to

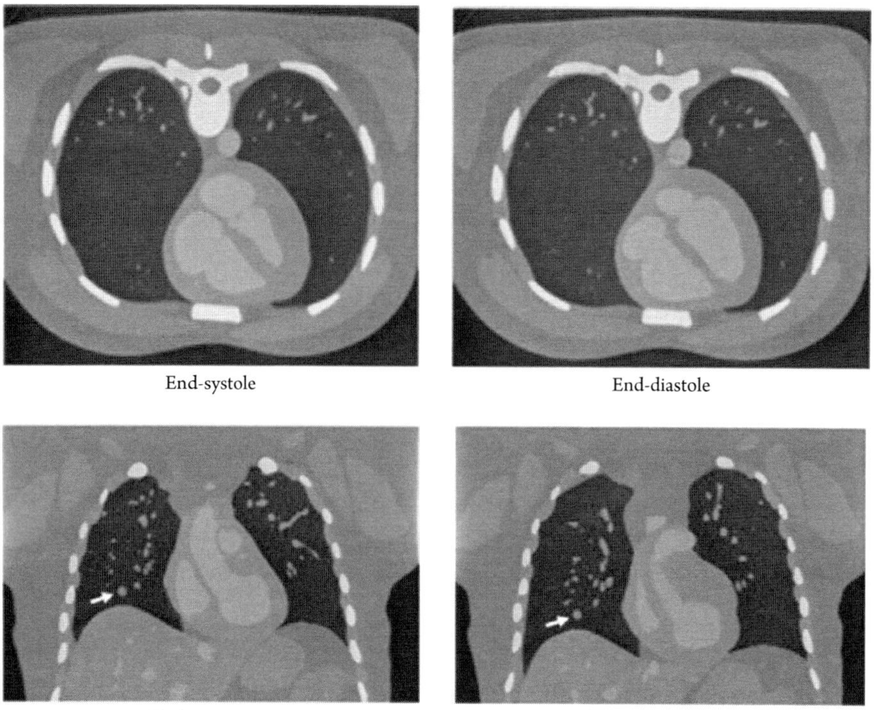

FIGURE 21.6 Cardiac-gated (*top*) and respiratory-gated (*bottom*) computed tomography (CT) images generated using the four-dimensional XCAT. A spherical lesion (*arrow*) was simulated in the respiratory-gated images. Reprinted from Segars WP, Mahesh M, Beck TJ, et al. Realistic CT simulation using the 4D XCAT phantom. *Med Physics.* 2008;35:3800–3808, with permission of the publisher, American Association of Physicists in Medicine.

simulate the chest wall of individual patients in order to produce a similar degree of beam hardening during CT measurements. Rods ranging from 0.4 to 6 cm in diameter were placed within the phantom to simulate the clinical location of a patient's nodule. As a result of this work, the CT number for calcification was established at 164 HU. As CT technology advanced, the phantom was no longer required to detect calcification.

The simulation of lung nodules for presentation on CT scan images is intimately related to the technology itself, particularly regarding collimation and spatial resolution. As CT scanner X-ray tube focal spots have become smaller, image resolution has improved, and thinner sections can now be reconstructed.[34] The nature of simulated nodules has continued to become correspondingly more complex. As stated above, in recent years, the sophistication of computer-based simulation techniques has increased the range of the methods for creating hybrid images for lung nodule perception research. Such images can now be used to train radiologists via computer-aided diagnosis (CAD) systems, thus increasing the opportunity for training programs and continuing education programs to provide efficient systems for deliberate practice. The well-known ACR B-Reader program for diffuse lung diseases is an example of such simulation-based training incorporating deliberate practice. In addition, it can be used for testing and certification.

LUNG NODULE PERCEPTION RESEARCH METHODOLOGY AND CLINICAL PRACTICE

The greatest advancement in the use of simulated lung nodules followed the paradigm shift from film-based CT images presented as "tiles" to the stacked metaphor that has become dominant in soft copy reading from computer archives without hard copy film. This revolutionary shift in radiology viewing was needed to cope with increasing numbers of images, particularly in MRI, and was facilitated by the increasing ability of computer technology to provide

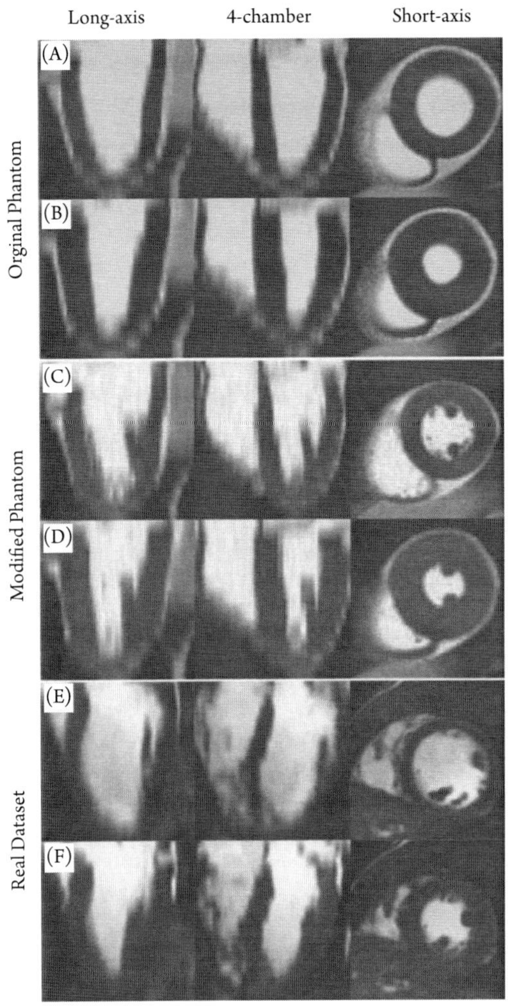

FIGURE 21.7 Examples of simulated images with the original phantom at end diastole (B) and end systole (B). Examples of simulated images with the modified phantom at end diastole (C) and end systole (D). Examples of a real cardiac magnetic resonance dataset at end diastole (E) and end systole (F). Reprinted from Tobon-Gomez C, Sukno FM, Huguet M, et al. Realistic simulation of cardiac magnetic resonance studies modeling anatomical variability, trabeculae, and papillary muscles. *Magn Reson Med.* 2011;65:280–288, with permission of the publisher, John Wiley and Sons.

desktop systems capable of providing images, thus eliminating the need for supercomputers.

In 1992, Seltzer et al,[35] researchers at Brigham and Women's Hospital (BWH), began a perception experiment using supercomputers and crude localization of pulmonary nodules that marked the cutting edge of technology at that time. Clinical CT scans performed on first-generation slip-ring technology scanners provided volumetric chest CT scans obtained with a single breath hold. Contiguous 10 mm images for clinical studies were routinely presented as 10 mm images at 10 mm intervals. For this study, normal chest CT scans were reconstructed with 10 mm images at 2 mm intervals for viewing on a supercomputer monitor and at 4 mm intervals for film-based viewing. The number of images for film-based display was reduced as a practical matter. The image profiles for electronically simulated nodules were added to the data in realistic locations by a physicist and were tested for acceptability by three radiologists prior to the randomized reader experiment, in which eight radiologist observers randomly read both conditions.

The simulated nodules measuring 3–5 mm in diameter were at the verge of visibility on CT scan images at that time. The limited resolution of the CT scan images allowed electronically simulated spheres with blurred edges to provide a realistic appearance accepted by radiologists as nodules interchangeably with tiny nodules present in the normal studies. This fact emerged from the data due to the instructions to the observers. While eight simulated nodules were placed for each case, the observers were asked to report ten locations of nodules. The purpose of this direction was to avoid satisfaction of search. The overwhelming selection of structures with characteristics of nodules rather than random blood vessels for the reports confirmed the realistic appearance of the simulated nodules. The detection of nodules from cine consistently exceeded that from film-based viewing. Although cine viewing decreased confusion regarding the continuity of blood vessels as tubular structures, a more powerful effect emerged—that of "nodule popping," whereby the radiologists eyes were drawn to the nodule by the motion between images. Motion is known to increase conspicuity of small and subtle objects. Optical illusions have long been built upon this principle. Following Seltzer's publication in 1995, radiologists quickly adopted soft copy reading, even in advance of clinical PACS. It was during this era that the initial lung cancer screening trials were performed in Japan and at Weill-Cornell Medical Center.[36] The pioneering work of the Early Lung Cancer Action Project (ELCAP) group taught the thoracic radiology community about previously inapparent features in small nodules, including solid and nonsolid components with irregular shapes associated with growing lesions and very characteristic appearances that are associated with adenocarcinoma. Three-dimensional reconstruction of 1 mm high-resolution CT (HRCT) images at 0.5 mm intervals allowed the study of interaction between volume and shape in a deformable structure. The change in conformation of small phantom nodules mimicked effects of respiration differences between scans, as well as nodule growth. The detection and volumetric measurement of nodules by Yankelevitz et al[37] extended the simulation of nodules beyond the use of simple spheres. The clinical application of the thin section volumetric imaging of a small lung cancer allowed detection of irregular changes in shape and growth in just 36 days.

The advent of multidetector CT scanning that allowed thin section imaging throughout the chest in a single breath hold, without added radiation, drove these observations from research to the clinical arena faster than the implementation of CAD systems and perceptual studies of nodule features.

The observations that lung cancer had a wide range in density, from a barely detectable attenuation difference compared with adjacent normal lung, and that the presence of both solid and nonsolid components had prognostic significance, with the possible potential of virtually perfect identification of malignancy, had a profound effect on the early identification of lung cancer. This led to intensive correlation between CT scan images with histology that culminated in an international study of bronchioloalveolar carcinoma and lung adenocarcinoma.[38,39]

As lung cancer screening followed in the historical development course of breast cancer screening, mammographic images were used to test the visibility of complex lesions in the BWH perception laboratory. The placement of simulated nodules on mammogram images could be performed randomly by a computer algorithm without regard for the parenchymal architecture. The availability of a well-studied mammogram library at the University of South Florida[40] provided pathologically proven images of cancer and normal mammogram images to use for background. Arthur Burgess[41] combined these images using interactive data language (IDL), a programming language, to place real pathologically proven lesions with mammographic images through a greater range of conditions than could be gathered directly. Two alternative forced-choice experiments for signal detection could then use pathologically proven lesions as the signal, and breast parenchyma served as anatomic noise.

The use of CT lung backgrounds for the creation of hybrid images to provide known ground truth benefitted from the advancements in software development and computer science embodied in multidetector CT scanning. To reduce the effort necessary to acquire suitable CT scan datasets for perception research and for education, five institutions formed the Lung Image Database Consortium (LIDC) to create a lung imaging database resource.[42] The development of commercial CAD systems benefitted from this and associated research endeavors, and resulted in the exposure of many radiologists to the applicability of these systems, although their clinical use today is still limited. Automated segmentation and measurement are desirable and can provide more consistent measurements over time than a radiologist using calipers on individual images. These systems, however, do so with variable degrees of accuracy, and that can affect classification of nodules by size for follow-up algorithms such as contained in the Fleischner Society guidelines for management of incidentally detected nodules.[43]

During the development of CAD systems, many software tools were developed that also facilitate research. These tools include methods for placing virtual nodules on chest CT images.[44] The creation of hybrid images using pathologically proven lesion image data with separately selected background CT images became accessible to radiologists through the efforts of the University of Iowa project led by Mark Madsen.[45] This effort has created a suite of interactive data language programs that allow importation of CT scan image datasets and provide tools to create libraries of both image backgrounds and lesions. The process by which the lesions are visually harvested also allows any distracting feature to be removed. Since state-of-the-art CT scanning of the lung reveals tiny nodules in almost every normal lung, the iterative use of this image revision provides a valuable method to purify normal backgrounds for study and teaching. These software programs provide database capability and visual inspection to create realistic images using nodules from patients and those created through mathematical simulation.

The architecture of lung parenchyma has also become a subject for computerized modeling, leading to new descriptions of diffuse lung disease features, and in turn increasing the precision of diagnosis and improvements in education and training for radiologists.[46] Attention to subtle opacities has led to the development of segmentation that can more adequately assess increases in nodule substance within areas of nodules that are not increasing in overall size (LMS Lesion Management System, Median Technologies, Valbonne, France). This bespeaks the further sophistication in lesion characterization that requires consideration in the creation of hybrid images for research and education.

CONCLUSION

With every advance, researchers see glimpses into future possibilities beyond current capabilities. The current work at BWH is designed to again repurpose experience with mammography to revolutionize the image display metaphor used for viewing chest CT. Stereoscopic digital mammography, envisioned by David Getty of BBN Technologies over 10 years ago, has now been developed into a clinically available tool used in a clinical trial led by Carl D'Orsi at Emory University.[47] The authors are currently developing and testing stereoscopic presentation of CT scan data to facilitate identification of pulmonary nodules.

At the more basic level, these advances in simulated image generation can now be used to train radiology residents and continuously train graduate radiologists through deliberate practice, as illustrated by programs such as the ACR Training Center. Technology is constantly changing; therefore, the understanding of it and the ability to use it must constantly advance.

REFERENCES

1. Gordon MS. Cardiology patient simulator. Development of an animated manikin to teach cardiovascular disease. *Am J Cardiol.* 1974;34: 350–355.

2. Gordon MS, Ewy GA, Felner JM, et al. A cardiology patient simulator for continuing education of family physicians. *J Fam Pract.* 1981;13:353–356.

3. Ewy GA, Felner JM, Juul D, et al. Test of a cardiology patient simulator with students in fourth-year electives. *J Med Educ.* 1987;62:738–743.

4. Minocha J, Yagmai V, Hammond N, et al. Cardiac imaging training in radiology residency programs: a survey of radiology chief residents. *Acad Radiol.* 2010;17:795–798.

5. American Board of Radiology. Accessed April 12, 2011, at http://www.theabr.org/ic/ic_dr/ic_dr_study.html9

6. Zaheer A, Raptopoulos V. Establishing a cardiac imaging rotation in radiology residency. *Acad Radiol.* 2006;13:871–873.

7. Towbin AJ, Paterson BE, Chang PJ, et al. Computer-based simulator for radiology: an educational tool. *Radiographics.* 2008;28:309–316.

8. Jacobs JE, Boxt LM, Desjardins B, et al. ACR practice guideline for the performance and interpretation of cardiac computed tomography (CT). *J Am Coll Radiol.* 2006;3:677–685.

9. Ripsweden J, Mir-Akbari H, Brolin EB, et al. Is training essential for interpreting cardiac computed tomography? *Acta Radiol.* 2009;50:194–200.

10. Society of Thoracic Radiology. Accessed April 12, 2011, at http://education.thoracicrad.org/cardiac_imaging.htm

11. Woodard PK, Bluemke DA, Cascade PN, et al. ACR practice guideline for the performance and interpretation of cardiac magnetic resonance imaging (MRI). *J Am Coll Radiol.* 2006;3:665–676.

12. Weidenbach M, Razek V, Wild F, et al. Computer-based training in two-dimensional echocardiography using an echocardiography simulator. *J Am Soc Echocardiogr.* 2005;18:362–366.

13. Weidenbach M, Razek V, Wild F, et al. Simulation of congenital heart defects: a novel way of training in echocardiography. *Heart.* 2009;95:636–641.

14. Bose R, Matyal R, Panzica P, et al. Transesophageal echocardiography simulator: a new learning tool. *J Cardiothorac Vasc Anesth.* 2009;23:544–548.

15. Bose RR, Matyal R, Warraich HJ, et al. Utility of a transesophageal echocardiographic simulator as a teaching tool. *J Cardiothorac Vasc Anesth.* 2011;25:212–215.

16. Kempny A, Piórkowski A. CT2TEE—a novel, internet-based simulator of transesophageal echocardiography in congenital heart disease. *Kardiol Pol.* 2010;68:374–379.

17. CT2EE simulator. Accessed April 12, 2011, at http://www.ct2tee.agh.edu.pl

18. Otero HJ, Steigner ML, Rybicki FJ. The "Post-64" era of coronary CT angiography: understanding new technology from physical principles. *Radiol Clin North Am.* 2009;47:79–90.

19. Rybicki FJ. Lower radiation dose coronary CT angiography with new imaging technologies. *Int J Cardiovasc Imaging.* 2009;25(S2):149–151.

20. Ulzheimer S, Kalender WA. Assessment of calcium scoring performance in cardiac computed tomography. *Eur Radiol.* 2003;13:484–497.

21. McCollough CH, Ulzheimer S, Halliburton SS, et al. Coronary artery calcium: a multi-institutional, multimanufacturer international standard for quantification at cardiac CT. *Radiology.* 2007;243:527–538.

22. McCollough CH, Primak AN, Saba O. Dose performance of a 64-channel dual-source CT scanner. *Radiology.* 2007;243:775–784.

23. Toepker M, Schlett CL, Irlbeck T, et al. Accuracy of dual-source computed tomography in quantitative assessment of low density coronary stenosis—a motion phantom study. *Eur Radiol.* 2010;20:542–548.

24. Flohr TG, Leng S, Yu L, et al. Dual-source spiral CT with pitch up to 3.2 and 75 ms temporal resolution: image reconstruction and assessment of image quality. *Med Phys.* 2009;36:5641–5653.

25. Groen JM, van der Vleuten PA, Grueter MJ, et al. Comparison of MRI, 64-slice MDCT and DSCT in assessing functional cardiac parameters of a moving heart phantom. *Eur Radiol.* 2009;19:577–583.

26. Horiguchi J, Fujoka C, Kiguchi M, et al. Prospective ECG-triggered axial CT at 140-kV tube voltage improves coronary in-stent restenosis visibility at a lower radiation dose compared with conventional retrospective ECG-gated helical CT. *Eur Radiol.* 2009;19:2363–2372.

27. Segars WP, Manesh M, Beck TJ, et al. Realistic CT simulation using the 4D XCAT phantom. *Med Phys.* 2008;35:3800–3808.

28. Segars WP, Lee TS, Tsui BMW. Simulation of motion defects in the 4D NCAT cardiac model. *J Nucl Med.* 2003;44:142P.

29. Tobon-Gomez C, Sukno FM, Huguet M, et al. Realistic simulation of cardiac magnetic resonance studies modeling anatomical variability, trabeculae, and papillary muscles. *Magn Reson Med.* 2011;65:280–288.

30. Kwan RK, Evans AC, Pike GB. MRI simulation-based evaluation of image-processing and classification methods. *IEEE Trans Med Imaging.* 1999;18:1085–1097.

31. Veress AI, Segars WP, Tsui BM, et al. Incorporation of a left ventricle finite element model defining infarction into the XCAT imaging phantom. *IEEE Trans Med Imaging.* 2011;30 :915–927.

32. Chakraborty DP, Breatnach ES, Yester MV, et al. Digital and conventional imaging: a modified ROC study of observer performance using simulated nodules. *Radiology.* 1986;158:35–39.

33. Zerhouni EA, Boukadoum M, Siddiky M, et al. A standard phantom for quantitative CT analysis of pulmonary nodules. *Radiology.* 1983; 149:767–773.

34. Kimme-Smith C, Hart EM, Goldin JG, et al. Detection of simulated lung nodules with computed radiography: effects of nodule size, local optical density, global object thickness, and exposure. *Acad Radiol.* 1996;3:735–741.

35. Seltzer SE, Judy PF, Adams DF, et al. Spiral CT of the chest: comparison of cine and film-based viewing. *Radiology.* 1995;197:73–78.

36. Henschke CI, McCauley DI, Yankelevitz DF, et al. Early Lung Cancer Action Project: overall design and findings from baseline screening. *Lancet.* 1999;354:99–105.

37. Yankelevitz DF, Reeves AP, Kostis WJ, et al. Small pulmonary nodules: volumetrically determined growth rates based on CT evaluation. *Radiology.* 2000;217:251–256.

38. Henschke CI, Yankelevitz DF, Mirtcheva R, et al. CT screening for lung cancer: frequency and significance of part-solid and nonsolid nodules. *AJR.* 2002;178:1053–1057.

39. Travis WD, Garg K, Franklin WA, et al. Bronchioloalveolar carcinoma and lung adenocarcinoma: the clinical importance and research relevance of the 2004 World Health Organization pathologic criteria. *J Thorac Oncol.* 2006;1(9 Suppl):S13-S19.

40.University of South Florida, DDSM Resource datasets. Accessed April 12, 2011, at http://marathon.csee.usf.edu/Mammography/DDSM/BCRP/bcrp.html44

41. Burgess AE, Jacobson FL, Judy PF. Human observer detection experiments with mammograms and power-law noise. *Med Phys.* 2001;28:419–437.

42. Armato SG, McLennan G, McNitt-Gray MF, et al. Developing a resource for the medical imaging research community. *Radiology.* 2004;232:739–748.

43. MacMahon H, Austin JH, Gamsu G, et al. Guidelines for management of small pulmonary nodules detected on CT scans: a statement from the Fleischner Society. *Radiology.* 2005;237:395–400.

44. Shin HO, Blietz M, Frericks B, et al. Insertion of virtual pulmonary nodules in CT data of the chest: development of a software tool. *Eur Radiol.* 2006;16:2567–2574.

45. Madsen MT, Berbaum KS, Ellingson AN, et al. A new software tool for removing, storing and adding abnormalities to medical images for perception research studies. *Acad Radiol.* 2006;13:305–312.

46. Pousse A, Pastor L, Manzoni P, et al. Pulmonary nodule distribution modeling as a diagnostic tool for HRCT images. *IEEE Trans Nucl Sci.* 2004;51:690–695.

47. Getty DJ, D'Orsi CJ, Pickett RM. Stereoscopic digital mammography: improved accuracy of lesion detection in breast cancer screening. *Lecture Notes in Computer Science, LNCS.* 2008;5116:74–79.

22

Simulation in Breast Imaging

LUIS F. SERRANO, SHIRLEY YODZIS, MIGNONNE BEAUDOIN MORRELL, AND LEONARD R. BOK

BREAST IMAGING is one of several subspecialties within radiology that requires comprehensive knowledge of multiple imaging modalities and technical skill in performing procedures within each of these modalities. In addition to being a crucial and integral part of surgical treatment, these procedures are often the first line in diagnosis of breast pathology. For this reason, it is important for those providing these services to be fully competent in performing the various interventions of the field. Medical training ideally promotes training with simulators to provide trainees with a safe, risk-free environment for learning procedural techniques. Simulation-based training (SBT) for technical skills acquisition in diagnostic and therapeutic image-guided breast procedures has been practiced with a variety of phantoms.[1–5] At Louisiana State University Health Sciences Center in New Orleans (LSUHSC-NO), we have adopted an SBT approach in training for breast intervention. For this purpose, we have created novel breast phantoms that have been successfully used with diagnostic and interventional modalities.

The Multilayer Phantom

Phantoms are specially designed objects that are utilized in medical imaging to evaluate, analyze, and tune the performance of imaging devices by simulating anatomical and pathologic tissues in various imaging modalities. These phantoms, which are typically used for quality assurance, are often expensive and not designed to play a role in procedural training.[3] Some selectively designed phantoms, however, are ideal for use by medical students, residents, and fellows to learn how to operate the imaging equipment and the technical aspects of interventional procedures. They provide an opportunity for trainees to undergo deliberate practice using SBT, and to succeed or fail without discomfort or harm to a patient. Phantoms are more readily available than a living subject or cadaveric specimen. In addition, they present a standardized, reproducible model for deliberate practice and uniform learner training.

A phantom used to evaluate an imaging device should respond in a similar manner to human tissues

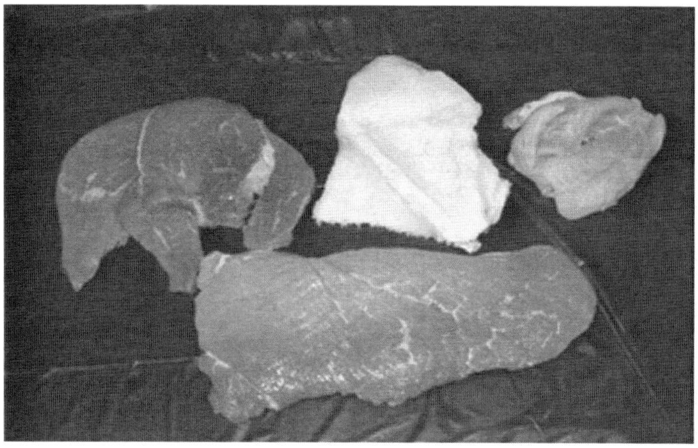

FIGURE 22.1 Multiple layers from different types of meat are placed on the table.

and organs when imaged by that modality. In breast imaging, a variety of breast tissue textures exist from one patient to another. They range from the softest and most fatty tissue, which is easily traversed with a biopsy needle, to the most resistant fibrotic parenchyma, which is significantly more difficult to cross with a needle to reach a target lesion. Based on these varying characteristics of patient tissues, a multilayer phantom was developed at LSUHSC-NO to simulate the different layers of tissue found in a human breast. The phantom is built up with different types of meat, stacked in an overlapping fashion to simulate the different tissue planes (Figures 22.1 and 22.2).

Additionally, such a construction allows the placement of "pseudo-lesions" at different depths within the phantom. A useful feature of this phantom is that, once the needle is inserted, opening the layers allows verification of the needle placement and positioning within the lesion. For ultrasound-guided procedures, this phantom can be freestanding on a table since tissue compression is not required to perform the biopsy procedure. For other image-guided procedures, such as stereotactic biopsy, needle localization, and magnetic resonance imaging (MRI)-guided biopsy, the phantom requires a plastic wrapping to maintain the multiple layers in place during compression. For ultrasound-guided interventions, the plastic wrap material is not used since significant artifact is created due to the presence of air beneath the plastic with limitation of tissue visualization (Figures 22.3 and 22.4).

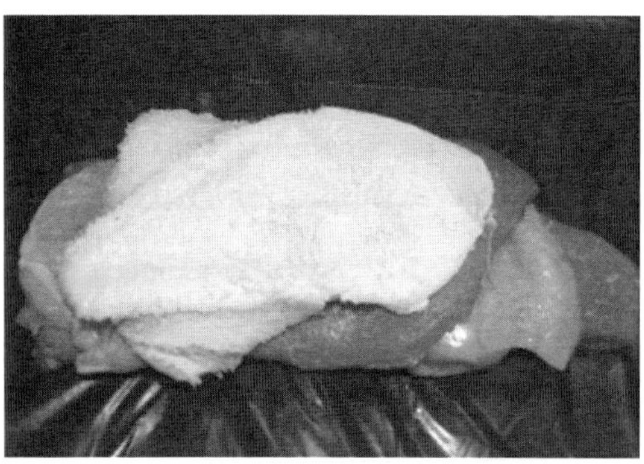

FIGURE 22.2 The multilayer phantom was assembled from top to bottom with layers of beef to give more density, flat steak, chicken breast, and on the bottom, round steak.

Phantom Construction

The ready availability and low cost of the breast simulation model materials, combined with the ease of preparation and reproducibility, make the training process simple, efficient, and highly effective. The excellent imaging characteristics of the multilayer phantom add to the realistic "feel" of the needle and biopsy devices in SBT. There are several advantages of using this particular phantom as a model, including the ability to perform several biopsies on the same phantom, the ability to place simulated lesions at multiple depths in the phantom, and the ability to replace the lesions without destroying the phantom.[4] This SBT format provides the opportunity for quick and efficient exposure of trainees to technical skills acquisition in the various modalities

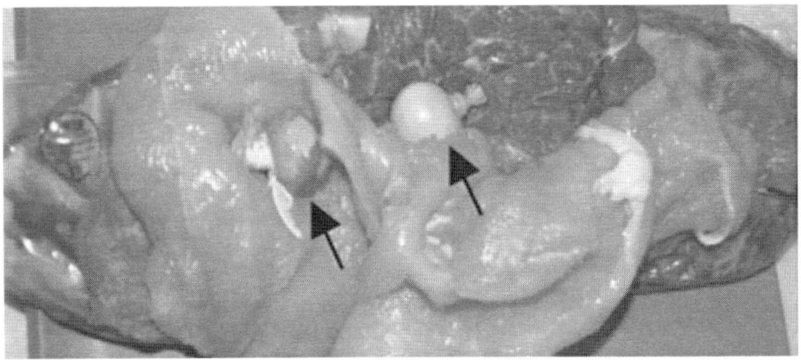

FIGURE 22.3 Multilayer phantom for breast ultrasound simulation with pseudo-lesions (*arrows*).

of image-guided biopsy for breast lesions. It allows the creation of a learning environment conducive to increasing skills confidence and proficiency in such techniques.

Our multilayer breast ultrasound phantom was assembled from top to bottom with layers of chicken breast with skin, chicken breast without skin, beef or cured pork, and ribs. The chicken breast with the skin mimics the skin of a real patient and creates a slight resistance when introducing the needle. The regular chicken breast simulates the subcutaneous tissue located in the pre-mammary zone. Any type of beef can be placed to create an area of resistance that mimics the more resistant mammary zone, formed from stroma. After this, we place a thin layer of any type of more firm meat that simulates the retromammary fascia and pectoral muscle, followed by ribs that represent the rib cage (Figure 22.5).

The key is to simulate, as much as possible, the pliability and resistance found in breast tissues, which vary with the extent of fibrosis or the involution of the fibroglandular tissue. In this way, the phantom may mimic as closely as possible the texture of an actual human breast.

Target Lesion Construction

The materials used to create the multilayer phantom for use in SBT of ultrasound-guided needle biopsies were chicken breast, pork, beef, and turkey breast. Each phantom was created in layers, and the simulated target lesions were placed between the layers at different levels within it to reproduce varying grades of needle biopsy difficulty, from basic to very difficult, based on the target lesion location. Extensive research of different kinds of materials for target lesions was performed in order to best reproduce different types of lesions, such as a solid mass, simple cyst, and complex cyst (Figures 22.6–22.10).

Pseudo-lesion Construction

The purpose for creating the pseudo-lesions is to provide a more realistic ultrasound imaging experience for learners during SBT. The simulated lesion should be developed based upon imaging modality compatibility, so as to be clearly visible in real time during the training. A key pseudo-lesion in breast radiology is the cyst, with multiple features that

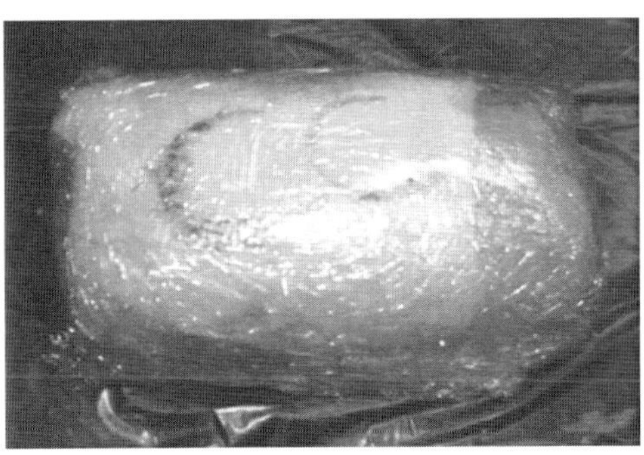

FIGURE 22.4 Multilayer phantom compacted with plastic wrap for ease of manipulation.

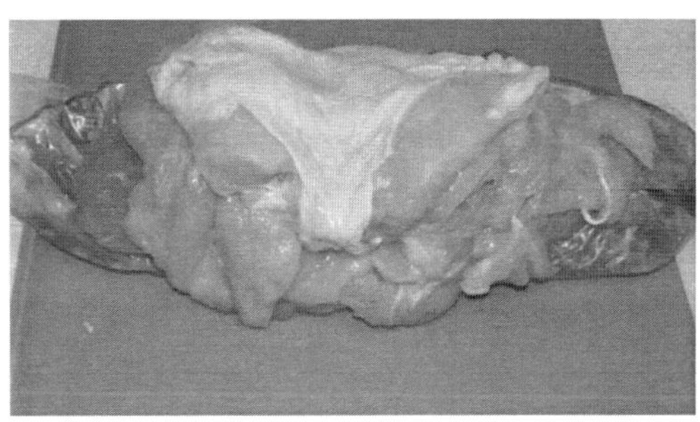

FIGURE 22.5 Breast ultrasound simulation. Multiple layers from different types of meat are assembled to form the multilayer phantom.

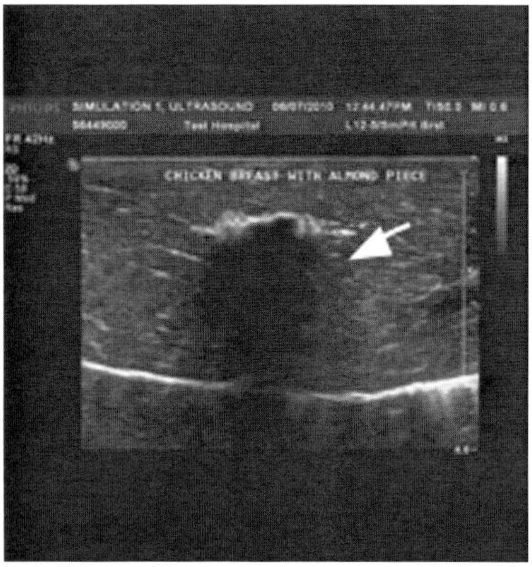

FIGURE 22.6 An almond (*arrow*) was folded into a chicken breast to simulate a hypoechoic mass.

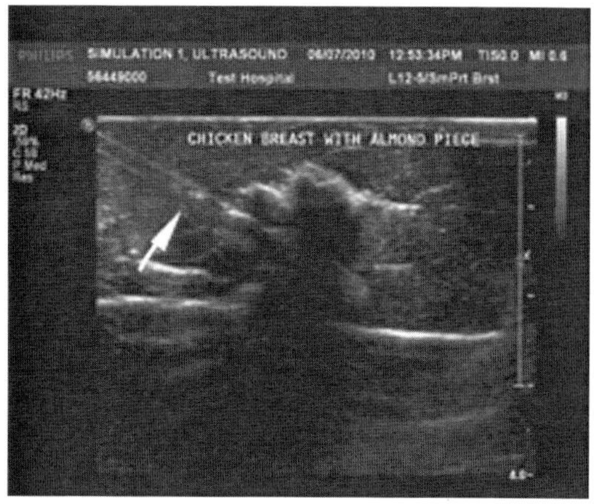

FIGURE 22.8 Vacuum-assisted biopsy with a 10-gauge needle (*arrow*) was performed with each of the simulators. After the tissue sample was obtained, it was transferred to a specimen container, allowing identification of the target material by direct vision.

range from simple to complex. With various materials and a little creativity, multiple target lesions can be created within the multilayer phantom that simulate a large variety of cystic lesions of different sizes and shapes. They can range from single to clustered, benign-appearing to suspicious for neoplasm, with fluid or solid content, and with or without septations, and can be of varying heterogeneity and wall thickness. Another useful feature is the ability to add color to the fluid inside these simulated pseudolesions to allow actual aspiration of the lesion during training.

To create a clear simple cyst, the finger of a disposable latex glove is filled with water and given the desired size and shape before closure of the

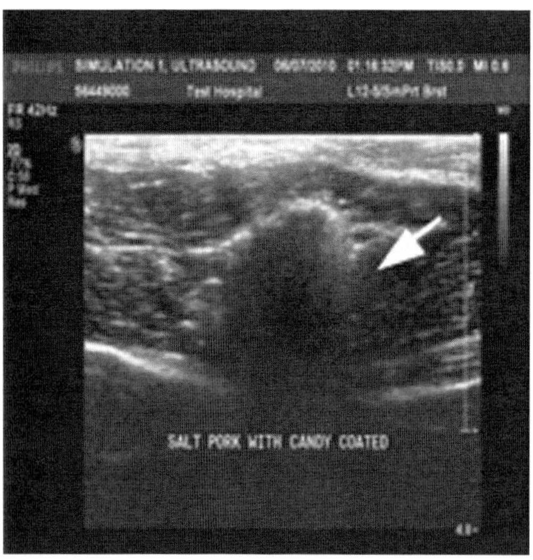

FIGURE 22.7 Salt pork was also used successfully as a lesion simulator with a candy-coated peanut placed inside seen as a hypoechoic mass (*arrow*). During simulation-based training, a small-gauge needle was used prior to performing the actual biopsy, in order to mimic the steps of local anesthetic administration.

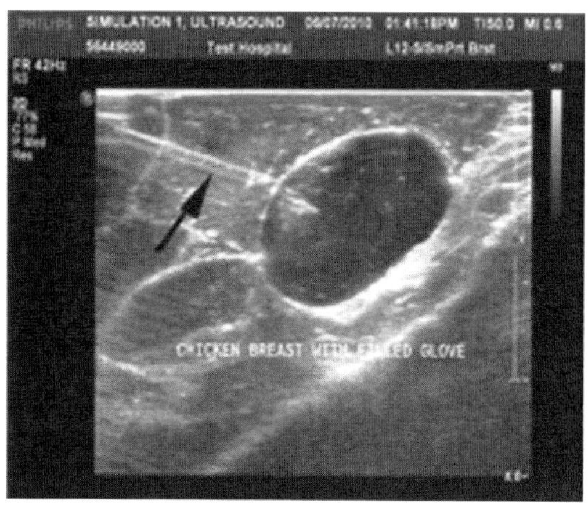

FIGURE 22.9 A latex glove finger filled with water was used to simulate a unilocular cystic lesion. The simulated cyst is punctured with the biopsy needle (*arrow*). Colored dye was added to the water in order to visualize the fluid collected from different targets within the phantom.

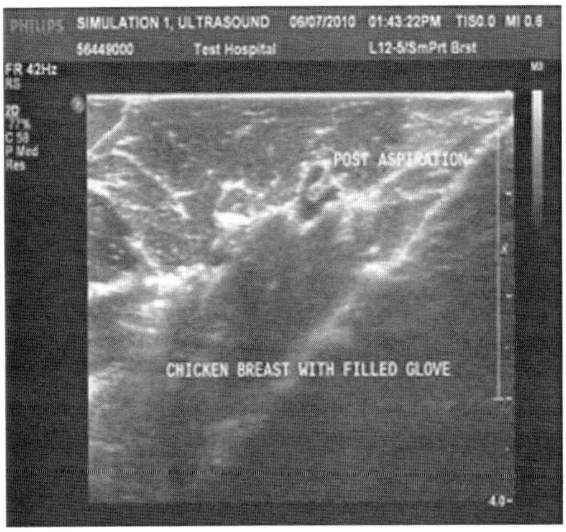

FIGURE 22.10 Chicken breast simulator with a water-filled glove finger as a target, status post fluid aspiration.

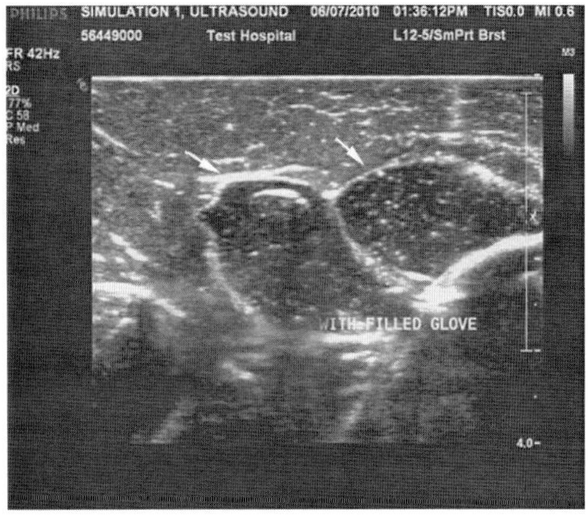

FIGURE 22.12 Breast ultrasound image of a multilayer phantom with latex glove finger filled with thick fluid simulating complex cyst (*arrows*) with thick septation and debris.

phantom. With ultrasound, it will appear sonolucent, well-circumscribed, oval or rounded, with thin wall. To give color to the fluid, we use water-soluble paints or any fluid of the desired color. For example, for a hemorrhagic cyst, ketchup or red wax can be used; for a brown-colored cyst, Betadine is used, so that at the moment of aspiration the colored fluid simulating the different types of cyst in breast disease is seen (Figure 22.11).

If a more viscous fluid is desired, a thick material can be added, such as water-insoluble gels, mustard, and ointments. This addition will show an echogenic material floating within the cyst, similar to that seen in simple cysts with high proteinaceous content, inflammatory cysts, or hemorrhagic cysts. To simulate wall thickening, the same cystic lesion is placed within the finger of another latex work glove. The more this last step is repeated, the greater the appearance of the wall thickening, so that more resistance will be felt at the moment of the needle insertion into the pseudo-cystic lesion. To create septations, the glove is filled with water and then multiple knots between every other finger of the glove are formed. With ultrasound, these lesion will

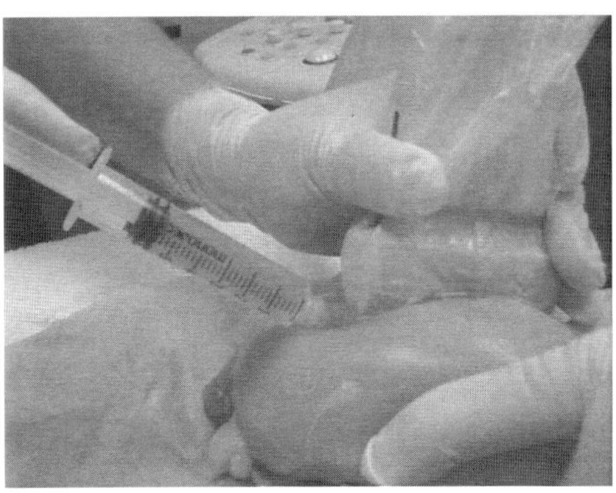

FIGURE 22.11 Simulation of breast fine needle aspiration (FNA) under ultrasound guidance. Note the colored fluid collected in the syringe simulating hemorrhagic fluid.

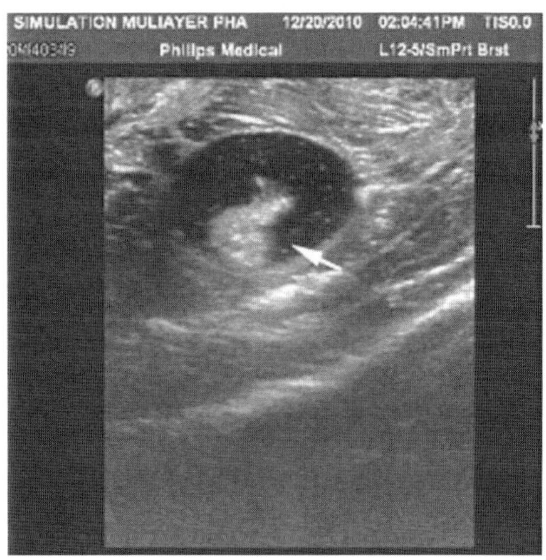

FIGURE 22.13 Simulation of a complex cyst with papillary lesion (*arrow*), made with a water-filled latex glove finger containing a piece of meat.

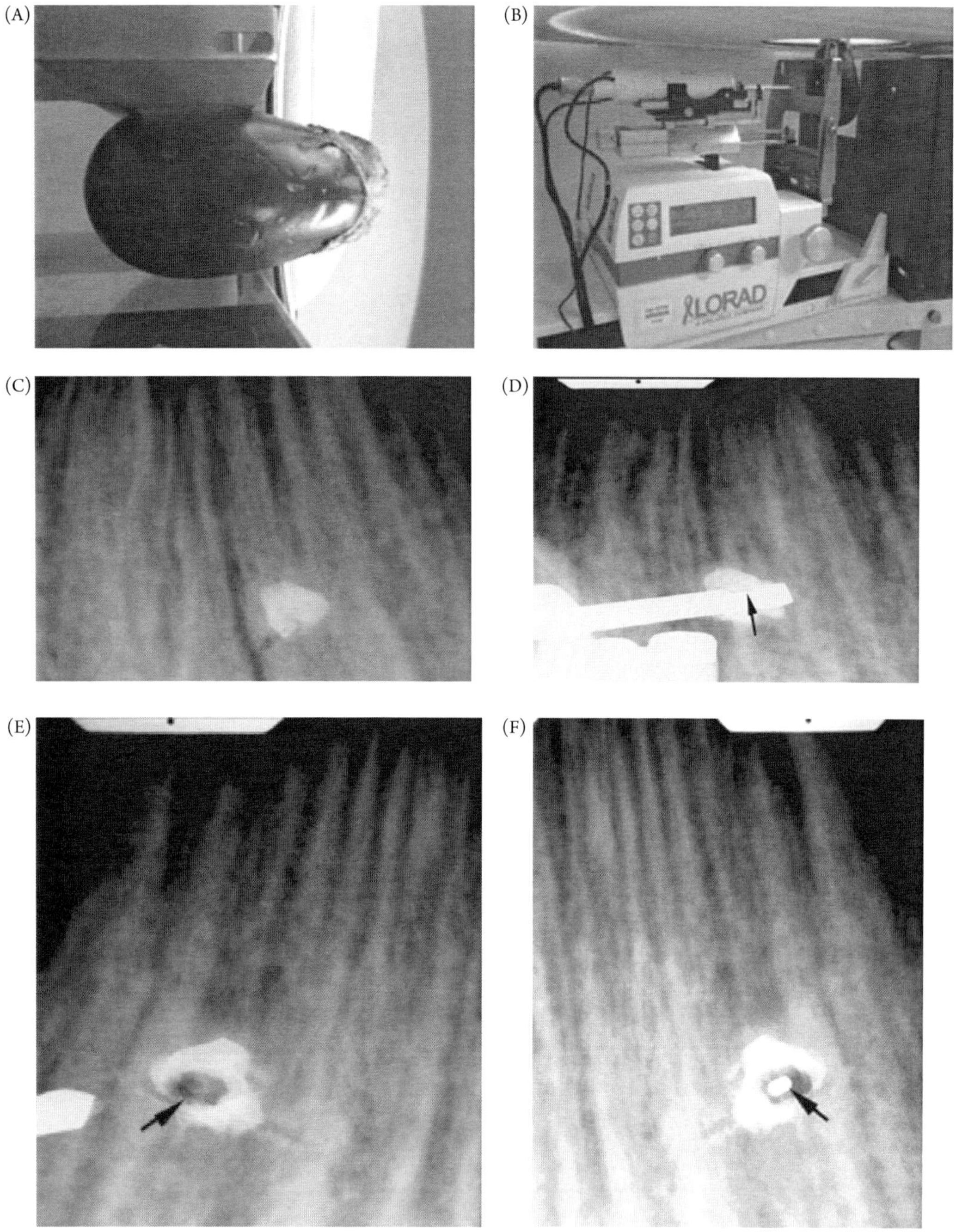

FIGURE 22.14 Simulation of a stereotactic breast biopsy on a prone table using an eggplant phantom, with vacuum-assisted biopsy device technology. (A) Eggplant phantom placed in the stereotactic compression device. (B) Vacuum-assisted device with 9-gauge needle (*arrow*) ready to penetrate the eggplant phantom. (C) A piece of almond within the eggplant phantom representing a lobulated solid lesion. (D) The 9-gauge needle notch is facing the lesion (*arrow*). (E) After core samples are taken, the central hypodense biopsy defect (*arrow*) within the residual lesion is visible. (F) A clip marker (*arrow*) was placed in the biopsied area within the lesion.

have the appearance of a cluster of cysts or multiple cysts with echogenic septations that need to be traversed during the simulated aspiration or biopsy. Finally, meat fragments can be added inside the glove to simulate papillary lesions within complex cysts (Figures 22.12 and 22.13).

ULTRASOUND-GUIDED NEEDLE BIOPSY

Ultrasound-guided needle biopsy is an attractive choice because it does not require ionizing radiation and also provides real-time imaging during the procedure. The major difficulty of the procedure is in maintaining a proper needle alignment. Simulation-based training can provide realistic hands-on ultrasound scanning to identify and examine different anatomic areas, as well as to recognize pathologic tissue.[6] The approach to learning ultrasound-guided biopsy starts with teaching the ultrasound theoretical physics basis. After this introduction, deliberate practice is undertaken. Only after repeated practice does the trainee proceed to hone skills in patient procedures.[7] Important techniques to include in any SBT program include fine needle aspiration (FNA), core-needle biopsy, and guided vacuum-assisted biopsy. Additionally, SBT should focus on the technical aspects of ultrasound scanning, including the manipulation of the ultrasound transducer and utilization of acoustic windows. Finally, SBT should include the study of sonographic cases with known tissue diagnosis to assist the learner in identifying different pathologies.[8] Commercial simulators for teaching breast biopsy procedure are available. Nevertheless, this chapter has concentrated on and described phantoms developed and used at LSUHSC-NO. These in-house simulators were selected for their ability to model tissue characteristics in imaging, particularly deformability; their ability to reproduce the varying texture patterns of the breast; and their affordability.

For the biopsy portion of SBT, a preloaded 10-gauge biopsy needle is placed in a biopsy gun apparatus. A freehand technique is used to guide the needle to the target at a 30- to 45-degree angle with one hand; meanwhile, the other hand manipulates the transducer to align the scanning plane and the needle.[9] After needle placement is confirmed by imaging, the sample is obtained by firing the biopsy gun, and the target material is identified within the core sample.

STEREOTACTIC BIOPSY SIMULATION

Stereotactic biopsy is requested when screening mammography reveals a suspicious lesion that is not palpable by clinical examination or readily visualized by ultrasound. Frequently, microcalcifications are present. Lieberman et al observed a learning curve for stereotactic breast biopsy. Significantly higher technical success rates and lower false-negative rates were noted after the first five 11-gauge vacuum-assisted biopsies.[10] Therefore, it is preferable to practice stereotactic breast biopsy on phantoms first, and progress to patient biopsy only after establishing a high skill level with the biopsy equipment and procedure. The ideal phantom for this procedure

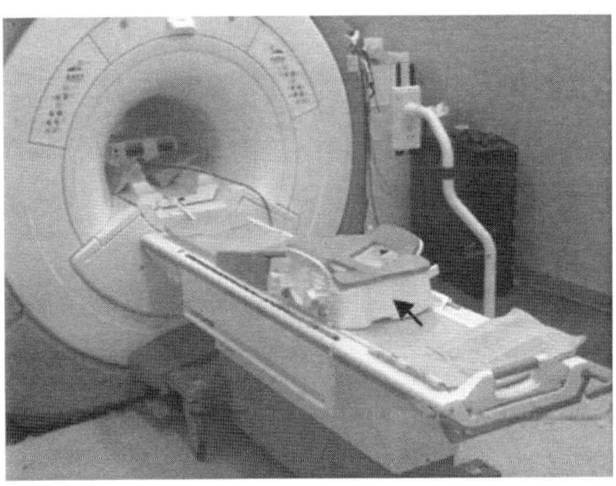

FIGURE 22.15 A 3-Tesla magnetic resonance imaging system with bilateral breast coil installed (*arrow*).

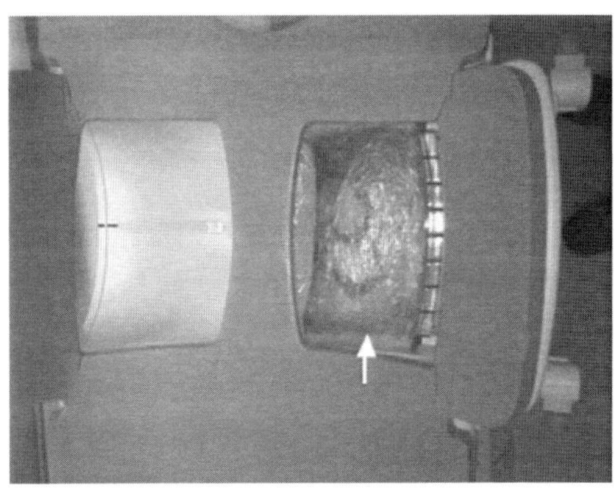

FIGURE 22.16 Simulation-based training for breast magnetic resonance imaging biopsy. Note the wrapped multilayer phantom (*arrow*) placed within the breast support.

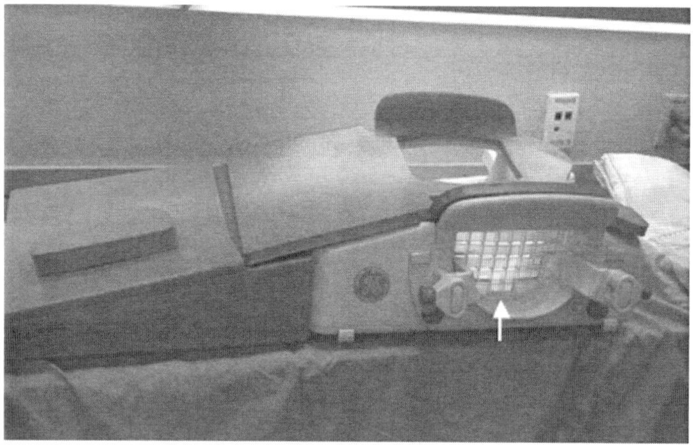

FIGURE 22.17 Simulation technique for breast magnetic resonance imaging biopsy with the dedicated breast coil (*arrow*) placed outside the magnet room.

should be low-priced, easily available, and of similar consistency to breast tissue.[11,12]

The stereotactic technique utilized in each radiology department is based at least in part upon the particular medical system used and the technology, applications, and standard protocol provided by the vendor. At LSUHSC-NO, stereotactic biopsies are performed using an automated dedicated prone table, with a vacuum-assisted biopsy device that supports 9- and 12-gauge needles. The equipment vendor's protocol is followed for both the stereotactic system and the vacuum-assisted device.

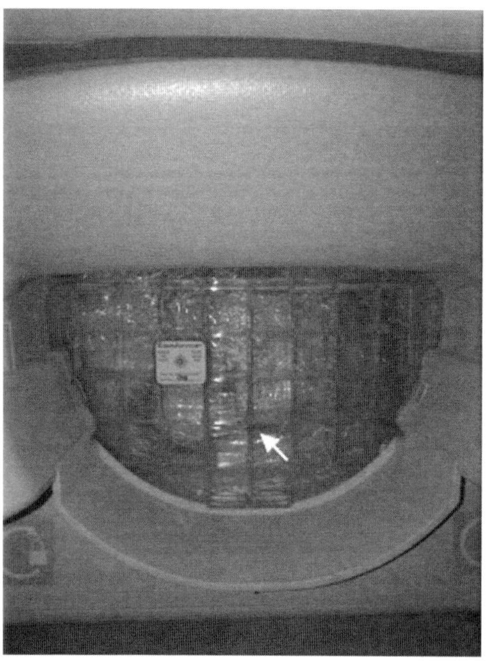

FIGURE 22.18 Simulation technique for breast magnetic resonance imaging biopsy. We use a grid technique (*arrow*). Note the plastic-wrapped multilayer phantom placed within the breast support behind the grid.

As previously described, our multilayer phantom is sufficiently versatile to be used with multiple modalities. It allows SBT for stereotactic biopsy, with the advantage of adding lesions, including calcifications, at different phantom depths. The use of either whole or fragmented almond is recommended in order to have immediate confirmation of lesion sampling by direct visualization of almond pieces within the core sample. This obviates the need for further mammographic imaging of the specimen to verify its contents, as would be performed for a standard stereotactic biopsy. Unlike the ultrasound-guided technique, the multilayer phantom for SBT of stereotactic biopsy requires an external plastic cover to compact the multiple layers and to maintain its form when compression by the stereotactic paddles is applied. Since the phantom is constructed with meat, its texture mimics compressed breast tissue.

An eggplant phantom also works well for SBT of stereotactic biopsy. It is probably the best choice for performing stereotactic biopsy simulation alone. The radiographic appearance of fibrous eggplant tissue closely resembles that of actual breast tissue. The eggplant fits easily into the biopsy device and can be repositioned without difficulty. We recommend the use of almond pieces for simulated solid lesions, which can be detected easily and thus allow the trainees to identify and localize the target

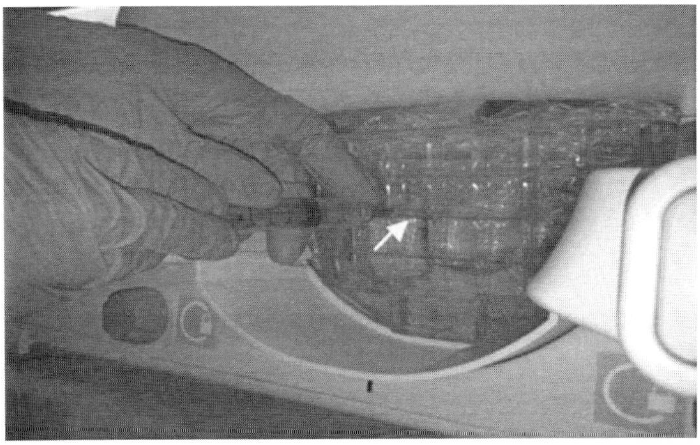

FIGURE 22.19 Infiltration of multilayer phantom by syringe with needle for local anesthesia simulation (*arrow*).

lesion. Larrison et al[13] described the utilization of water-soluble sonographic transmission gel combined with fragmented particles of barium sulfate tablet to simulate microcalcifications. Injecting this combination into the eggplant through an 18-gauge needle, while making several passes through the eggplant perpendicular to its long axis, can create the appearance of microcalcifications. The introduction of the gel mixture into the eggplant provides multiple targets for biopsy training. The use of sonographic gel also reduces the amount of air introduced into the phantom. The multilayer phantom may be used in conjunction with the eggplant phantom, as each phantom provides different textures and handling during the biopsy procedure (Figure 22.14).

MAGNETIC RESONANCE IMAGING-GUIDED BIOPSY SIMULATION

The MRI-guided technique varies within each radiology department based upon the particular medical system, technology, applications, and standard protocols used by each vendor. At LSUHSC-NO, SBT of MRI-guided breast biopsies is performed in a 3-Tesla magnet with dedicated bilateral breast coils, using a grid technique with a vacuum-assisted device that supports 9- and 12-gauge needles. The vendor's protocol for both the MRI system and vacuum-assisted device are followed during the procedure (Figure 22.15).

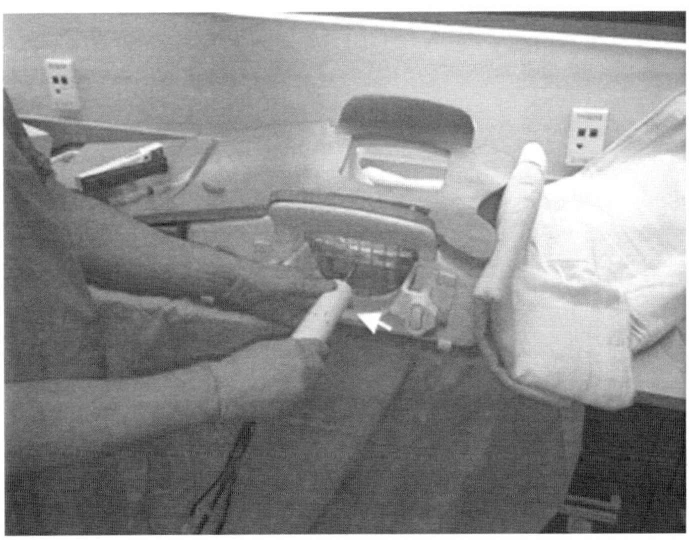

FIGURE 22.20 Vacuum-assisted biopsy being performed (*arrow*).

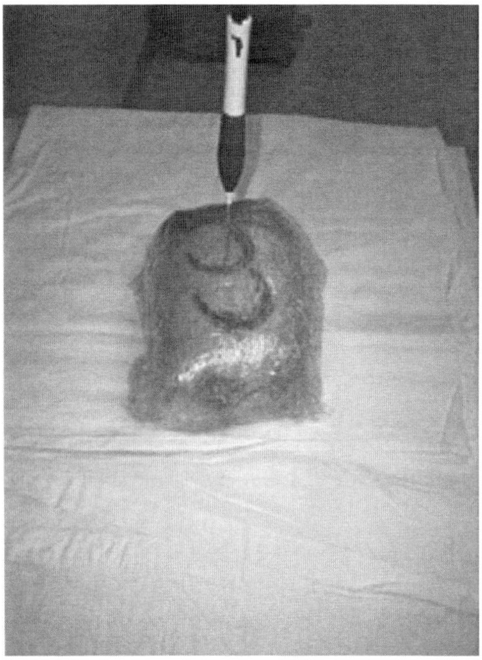

FIGURE 22.21 Wrapped multilayer phantom for needle localization simulation procedure. Note the "CC" marks on top and the needle used to introduce a metal clip.

The multilayer phantom, with plastic cover, is the primary model used because of its varying tissue layers, ease of target placement, and capacity for placing multiple lesions in the phantom at the same time. It is used in a similar fashion to SBT for ultrasound-guided breast biopsy, except for the addition of a plastic cover to give the phantom shape, firmness, and consistency (Figure 22.16).

The addition of complex cystic lesions as targets is a good option since this allows verification of the core content of the sample, with colored fluid retrieved in the vacuum chamber. In this way, the trainees can correlate image findings with core samples. As the learning curve progresses, the lesions can be made more complex, such as using vitamin E capsules with fragmented nuts stuck to the coated capsule. Since this procedure requires magnet availability, which is difficult in most institutions, the SBT can also be divided into two steps: without and with imaging.

The dedicated breast coil may be taken out of the magnet room and placed on a table, with assembly of the guidance system and practice of needle introduction into the phantom, following departmental standard protocol. This initial training gives the learner a better feeling of how the needle penetrates the phantom tissue. Following this step, the complete procedure, including imaging protocol, can be conducted using the MRI scanner (Figures 22.17–22.20).

NEEDLE LOCALIZATION WITH MAMMOGRAPHIC GUIDANCE

After image-guided direct needle biopsy, some lesions may require diagnostic or therapeutic surgical biopsy. If a malignant or indefinite diagnosis is obtained, surgical excision is indicated. The excision, in turn, will require accurate localization of the lesion. High accuracy of such localization is necessary to ensure correct and adequate removal of the lesion and to minimize the degree of cosmetic disfigurement. To obtain successful results, it is important for the operator to undergo adequate SBT training and demonstrate ability and skill prior to performing the procedure on an actual patient. The surgical outcome is largely dependent on the radiologist's accuracy in localization of lesions, which are usually grossly imperceptible at surgery. The radiologist may be required to accurately locate the lesion and expeditiously perform the localization in order to keep operating schedules on time.

Needle localization is performed using a standard protocol technique with mammographic guidance. Ultrasound guidance may be used on occasion in special cases, such as intraductal lesions, but the technique is institution-specific based upon the particular medical system, technology, applications, and standard vendor protocols. The multilayer phantom offers a good opportunity for trainees to practice since it simulates the texture of the breast tissue. Wrapping the phantom is recommended since change in positioning from craniocaudal (CC) to lateral position, or vice versa, must be performed. An adhesive sticker or mark is placed in the plastic cover to label the direction for the first approach (e.g., CC or lateral) (Figure 22.21).

In normal practice, localization of post-biopsy clip markers is performed frequently. For this reason, simulated clips are inserted within the phantom. Any small metallic device can be used to simulate a clip and can be introduced into the phantom. Attention should be paid to landmarks for easier placement and faster visualization on imaging. Fragments of standard paperclips are ideal and are readily available. Multiplanar views are taken to verify the wire placement related to the metal clip (Figure 22.22).

Although a variety of options may be successfully used for SBT, the experience at LSUHSC-NO with the multilayer phantom has provided a versatile

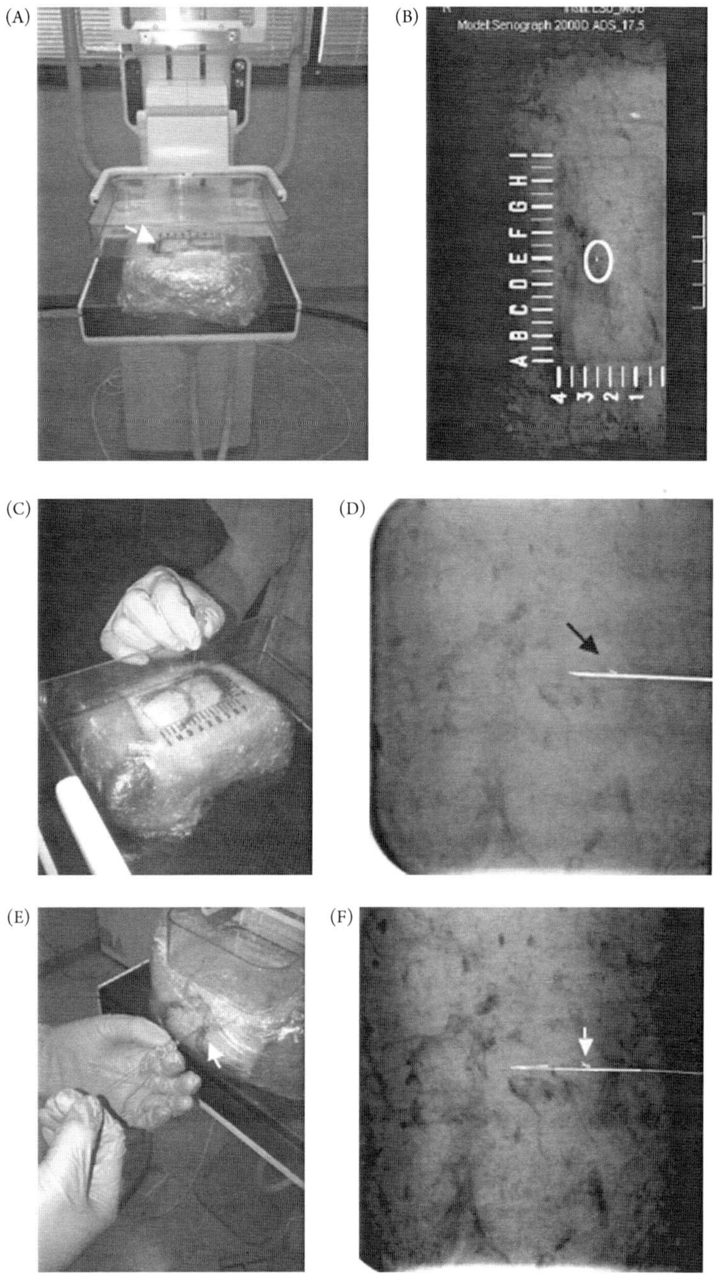

FIGURE 22.22 Simulation of breast wire needle localization with multilayer wrapped phantom. (A) Conventional upright mammography system with the multilayer phantom compressed between the digital receptor plate and the compression paddle. Note the CC marks (*arrow*) on top of the phantom indicating craniocaudal (CC) approach. (B) Mammographic view of the phantom with alphanumeric reference to localize the clip within the phantom (*circle*) and plan the needle approach. (C) Introduction of the wire needle (*arrow*) through the phantom on CC approach using a compression paddle with alphanumeric nomenclature. (D) Mammographic view after needle placement to verify the needle position in relation to the metal clip (*arrow*). (E) The multilayer phantom was turned into a lateral position with the CC marks (*arrow*) facing the operator. The resident pulls back the needle with the left hand while keeping the wire steady with the right hand. (F) Mammographic verification view shows the wire placed in good position, with the clip located adjacent to the middle part of the thick needle localizer cylinder (*arrow*).

model for training in multiple breast interventional modalities. It is inexpensive and easily reproducible, allowing standardized proficiency-based training of learners until the preestablished objective end points of expertise have been attained.

SIMULATION IN BREAST IMAGE INTERPRETATION TRAINING

This chapter has focused on SBT in technical skills related to image-guided breast interventional procedures as it has evolved in the teaching curriculum at LSUHSC-NO. This is an ideal SBT curriculum for medical students, residents, and fellows. Two additional points should be noted. First, SBT is most useful when integrated into a meaningful curriculum. Without a curriculum serving as a foundation, it can devolve into a game-like activity. Second, the concept of "simulation" in the field of breast imaging is much broader and has greater significance than may be apparent. At the 2009 meeting of the Accreditation Council on Graduate Medical Education (ACGME), K. Anders Ericsson, sometimes known as "the expert on experts," proposed the question, "can we make superior doctors through deliberate practice"?[14,15] He discussed at some length the belief, based on extensive study, that so-called *expert performance* is acquired through years of deliberate practice. Ericsson pointed out that some areas of medicine have researched the difference between novice practitioners, competent practitioners, and expert practitioners. Mammography interpretation and chest film interpretation are two of those areas in which the nature of expertise has been explored.[16–18] Applying these principles of deliberate practice in developing and validating simulation-based curricula in mammographic image interpretation is another means of introducing SBT into breast imaging. In summary, SBT techniques will prove increasingly useful in both breast imaging and breast interventional procedure training.

SIMULATION VIDEO

Diagnostic and interventional video may be accessed at:http://www.medschool.lsuhsc.edu/radiology/

REFERENCES

1. Harvey JA, Moran RE, Hamer MM, et al. Evaluation of a turkey-breast phantom for teaching freehand, US-guided core-needle breast biopsy. *Acad Radiol.* 1997;4:565–569.

2. Sisney GA, Hunt KA. A low-cost gelatin phantom for learning sonographically guided interventional breast radiology techniques. *AJR.* 1998;171:65–66.

3. Quinn AD, Smiddy PF, Duggan M, et al. Technical Report: a training phantom for stereotactic breast biopsies. *Clin Radiol.* 1997;52:149–150.

4. Fujisaki T, Kimura M, Saitoh H, et al. Production design and evaluation of a novel breast phantom with various breast glandular fractions. *Radiat Med.* 2006;24:647–652.

5. Friedrich MJ. Practice makes perfect: risk-free medical training with patient simulators. *JAMA.* 2002;288:2811–2812.

6. Fernandez-Frackelton M, Peterson M, Lewis RJ, et al. A bedside ultrasound curriculum for medical students: prospective evaluation of skill acquisition. *Teach Learn Med.* 2007;19:14–19.

7. Prager RW, Rohling RN, Gee AH, et al. Rapid calibration for 3-D freehand ultrasound. *Ultrasound Med Biol.* 1998;24:855–869.

8. Burke T, Madsen E, Zagzebski J. X-Ray linear attenuation coefficients in the mammographic range for ultrasonic breast phantom materials. *Radiology.* 1982;142:755–757.

9. Mendiratta-Lala M, Williams T, Quadros N, et al. The use of a simulation center to improve resident proficiency in performing ultrasound-guided procedures. *Acad Radiol.* 2010;17:535–540.

10. Lieberman L, Benton CL, Dershaw DD. Learning curve for stereotactic breast biopsy: how many cases are enough? *AJR.* 2001;176:721–727.

11. Liney G, Tozer D, Turnbull L. A simple and realistic tissue-equivalent breast phantom for MRI. *J MRI.* 1999;10:968–971.

12. Fischmann A, Siegmann KC. Low-cost phantoms for training of stereotactic vacuum-assisted biopsy of the breast. *Clinical Imaging.* 2010;34:97–99.

13. Larrison M, DiBona A, Hogg D. Low-cost phantom for stereotactic breast biopsy training. *AJR.* 2006;187:972–974.

14. Ericsson KA. Marvin Dunn Keynote Address. Presented at the ACGME Annual Educational Meeting; March 7, 2009, Grapevine, TX.

15. Ericsson KA, Krampe, RT, Tesch-Romer C. The role of deliberate practice in the acquisition of expert performance. *Psych Review.* 1993;100:363–406.

16. Nodine CF, Mello-Thomas C, Kundel, HL, et al. Time course of perception and decision making during mammographic interpretation. *AJR.* 2002;179:917–923.

17. Christensen EE, Murray RC, Holland K, et al. The effect of search time on perception. *Radiology.* 1981;138:361–365.

18. Nodine CR, Kundel HL, Lauver SC, et al. Nature of expertise in searching mammograms for breast masses. *Acad Radiol.* 1996;3:1000–1006.

23

Simulation in Abdominal Radiology

ROCIO PEREZ JOHNSTON, ARAN TOSHAV, AND DAVID L. SMITH

FROM THE earliest days of radiography, imagers have kept films of interesting cases. With increasing numbers of training institutions, film teaching file libraries emerged, many of which exist to this day. Such film libraries served as a cornerstone for training radiology residents to recognize rare and important radiographic findings. As such, they represented a basic form of simulation-based training (SBT) founded on the principle of deliberate practice. The development and general use of digital radiography, however, has largely rendered these hardcopy libraries obsolete, or at least inconsistent with today's digital workplace mentality. These teaching film libraries are being replaced by digital teaching files.

Today, selected digital images are archived and made available to radiologists for educational purposes.[1] Such archives often have interactive teaching points. This approach has resulted in some large, commercial, web-based teaching files, such as Statdx™ (Amirsys, Inc., Salt Lake City, Utah).

Some groups have utilized digital imaging to simulate the work environment of the radiologist in order to train and/or assess the interpretive skills of residents.[2–5] In such studies, individual and personal data are deleted from complete sets of imaging series, then recompiled and presented to a trainee in SBT, often for pre-call assessment.

Other groups are using imaging data to simulate the anatomic experience of a radiologist. This approach to SBT has well-established roots. Mannequin-based simulators, such as those used in training health care workers in basic life support, advanced cardiac life support, and basic procedural skills (e.g., intubation) have long been widely used. The Harvey™ cardiopulmonary patient simulator (Laerdal Medical AS, Stavanger, Norway) has been used in teaching institutions for nearly 40 years.[6]

Cross-sectional imaging data can be utilized to simulate the imaging findings a radiologist can expect to encounter in an actual patient. A collaborative effort centered in Boston has utilized a sonographic simulator to assess residents before overnight call[5] and to improve resident proficiency in ultrasound-guided procedures.[7] Another group has used a simulator to aid in training for gynecologic ultrasound applications.[8]

Additional literature details efforts in utilizing simulation in interventions using two-dimensional (2-D) fluoroscopic imaging. Much of this work has been done in vascular imaging and endovascular intervention. Some studies have simulated carotid artery stenting[9,10] and angioplasty[11] using computerized tomographic angiography (CTA) data of specific patients for the purpose of preprocedural planning and rehearsal. Other studies have developed simulations for the purposes of learning the Seldinger technique[12] and for training to improve endovascular procedural skills and cannulation times.[13,14]

Cross-sectional imaging has also been used to simulate the anatomy or pathology that a surgeon or endoscopist could find during a procedure. The emerging field of virtual colonography is a good example of this approach.[15] Similarly, SBT for upper gastrointestinal endoscopy and virtual bronchoscopy could be useful in both procedural training and diagnosis.

One area of abdominal imaging in which the use of simulation has become an important part of training is virtual colonography. Computed tomography colonography (CTC) is a rapidly evolving noninvasive imaging technique that relies on the performance of thin-section computed tomography (CT) of the colon, providing both 2-D and three-dimensional (3-D) images. It has recently been used for screening for colonic polyps and detecting colorectal cancers. Computed tomography colonography is a complex study that requires radiologists to know the theory behind polyp/cancer detection, the technical factors related to the imaging, and any pitfalls that may affect accurate study interpretation.

CURRENT SCREENING TESTS FOR COLON CANCER

Current screening tests for colon cancer are compared in Table 23.1. Colon cancer screening in asymptomatic patients with average, nonfamilial risk for colorectal cancer is currently recommended to begin at age 50 years.

Current colon screening options have important limitations. Although the performance of yearly fecal occult blood testing has demonstrated a reduction in mortality due to colorectal cancer, fecal occult blood testing is not a direct evaluation of the colonic mucosa.[16] Large adenomatous polyps or, less commonly, cancers, may not bleed, resulting in false-negative results for occult blood testing.

Screening sigmoidoscopy has been shown to decrease mortality due to colorectal cancer.[17] Sigmoidoscopy visualizes only the rectum and sigmoid colon, and complete colon screening is not achieved.[18]

Table 23.1 Current available screening tests for colon cancer

TEST	SENSITIVITY/SPECIFICITY	RISK COMPLICATION	ADVANTAGES
Fecal occult blood testing	72%–78%/98%	None	Noninvasive
Sigmoidoscopy	85%	Perforation 1–25,000 to 1–50,000	No sedation
Double contrast barium enema	48% >10mm polyps/90%	Perforation 0.02% to 0.04%	No sedation
Colonoscopy	87%–92%	Perforation: 1–500 to 1–1300	Biopsy, polypectomy
Computed tomography colonography	75%–100% /79%–96%	Perforation: no definite data, only case reports in patients with existing pathology (adenocarcinoma or irritable bowel disease)	Visualization of segments not seen on colonoscopy Extracolonic findings

Courtesy of Rocio Perez-Johnson, MD.

The double-contrast barium enema (DCBE) has been widely used for evaluation of colonic pathology. Rockey et al,[19] however, demonstrated in a prospective trial that, although DCBE specificity could approach 90%, sensitivity was low, with only a 48% detection rate for colonic polyps larger than 10 mm in diameter. Such low sensitivity limits DCBE use.

Complete endoscopic colonoscopy allows the most thorough evaluation of the colon, with the added benefit of the endoscopist's ability to perform selective biopsy or excision of polyps and some other lesions. Colonoscopy is thus considered the reference standard for colonic evaluation.[20] Some important limitations exist, however, to the widespread use of screening colonoscopy, including the need for sedation, the potential risk of colon perforation and bleeding, the costs of the procedure (including sedation), and the inability to complete the examination in 5%–10% of patients.[21]

COMPUTED TOMOGRAPHY COLONOGRAPHY VS. COLONOSCOPY: RELATIVE ADVANTAGES/DISADVANTAGES

Clinical evaluation of CTC has shown promise for the detection of polyps and cancers of the colon and rectum, with polyp detection sensitivity values ranging from 75% to 100% for polyps 10 mm and larger.[22]

Computed tomography colonography could provide a useful alternative for widespread screening, since it requires no intravenous administration of sedatives and analgesia or recovery time. It allows the evaluation of all of the colonic segments, especially important in the setting of an incomplete colonoscopy. Computed tomography colonography also allows localization and staging of carcinomas by detecting tumor extension through the colon or rectal wall, by identifying enlarged lymph nodes, and by determining the presence of distant metastases within the abdomen.

There are some disadvantages to CTC. Patients are exposed to X-radiation. In addition, CTC requires bowel preparation and gas insufflation, which can be uncomfortable. It requires expensive computer hardware for interpretation, and has been shown to have false-positive findings, especially in the presence of residual fecal material and underdistended colon segments. False negative findings can also occur, especially for flat lesions protruding less than 3 mm into the colon lumen, which are difficult to visualize.

INDICATIONS FOR COMPUTED TOMOGRAPHY COLONOGRAPHY

Common indications for CTC are described in Table 23.2.

Table 23.2 Indications for computed tomography colonography, and technical factors

CRITERIA	INDICATION-TECHNIQUE
Patients over 50 years, asymptomatic	Screening:
Patients with known tortuous colon	– Low-dose supine and prone (kV 120, mAs 70)
History of polyps	– No IV contrast
Symptomatic patients (guaiac-positive stools, bleeding per rectum, weight loss)	Diagnostic:
	– Low-dose supine (kV120, mAs 70)
History of colon cancer	– Prone: kV 120, mAs automated (min 150, max 400); IV contrast
History of prior colon surgery	
History of extracolonic malignancy	
Tortuous colon	Incomplete colonoscopy:
Sharp angulation, hernia	– Low-dose supine (kV120, mAs 70)
Extrinsic compression	– Prone: kV 120, mAs automated (min 150, max 400); IV contrast indicated only if mass, large polyp seen on OC, or if history of malignancy (colonic or extracolonic)
Stricture (benign or malignant)	
Search for synchronous tumors	

Courtesy of Rocio Perez-Johnson, MD.

Key Steps in Computed Tomography Colonography

It is important for all radiologists to know the different technical steps and factors that influence the outcome of the study and indirectly impact on the reporting of the study. In addition, radiologists performing CTC need to be familiar with the tools used to facilitate the interpretation of CTC.

STEP 1: PATIENT PREPARATION

Several different techniques may be used for bowel preparation, and controversy remains as to how to optimize patient preparation. The goal is to have a well-prepared, well-distended colon that will facilitate polyp detection and minimize false-positive findings, thereby maximizing the ability to differentiate polyps, folds, and residual fecal material in the colon.

Commercially available bowel preparations include cathartics, such as magnesium citrate and phosphosoda, and colonic lavage solutions, such as polyethylene glycol. At Massachusetts General Hospital (MGH), HalfLytely™ & Bisacodyl Bowel Prep Kit (sodium chloride, sodium bicarbonate, and potassium chloride oral solution, plus bisacodyl tablets; Braintree Laboratories, Massachusetts), has demonstrated good patient tolerance and resulted in good image quality for CTC interpretation.

Residual fecal material can make interpretation difficult. Tagging the fecal residue with contrast material helps to reduce false-positive findings on CTC. Fecal tagging is achieved by having the patient ingest small amounts of iodine containing contrast medium prior to imaging. The high-attenuation contrast material will be incorporated into residual fecal matter, thus facilitating differentiation from polypoid mucosal lesions.

STEP 2: PROCEDURE PERFORMANCE

For colonic insufflation, either room air or carbon dioxide (CO_2) can be used. The use of room air is easy, clean, and inexpensive. In our experience, CO_2 use is preferred because it is readily absorbed from the colon and causes less cramping after the

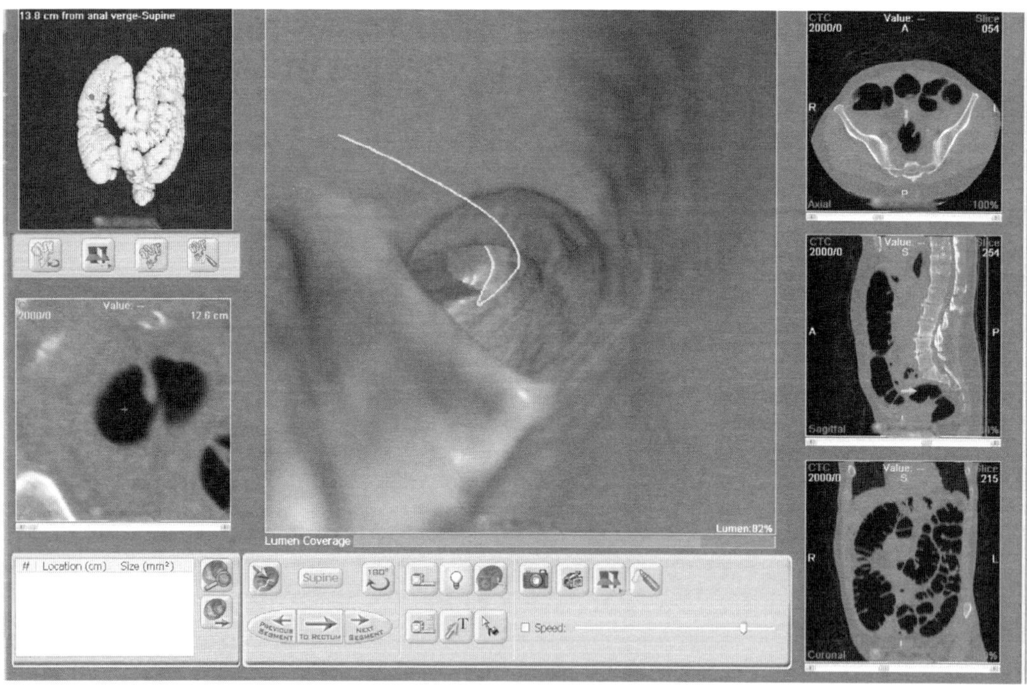

FIGURE 23.1 Display of the software used for interpretation of computed tomography colonography. The simulation cases are rendered anonymous; the only information left is the gender and age of the patient (as seen on the top of the screen). The software allows correlation in the three-dimensional endoluminal view (center of the screen) with two-dimensional axial, sagittal and coronal (right side of screen). Courtesy of M. Zalis, Mass General Imaging and Viatronix, Stony Brook, New York.

procedure than does room air insufflation.[23] A small flexible rectal catheter is inserted, and pneumocolon is achieved through the patient-controlled insufflation of CO_2 immediately before scanning. The patient holds the breath while rapid CT scanning is performed in both supine and prone positions. The acquisition of supine and prone scans improves overall colonic distention and leads to a diagnostically important redistribution of gas, residual fluid, and stool. A lesion hidden in a collapsed colon segment with the patient in supine position may be visible with the patient in the prone position.[24]

STEP 3: STUDY PROCESSING/READING

Image processing and interpretation are performed on a 3-D workstation with the use of a commercially available CTC software system (e.g., Viatronix V3-D Colon version 4™, Viatronix, Stony Brook, New York). This software program extracts the images of the gas-filled colon, generates an automated centerline for luminal navigation, and electronically removes residual tagged material from the images in a routine postprocessing step. The diagnostic interface allows for a virtual "fly through" tour of the 3-D image and rapid correlation with the 2-D images for any suspected abnormality (Figure 23.1).

Two approaches exist for CTC interpretation: primary 2-D reading with 3-D corroboration, and 3-D primary reading with 2-D correlation. At MGH, intraluminal 3-D primary reading is preferred to allow better visualization of small lesions. Two-dimensional cross-sectional images are then used to corroborate the density and any fixed point of

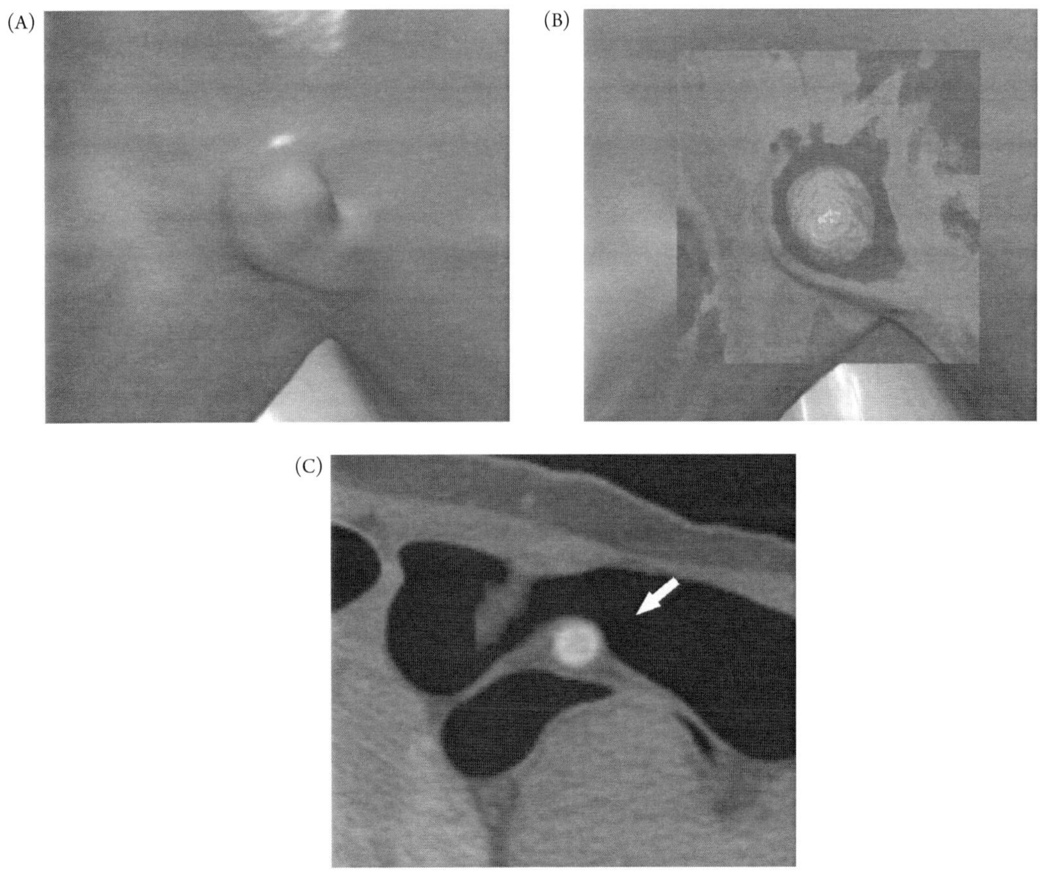

FIGURE 23.2 Screening computed tomography colonography in a 56 year old patient, in which in three-dimensional endoluminal view (A) a polypoid lesion is seen in the sigmoid colon. However, with the translucency tool (B), high-density material is seen (*white color*), which is corroborated on the two-dimensional image (C) and is seen extending outside of the colonic wall in relation to an inverted diverticulum. Courtesy of M. Zalis, Mass General Imaging.

attachment of the finding. The translucency rendering tool, which consists of an attenuation-dependent color map that complements the 2-D density assessment of the internal features of polypoid lesions, is commonly used (Figure 23.2).[25]

The use of a computer-assisted device (CAD), either concurrently or as a second reader, improves detection of sessile and polypoid lesions 6 mm and larger in diameter.[26] In screening patients, it has been demonstrated that CAD's sensitivity is comparable to optical colonoscopy for adenomas over 8 mm in diameter.[27] Further study is needed to determine CAD's performance in different settings. At MGH, CAD is not used for primary reading and is not available for teaching purposes.

STEP 4: INTERPRETATION

Computed tomography colonography relies for accuracy of interpretation on several technical factors, such as adequate colon preparation and distension. It is important to review the possible pitfalls that can be encountered during the CTC reading.

A technically inadequate CTC study is defined by the CT Colonography Reporting and Data System (C-RADS), as C0, an examination in which confident interpretation of the colonic findings is not possible owing to technical limitations, and the radiologist cannot exclude the presence of polyps (see Table 23.4). Incomplete bowel preparation (leading to large amounts of retained fecal material) and insufficient bowel gas insufflation (leading to segmental collapse in both prone and supine positions) can severely limit the performance of CTC (Figure 23.3).[28]

Residual stool can either simulate or obscure colonic lesions, leading to interpretation errors. On 3-D views, stool can often have irregular, geometrical, angulated borders, or an oval or rounded "pseudopolypoid" configuration. Therefore, careful analysis of the 2-D images is necessary to evaluate the density of a finding. Residual fecal material typically contains gas, is heterogeneous, and moves with patient change in position.

Fecal tagging usually helps in this setting, by mixing the high-density iodine-containing contrast material with stool, thus differentiating it from the bowel wall and colonic lesions.[29] Solid collections of contrast material can simulate a polypoid lesion on 3-D endoluminal images. Retained contrast material may be uniformly hyperattenuating and may be mixed with stool in various patterns, and, in order to be distinguished from a polyp, the 2-D images need to be correlated (Figure 23.4).

Sudden respiratory motion during CTC results in data misregistration and degrades image quality. In 2-D and on 3-D images, respiratory motion appears as colon wall defects. Metallic structures, like hip prostheses, cause beam-hardening artifacts that degrade the image quality and obscure portions of the bowel wall, especially in the pelvis.

Computed tomography colonography interpretation can be difficult and has a steep learning curve to proficiency. Before a CTC study can be interpreted, the 3-D software package must be mastered, and the interpreter must learn to manipulate the dataset to evaluate the entire colon. The interpreter must become skilled at passing back and forth between the 3-D and 2-D images and learn how to manipulate the software, so that all data is interpreted. Thereafter, even experienced readers may not be familiar with the finer details of interpretation of CTC studies. In general, readers are confronted with huge datasets from which they are required to locate random and uncommon tiny bumps on the colon mucosal surface. Such a situation makes interpretation very difficult, especially in a screening population in which it is assumed that the total number of patients with true disease is low.[30]

In part because of the difficulty in mastering interpretation, marked variation occurs in reported diagnostic accuracy of CTC. A large screening study by Pickhardt and colleagues[31] demonstrated that CTC can detect polyps with sensitivity similar to optical colonoscopy. Other large studies, however, have shown that observer detection rates can vary widely.[32]

The American College of Radiology Imaging Network (ACRIN) trial was developed to investigate the potential for CTC to be applied as a screening methodology. The readers chosen to interpret the studies were required to be proficient readers of CTC, and specific reader selection criteria were established. Each participating radiologist was required to submit confirmation of having interpreted at least 500 CTC examinations or of having participated in a specialized 1.5-day CTC training session. All participating radiologists were required to complete a qualifying examination in which they achieved a detection rate of 90% or more for polyps measuring 10 mm or larger in diameter in a reference image set. Of the 20 radiologists who met

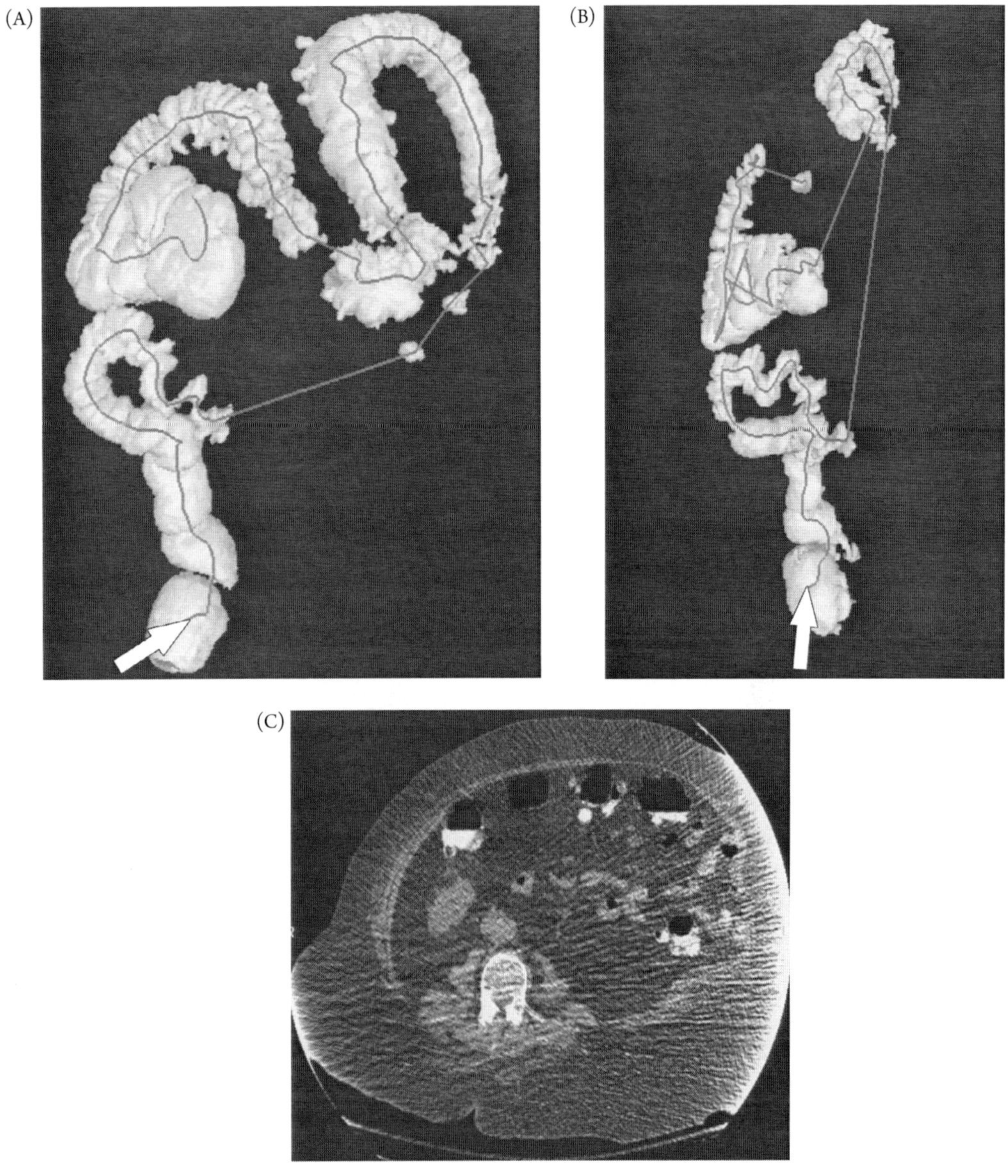

FIGURE 23.3 Completion computed tomography colonography in a 280-pound, 79-year-old patient, with inadequate insufflation. A large segment of descending colon was not visualized on both supine (A) and prone (B) views. Additionally, the quality of the cross-sectional images was considerably degraded by noise and streak artifact. The study was categorized as technically inadequate C0. Courtesy of M. Zalis, Mass General Imaging.

the initial entry criteria, 15 with the highest scores on the qualifying examination were subsequently invited to participate in the study.[33,34] The rigorous selection criteria for readers were necessary for credibility of this study. The eventual study results were similar to those of Pickhardt et al[34]

The ACRIN trial required strict adherence to protocol, including stool tagging regimens, mechanical insufflation of the colon, and thin-section and low-dose CT techniques.[33] Quality control is an essential and recognized aspect of all CTC and colon cancer screening regimens. The American College of Radiology (ACR) practice guidelines state that colon cleansing and distention should allow adequate visualization of the colon and rectum. Each segment should be distended and free of

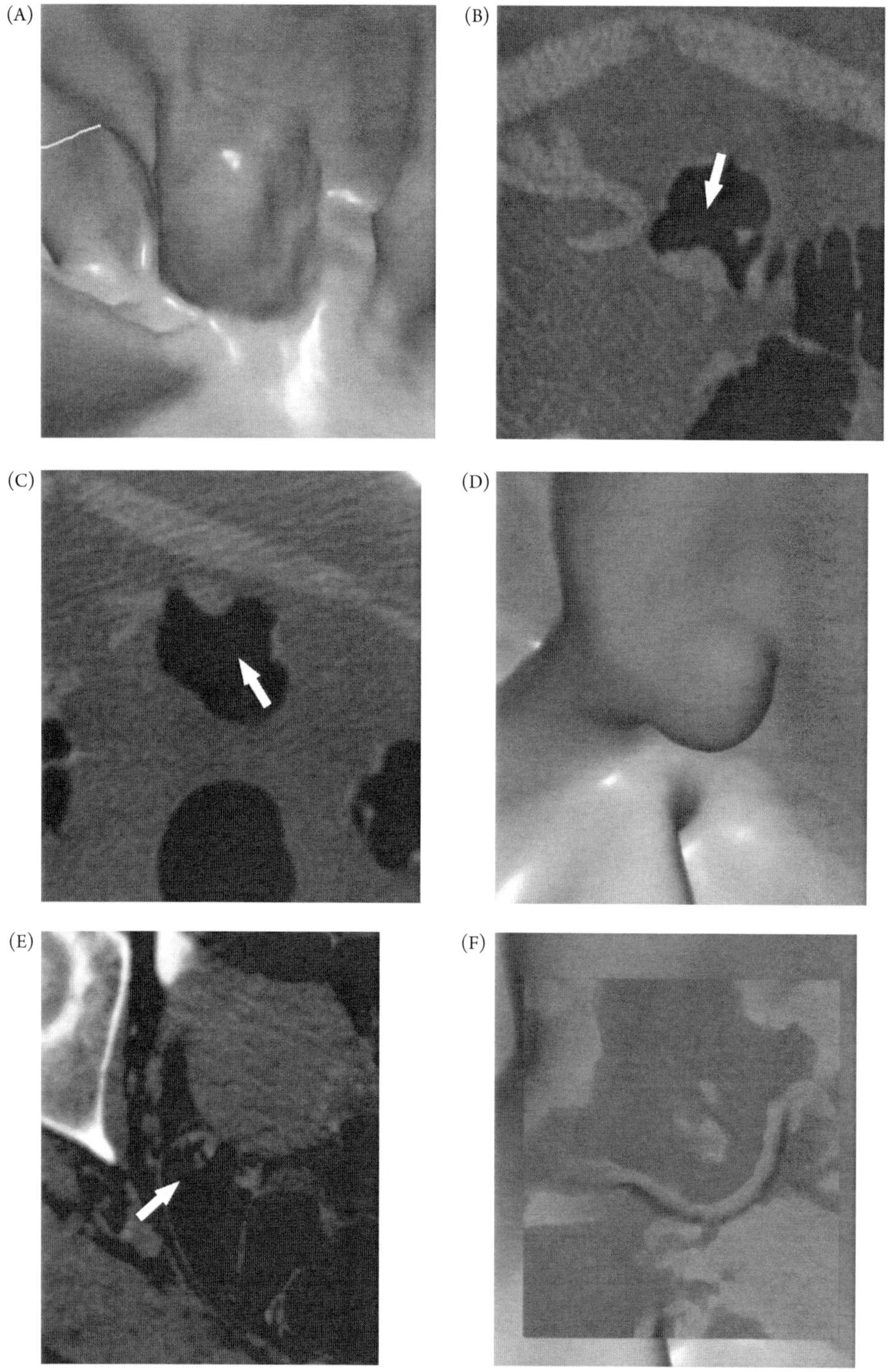

FIGURE 23.4 Two different cases of retained fecal material. The top images represent a patient with untagged fecal material in the sigmoid colon. As seen on three-dimensional (3-D) image (A) fecal material can mimic a mass, which on two-dimensional (2-D) supine image (B) shows soft tissue density. However, on 2-D prone image (C), displacement to the dependent wall is observed. On the bottom images, a polypoid lesion is observed in the sigmoid colon on the 3-D image (D). On the 2-D supine image (E), air is seen inside the polypoid finding, which can be correlated with the translucency image (F), which shows central air "green bubble," consistent with fecal material. Courtesy of M. Zalis, Mass General Imaging.

(A) (B)

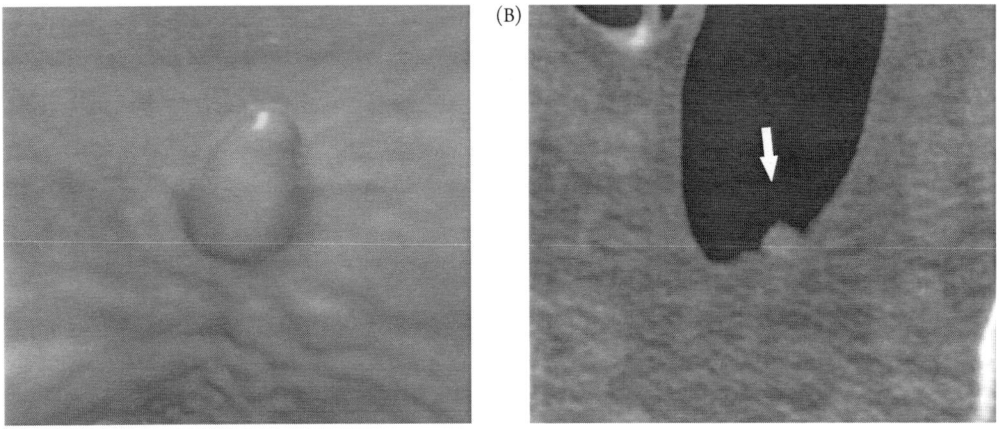

FIGURE 23.5 Example of polyps. A 61-year-old patient underwent screening computed tomography colonography, in which a 10 mm sessile polyp was seen on three-dimensional endoluminal image (A),which on two-dimensional image (B) shows soft tissue density. The polyp was removed at optical colonoscopy. The pathology report was tubular adenoma. Courtesy of M. Zalis, Mass General Imaging.

most fluid. Suboptimal visualization of any segment of the colon requires a repeat scan.[35]

The ACR and other organizations have developed guidelines and consensus statements regarding the minimum training necessary to interpret CTC. The ACR recommends that physicians supervising and interpreting CTC should have reviewed at least 50 endoscopically confirmed CTC cases performed for a variety of indications (e.g., screening, symptomatic, incomplete endoscopy), using a variety of scanning methods (e.g., with and without oral tagging and intravenous contrast).[35]

At MGH, an SBT module using a workstation simulator was created to teach clinical fellows and residents the basics of CTC performance and interpretation. The training module consists of 50 preselected studies, including normal studies and studies with artifact mimicking disease, as well as studies with pathology validated with optical colonoscopy and tissue pathology. The SBT model presented below is based upon the experience of the authors with the training module at MGH.

Prior to beginning practice on the workstation simulator, the reader receives a short didactic

Table 23.3 Basic characteristics of the different findings that radiologists encounter during simulation.

	MORPHOLOGY	DENSITY	FIXED POINT OF ATTACHMENT
Polyp	Flat, sessile, pedunculated	Soft tissue density	Yes
Mass/stricture	Circumferential Polypoid Shouldering	Soft tissue density Enhancement	Yes
Stool	Polypoid, irregular, sharp margins	Heterogenous May contain air	No
Tagging	Polypoid, irregular, layering	High density	No
Lipoma	Flat or sessile (submucosal)	Fat density	Yes

Courtesy of Rocio Perez-Johnson, MD.

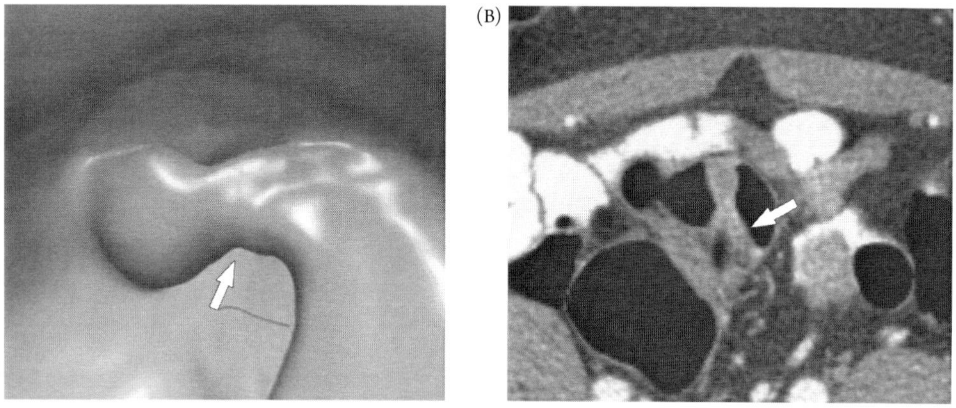

FIGURE 23.6 Three-dimensional endoluminal view of a 12 mm pedunculated polyp of a 54-year-old patient (A). On the two-dimensional image (B), the soft tissue density of the lesion is corroborated, and enhancement is observed. The arrows point to the stalk of the polyp, which should not be included when measuring the polyp. Polypectomy was performed and pathologically the lesion showed high-grade dysplasia and carcinoma in situ arising from a tubular adenoma. Courtesy of M. Zalis, Mass General Imaging.

session in which the various features of the workstation are described and the reader is shown an example of their uses. Function keys are labeled on the keyboard to describe the various key functions. Fifty preselected cases are loaded onto the Viatronix stand-alone workstation, with all bookmarked areas of concern, patient information, and measurements removed. The study is interpreted in 3-D format and

Table 23.4 C-RADS, as established in 2005 by the Working Group on Virtual Colonoscopy (includes members of the American College of Radiology Colon Cancer Committee)

C-RAD		EXAMPLES
C0	Inadequate study awaiting prior comparisons	– Inadequate prep: cannot exclude >10 mm owing to presence of fluid/feces – Inadequate insufflation: one or more colonic segments collapsed on both views – Awaiting prior colon studies for comparison
C1	Normal colon or benign lesions Next screening in 5 years	– No visible abnormalities of the colon – No polyp >6 mm – Lipoma – Non-neoplastic findings: diverticula
C2	Intermediate polyp/ indeterminate finding Surveillance (up to 3 years) or colonoscopy recommended	– Polyp 6–9 mm, less than three in number – Cannot exclude polyp > 6 mm in technically adequate exam
C3	Polyp, possibly advanced adenoma. Colonoscopy recommended	– Polyp > 10 mm – More than three polyps, 6–9 mm each
C4	Colonic mass, likely malignant Surgical consultation recommended	Lesion compromises bowel lumen, demonstrates extracolonic invasion

can be correlated with 2-D images in either axial, coronal, or sagittal planes. Both supine and prone series are interpreted. The cases are labeled case number 1 through 50 and are presented in random order to avoid reader bias. Each case is presented exactly as it would be if the study was a patient diagnostic case.

The reader interprets the study, notes the findings, and compares it to a portable document format (PDF) document that contains the pertinent findings, as well as pictures of the lesions on 2-D and 3-D imaging. The system is designed for individual self-evaluation, but it could easily be adapted to a test format, so that an individual's performance could be logged and improvement quantified.

CTC Interpretation

POLYPS

The most important part of the training in CTC is to acquire the basic knowledge to detect polyps. On CTC, polyps are defined as round, oval, or lobulated intraluminal filling defects, with homogeneous soft-tissue density and a fixed point of attachment to the colon wall (Figure 23.5).

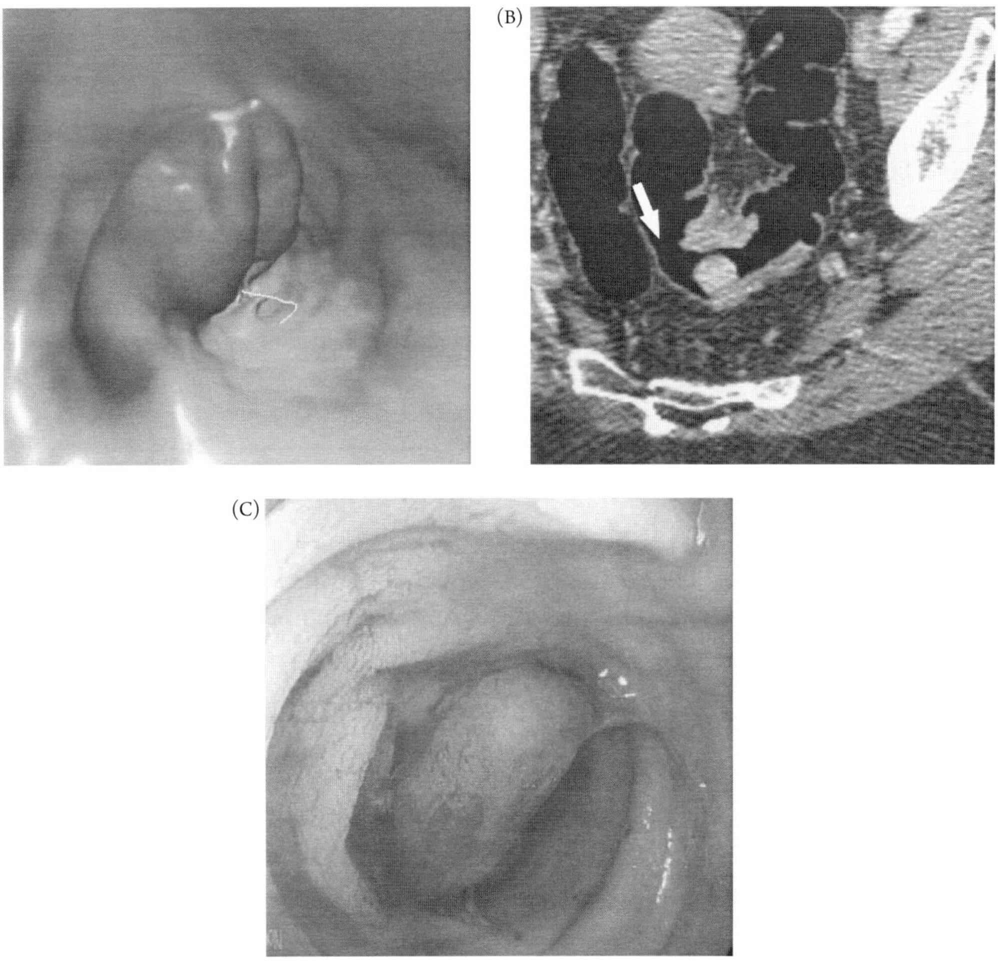

FIGURE 23.7 Completion computed tomography colonography in an asymptomatic 57-year-old female patient. On three-dimensional endoluminal view (A), a large, partially obstructing mass is seen arising from the sigmoid colon wall. The finding is corroborated on two-dimensional image (B), in which a circumferential enhancing mass is seen in the sigmoid colon. On optical endoscopy (C), the lesion was biopsied, displaying adenocarcinoma on pathology. Courtesy of M. Zalis, Mass General Imaging.

Polyps can be flat (i.e., plaque morphology, with less than 3 mm of vertical elevation, or with height no more than one-half the width), sessile, or pedunculated. With intravenous contrast administration, polyps will usually enhance (Table 23.3).

As defined by C-RADS, polyp size remains the most important criterion by which a given lesion should be categorized, according to the inherent risk of developing subsequent malignancy.[28] Lesion size is defined as the largest diameter of the polyp head, excluding the stalk when present. The majority of polyps 5 mm or less in diameter are mostly hyperplastic and are considered unlikely to have an increased risk of developing carcinoma. Consequently, they are not reported as a finding on CTC.[36]

Polyps measuring between 6 and 9 mm in diameter are mostly benign, and up to 30% are not adenomas. The likelihood that a polyp of this size range contains high-grade dysplasia is 3%–5%. The likelihood that such a polyp contains invasive carcinoma is less than 1%.[37] Patients with lesions 10 mm or larger in diameter should be referred for colonoscopy, since 10%–25% can harbor either high-grade dysplasia or carcinoma.[38] Masses are defined as lesions 30 mm or larger in diameter or lesions that either compromise the bowel lumen or demonstrate extracolonic invasion (Figure 23.6).

Lesion location is described according to the colonic segment (i.e., rectum, sigmoid, descending colon, transverse colon, ascending colon, or cecum). At MGH, the radiologist in training who is working

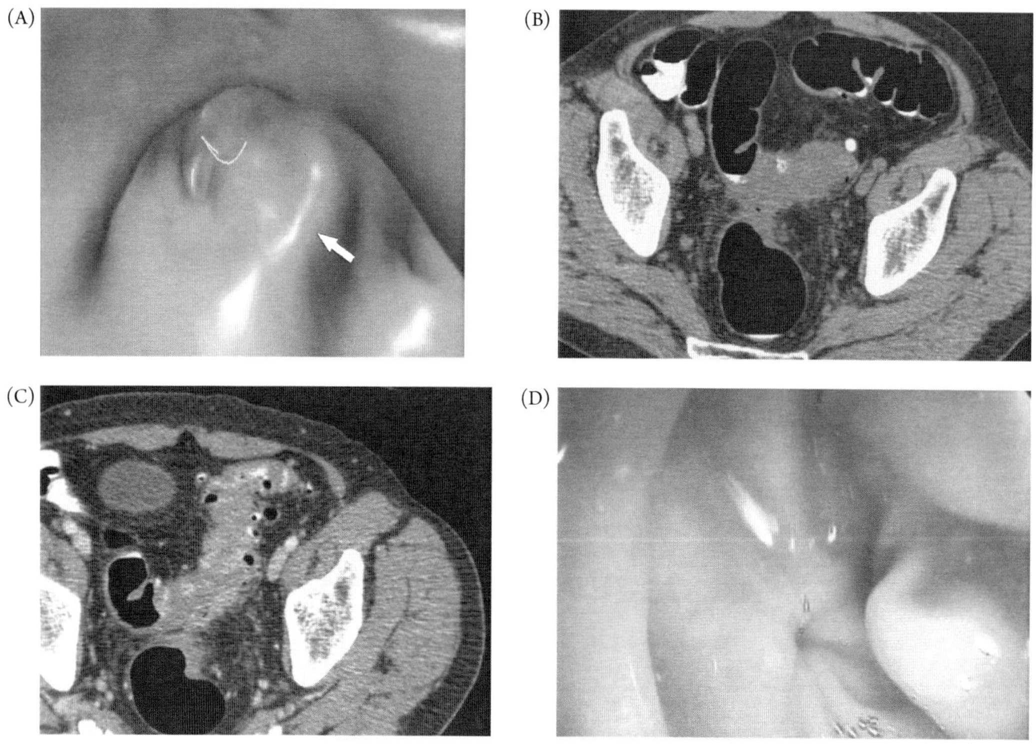

FIGURE 23.8 Completion computed tomography colonography of a 58-year-old male, with a history of diverticular disease and currently referred for constipation and abdominal distension. The patient underwent optical colonoscopy, with a report of a benign-appearing stricture in the sigmoid colon. (A) A three-dimensional endoluminal view in which narrowing of the lumen was encountered. Note the bulky mucosa at the site of narrowing (*arrow*). The differential diagnosis includes neoplastic or inflammatory stricture. (B) Supine unenhanced two-dimensional (2-D) axial image, demonstrating thickening of the sigmoid wall and diverticula, with stranding of the mesosigmoid. (C) Prone, contrast-enhanced axial 2-D image with mild enhancement of the sigmoid colon wall. (D) Optical colonoscopy correlation. Biopsy pathology examination showed a benign inflammatory process, presumed secondary to diverticulitis. Courtesy of M. Zalis, Mass General Imaging.

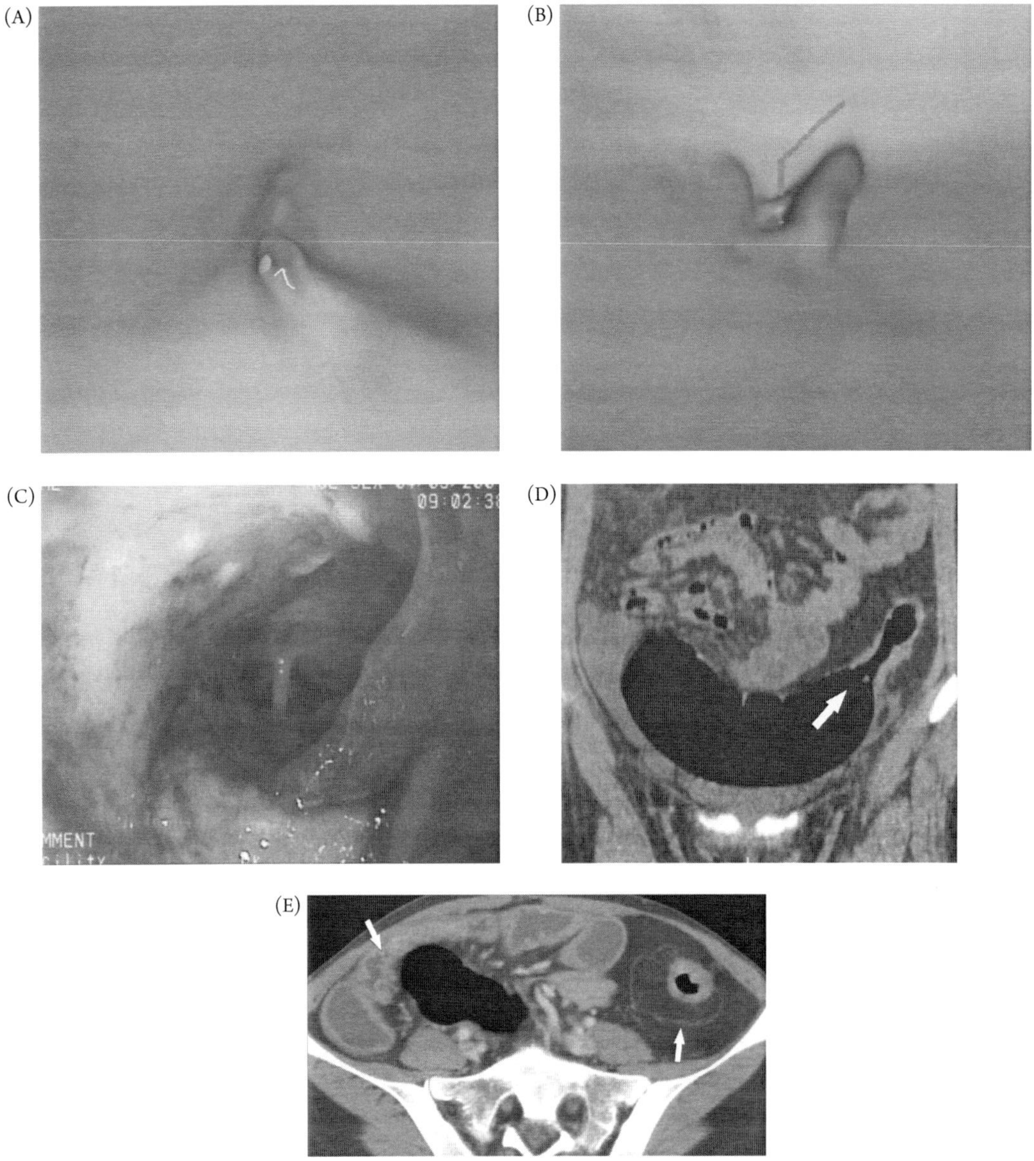

FIGURE 23.9 Completion computed tomography colonography in a 27-year-old female patient with a history of Crohn's disease. (A) and (B) prone and supine three-dimensional endoluminal views of a stricture. Note the smooth tapering of the lumen. (C) Optical endoscopy correlation. (D) Coronal noncontrast two-dimensional (2-D) prone image showing narrowing of the lumen of the ascending colon. (E) Axial contrast-enhanced supine 2-D image showing additional signs of Crohn's disease, with concentric thickening of the wall of the colon and the terminal ileum (*short arrow*), mild enhancement, and fatty proliferation (*arrow*). Courtesy of M. Zalis, Mass General Imaging.

on the workstation simulator specifies the lesion distance from the anal verge and the colon segment in which the lesion is located.

The radiologist trainee learns the standardized C-RADS reporting system for CTC. Standardized reporting assists the referring physician in making management decisions on the basis of the results of the study. C RADS is described in Table 23.4.[28]

At MGH, the SBT incorporates various examples of benign and malignant colonic and extracolonic pathology. Anatomical variants (e.g., malrotation, different morphological appearances of the ileocecal

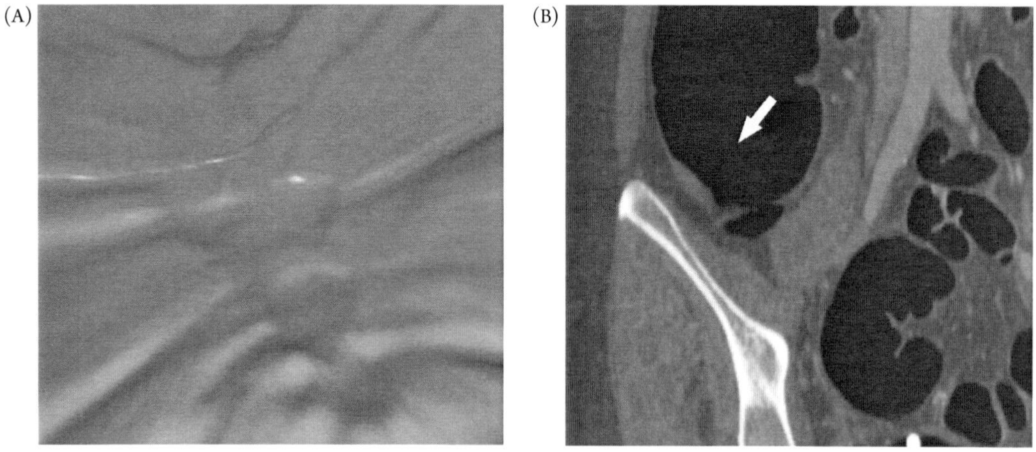

FIGURE 23.10 Completion computed tomography colonography in which a submucosal lesion, presumed to be a lipoma, was seen in the optical colonoscopy in the cecum. On the three-dimensional endoluminal view (A), a submucosal lesion was seen, and the coronal two-dimensional image (B) shows a soft tissue lesion arising from the cecal wall. This lesion was found to be a stromal tumor (GIST). Courtesy of M. Zalis, Mass General Imaging.

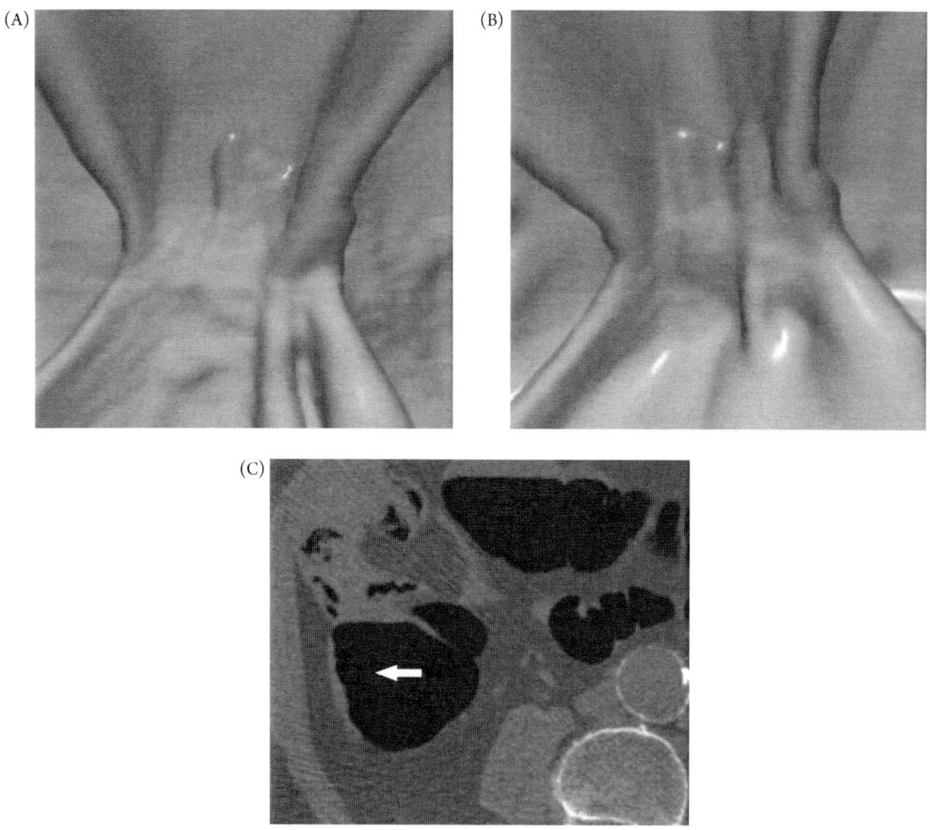

FIGURE 23.11 Completion computed tomography colonography done due to looping of the colon, in a 71-year-old patient. A flat, irregular lesion in the cecum is seen on both supine and prone three-dimensional endoluminal views (A) and (B). The origin of the lesion remained uncertain since a submucosal lesion could have the same morphology. On two-dimensional axial image (C), a soft tissue flat lesion arising from the cecal wall is seen, without clearly identifying the origin of the lesion. The patient underwent right hemicolectomy, and cecal adenocarcinoma was reported on pathology examination. Courtesy of M. Zalis, Mass General Imaging.

valve) and pitfalls that should be accurately recognized are an important part of the training. Additionally, the cases with pathology are mixed in random order with normal studies. Before starting a simulation-based course, it is important for the radiologist to know the different pathologies that may be encountered in the actual clinical setting.

COLON AND RECTOSIGMOID CARCINOMA

Colorectal adenocarcinoma can have various morphologic presentations. It can present as a polypoid mass, as a flat lesion with or without ulceration, as an annular constricting lesion, or as an invasive, obstructing tumor with extension through the colonic wall (Figure 23.7).

Some benign pathologies can mimic neoplasm. For example, long-standing diverticular disease with chronic strictures can be very difficult to differentiate from obstructing malignant neoplasm. Additionally, patients with inflammatory bowel disease can present with stricture, usually presenting as a smooth tapering of the lumen. When a stricture is diagnosed on CTC, it is important to look for such additional signs suggestive of inflammatory disease as diverticulosis, stranding of the pericolonic fat, mesocolic fat proliferations, and extracolonic areas of inflammation to correlate with the clinical history. For diagnostic confirmation, however, these patients may require biopsies and/or follow-up studies (Figures 23.8 and 23.9).

SUBMUCOSAL AND "FLAT" LESIONS

A variety of submucosal lesions can elevate the overlying epithelium and mimic a smooth, intraluminal polypoid appearance. Although most submucosal lesions have a nonspecific soft-tissue appearance at CTC, some characteristic benign entities, such as lipoma and pneumatosis, can be specifically identified at CTC. Gastrointestinal stromal tumors often arise from the stomach or small bowel, but can be of colorectal origin. These mural-based lesions are often large and obvious on cross-sectional 2-D images, but can be subtle when viewed as 3-D images.

Some adenocarcinomas may present as large sessile lesions, which can appear submucosal in origin. Colonic metastasis and serosal implants from extracolonic primary malignant neoplasm can mimic colorectal cancer (Figures 23.10 and 23.11).

At MGH, the CTC simulation-based library has considerably helped residents and fellows in training to learn the variable appearances of different pathologic processes of the colon and the multiple factors that influence the reading of a CTC.

CONCLUSION

Computed tomography colonography is one aspect of abdominal imaging in which SBT can play an important role, and SBT will be progressively incorporated into radiology resident education. In abdominal radiology, a simulator for fluoroscopy will be useful for the education of residents. Fluoroscopic studies are currently performed with decreasing frequency, and it is becoming increasingly difficult for trainees to acquire the necessary technical skills. Such SBT would assist the resident in learning the techniques necessary to become proficient. It would also provide a framework to work on decreasing radiation dose and improving image quality. Clearly, the use of simulation in abdominal radiology will continue to evolve.

REFERENCES

1. Goldberg DJ, DeMarco JK, Parikh T. Computers in radiology: internet-based interactive teaching file for neuroradiology. *Am J Roentgenol* 2000;175: 1371–1373.
2. Towbin AJ, Paterson BE, Chang PJ. Computer-based simulator for radiology: an educational tool. *Radiographics.* 2008;28:309–316.
3. Towbin AJ, Paterson B, Chang PJ. A computer-based radiology simulator as a learning tool to help prepare first-year residents for being on call. *Acad Radiol.* 2007;14:1271–1283.
4. Ganguli S, Pedrosa I, Yam CS, et al. Part I: Preparing first-year radiology residents and assessing their readiness for on-call responsibilities. *Acad Radiol.* 2006;13:764–769.
5. Ganguli S, Camacho M, Yam CS, et al. Preparing first-year radiology residents and assessing their readiness for on-call responsibilities: results over 5 years. *Am J Roentgenol.* 2009;192:539–544.
6. Gordon MC. Cardiology patient simulator. Development of an animated manikin to teach cardiovascular disease. *Am J Cardiol.* 1974;34: 350–355.
7. Monsky WL, Levine D, Mehta TS, et al. Using a sonographic simulator to assess residents before overnight call. *Am J Roentgenol.* 2002;178:35–39.
8. Mendiratta-Lala M, Williams T, de Quadros N, et al. The use of a simulation center to improve resident proficiency in performing ultrasound-guided procedures. *Acad Radiol.* 2010;17:535–540.

9. Heer IM, Middendorf K, Müller-Egloff S, et al. Ultrasound training: the virtual patient. *Ultrasound Obstet Gynecol.* 2004;24:440–444.

10. Roguin A, Beyar R. Real case virtual reality training prior to carotid artery stenting. *Catheter Cardiovasc Interv.* 2010;75:279–282.

11. Hislop SJ, Hedrick JH, Singh MJ, et al. Simulation case rehearsals for carotid artery stenting. *Eur J Vasc Endovas Surg.* 2009;38:750–754.

12. Willoteaux S, Lions C, Duhamel A, et al. Virtual interventional radiology: evaluation of performances as a function of experience. *J Radiol.* 2009;90(Pt 1):37–41.

13. Luboz V, Hughes C, Gould D, et al. Real-time Seldinger technique simulation in complex vascular models. *Int J Comput Assist Radiol Surg.* 2009;4:589–596.

14. Narra P, Kuban J, Grandpre LE, et al. Videoscopic phantom-based angiographic simulation: effect of brief angiographic simulator practice on vessel cannulation times. *J Vasc Interv Radiol.* 2009;20:1215–1223.

15. Seymour NE, Gallagher AG, Roman SA, et al. Virtual reality training improves operating room performance: results of a randomized, double-blinded study. *Ann Surg.* 2002;236:458-463; discussion 463–464.

16. Kronborg O, Fenger C, Olsen J, et al. Randomized study of screening for colorectal cancer with fecal occult blood test. *Lancet.* 1996;348:1467–1471.

17. Selby JV, Friedman GD, Quesenberry PC, et al. A case control study of screening sigmoidoscopy and mortality from colorectal cancer. *N Engl J Med.* 1992;326:653–657.

18. Imperiale TF, Wagner DR, Lin CY. Risk of advanced neoplasms in asymptomatic adults according to the distal colorectal findings. *N Engl J Med.* 2000;343:169–174.

19. Rockey DC, Paulson E, Niedzwiecki D, et al. Analysis of air contrast barium enema, computed tomographic colonography and colonoscopy: prospective comparison. *Lancet.* 2005;365:305–311.

20. Ransohoff DF, Sandler RS. Clinical practice: screening for colorectal cancer. *N Engl J Med.* 2002;346:40–44.

21. Anderson ML, Heigh RI, McCoy GA, et al. Accuracy of assessment of the extent of examination by experienced colonoscopists. *Gastrointest Endosc.* 1992;38:560–563.

22. Johnson CD, Dachman AH. CT colonography: the next colon screening examination. *Radiology.* 2000;216:331–341.

23. Stevenson GW, Wilson JA, Wilkinson J, et al. Pain following colonoscopy: elimination with carbon dioxide. *Gastrointest Endosc.* 1992;38:564–567.

24. Yee J, Kumar NN, Hung RK, et al. Comparison of supine and prone scanning separately and in combination at CT colonography. *Radiology.* 2003;226:653–661.

25. Pickhardt PJ. Translucency rendering in 3D endoluminal CT colonography: a useful tool for increasing polyp specificity and decreasing interpretation time. *Am J Roentgenol.* 2004;183:429–436.

26. Burling D, Moore A, Marshall M, et al. Virtual colonoscopy: effect of computer-assisted detection (CAD) on radiographer performance. *Clin Radiol.* 2008;63:549–556.

27. Summers RM, Yao J, Pickhardt PJ, et al. Computed tomographic virtual colonoscopy computer-aided polyp detection in a screening population. *Gastroenterology.* 2005;129:1832–1844.

28. Zalis ME, Barish MA, Chol JR, et al. CT colonography reporting and data system: a consensus proposal. *Radiology.* 2005;236:3–9.

29. Lefere PA, Gryspeerdt SS, Dewyspelaere J, et al. Dietary fecal tagging as a cleansing method before CT colonography: initial results—polyp detection and patient acceptance. *Radiology.* 2002;224:393–403.

30. Johnson CD. CT colonography: coming of age. *Am J Roentgenol.* 2009;193:1239–1242.

31. Pickhardt PJ, Choi JR, Hwang I, et al. Computed tomographic virtual colonoscopy to screen for colorectal neoplasia in asymptomatic adults. *N Engl J Med.* 2003;349:2191–2200.

32. Cotton PB, Durkalski VL, Pineau BC, et al. Computed tomographic colonography (virtual colonoscopy): a multicenter comparison with standard colonoscopy for detection of colorectal neoplasia. *JAMA.* 2004;291:1713–1719.

33. Fletcher JG, Chen M, Herman BA, et al. Can radiologist training and testing ensure high performance in CT colonography? Lessons From the national CT colonography trial *Am J Roentgenol.* 2010;195:117–125.

34. Johnson CD, Chen MH, Toledano AY. Accuracy of CT colonography for detection of large adenomas and cancers. *N Engl J Med.* 2008;359:1207–1217.

35. American College of Radiology. ACR practice guideline for the performance of computed tomography (CT) colonography in adults. Accessed December 5, 2011, at http://www.acr.org/SecondaryMainMenuCategories/quality_safety/guidelines/dx/gastro/ct_colonography.aspx

36. Bond JH. Clinical relevance of the small colorectal polyp. *Endoscopy.* 2001;33:454–457.

37. Van Stolk RU, Beck GJ, Baron JA, et al. Adenoma characteristics at first colonoscopy as predictors of adenoma recurrence and characteristics at follow-up. The Polyp Prevention Study Group. *Gastroenterology.* 1998;115:13–18.

38. Bond JH. Polyp guideline: diagnosis, treatment, and surveillance for patients with colorectal polyps. Practice Parameters Committee of the American College of Gastroenterology. *Am J Gastroenterol.* 2000;95:3053–3063.

24

Simulation-Based Training for Pediatric Radiology

PAUL BABYN AND JENNIFER STIMEC

THE LITERATURE for simulation-based training (SBT) for pediatric radiology shares many similarities to that for adult radiology. These studies have focused on a number of specific pediatric interventional procedures and in training medical staff to respond rapidly and appropriately to emergent life-threatening situations in children. This chapter focuses on the role SBT can play for certain aspects and issues unique to pediatric management in radiology. In daily pediatric practice, a range of patient sizes are encountered, from the premature neonate to adolescent. This fact necessitates a knowledge of appropriate medication dosage and the technical skills needed to manage life-threatening emergencies across a diverse pediatric population. Maintenance of these skills presents an ongoing challenge given the low frequency of such events in routine practice. Fortunately, specifically designed pediatric mannequins are available to help the trainee develop and maintain these essential skills for caring for small patients (Figure 24.1).

Children are also more likely than adult patients to require sedation to ensure quality diagnostic studies. Thus, radiologists must be able to manage complications that may arise related to such sedation. One emerging area of pediatric SBT in radiology has focused on the administration of sedation by radiologists.

Other areas of practice that present challenges that are very important to the pediatric patient include proper monitoring of radiation usage and management of patient anxiety. Simulation-based training has been used to address radiation dose concerns and investigate methods to reduce dose while obtaining an adequate diagnostic quality study, particularly in computed tomography (CT). Simulation-based training has also been used in helping radiologists hone skills needed for pediatric-specific procedures, such as intussusception reduction. In fact, its role has been explored in maintaining competency for performing such examinations.

Furthermore, a role for SBT has emerged beyond the levels of the radiologist or trainee, involving the patient directly. The development of magnetic resonance imaging (MRI) toy models and mock

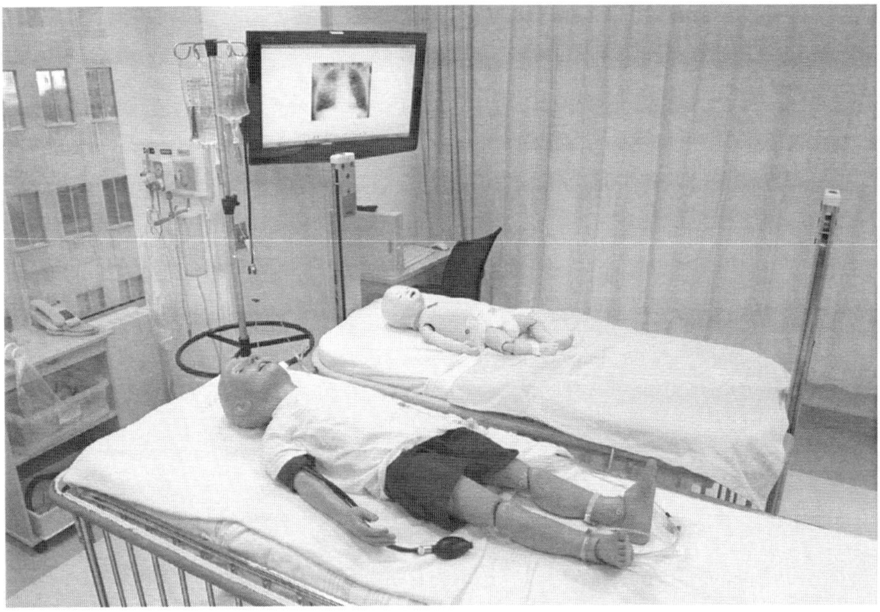

FIGURE 24.1 Center for pediatric simulation at the Hospital for Sick Children, where several pediatric subspecialties are able to learn and practice patient management skills. Preadolescent child and infant mannequins are provided for simulation-based learning.

scanners has been aimed at improving pediatric patient acceptance of MRI studies. This chapter focuses on all of these aspects of the practice of radiology that are unique to the pediatric population and on SBT for nontechnical skills (NTS)—managing pediatric crises.

PEDIATRIC EMERGENCY SITUATIONS ENCOUNTERED IN RADIOLOGY

Life-threatening emergency situations requiring resuscitation skills arise quite rarely in daily practice in pediatric radiology, resulting in limited exposure to such episodes for radiology residents as they rotate on the pediatric radiology service during residency training. Consequently, NTS in crisis management need to be developed and practiced during training; additionally, appropriate acquisition of resuscitation-related technical skills is also required. Several studies have demonstrated that pediatric residents have major deficits related to key technical skills needed for proper airway management,[1] cardiopulmonary and trauma resuscitation skills,[2–4] and endotracheal intubation.[5] The pediatric patient presents distinct anatomical and physiologic[6] differences due to a wide range of patient size.[7] For instance, intubation of the neonate demands a different technical skill set than performing the same technique in an adolescent. Furthermore, behavioral and psychological differences in managing crises in children arise from the practitioners' own personal anxiety, deeply rooted underlying social expectations to protect children, and the additional stress related to working with a parental presence in the room.

Pediatric radiologists most frequently encounter adverse events requiring airway management or cardiopulmonary resuscitation when dealing with very complex, severely ill patients in the setting of conscious sedation administered for clinical diagnostic or therapeutic studies or in children exhibiting a severe intravenous (IV) contrast reaction. Fortunately, the incidence of moderate to severe contrast reactions is rare, reportedly as low as 0.05%–0.08% in the general population,[8,9] and they occur even less frequently in children.[10] Consequently, spontaneous episodes arising from a radiology resident trainee's clinical experience or even staff pediatric radiologist exposure to such events is severely limited at best. The appropriate triage and management of an emergency, however, remains essential for successful outcomes, especially during the stressful time prior to arrival of a hospital-wide code team since performance in the first few minutes of a crisis may critically impact outcome.[11] A 2003 survey of radiologists and trainees highlighted significant deficiencies in severe contrast reaction management; only 43% of respondents were familiar with the current recommended epinephrine dose. Most responses resulted in an epinephrine overdose. Given that pediatric doses vary with patient weight, accuracy of dosing becomes even more complex in the neonatal or younger pediatric setting. In fact, none of those surveyed in a pediatric hospital was able to provide the correct dose of epinephrine. The study concluded that adequate experience could only arise from regular and compulsory training.[12]

BENEFIT OF SIMULATION-BASED TRAINING TO THE PARTICIPANT

The simulated environment provides a safe forum for a participant to encounter a realistic clinical crisis scenario and develop crucial technical and non-technical skills without either harm to the patient or damage to academic status.[13] Published studies have described simulated scenarios that closely mimic real crises. Similar to reality, participants enter a room and are expected to react appropriately and efficiently given standard resources, just as they would with a live patient. Scenario-based training allows one to practice the important skill of gathering information quickly, both from verbal feedback from other team members and from integration of physical examination cues from the high-fidelity simulation (HFS) computerized mannequin and support monitors. The HFS mannequin is typically capable of demonstrating a diverse range of physiologic responses including the presence or absence of cardiac pulses, respiratory sounds, and chest expansion. In addition, it also allows placement of IV access and mimicking of drug administration.[11] All of these features have been shown to contribute to the perception of realism by individuals interacting with them.[14]

Simulation-based training using the HFS mannequin allows the opportunity for a participant to be immersed in a designated leadership role to develop critical NTS. In such a situation, participants must hone their decision-making skills, work with team members to articulate and plan an appropriate strategy, have knowledge of the environment, utilize resources, and maintain professionalism.[15]

Simulation-based training can also be tailored to each individual participant, allowing targeting of personal strengths and weaknesses. Observation of simulated pediatric trauma stabilization training exercises has revealed a number of crucial knowledge-based and technical skills in need of improvement, including estimating a child's weight, proper ordering of IV fluid boluses, and the appropriate application of warming measures.[16] Such high-fidelity SBT also provides standardized and frequent educational experiences that cannot be achieved through an apprenticeship model of learning alone.[1] Learners can be exposed to training scenarios of varying degrees of difficulty, thus promoting the acquisition and maintenance of key technical skills.[6]

Moreover, SBT provides a forum to observe and teach while residents are engaged in an active learning process. It has uncovered concerns not previously recognized. For example, simply having resuscitation materials readily available does not translate to their proper utilization or their proper sequence of use.[17,18] In another study, observation of pediatric resident management of acute airway obstruction simulated scenarios revealed that certain steps involved in the process of intubation were omitted.[1] More troubling was the observation of other potentially harmful actions. They included not connecting the bag-valve-mask to oxygen, choosing an inappropriate endotracheal tube size, pulling a cuffed tube out while inflated, and placing the laryngoscope blade on backward.[1] Thus, a simulated environment generates teachable moments that can be discussed during a post-action debriefing session. Even though most physicians have acquired a checklist of skills through previous didactic training and examination, using these skills in proper chronologic order and in an effective manner under high pressure is often when didactic teaching falls short.

In pediatric radiology, a study by Gaca et al[18] revealed that only 5 of 19 junior radiology residents were able to recognize a simulated scenario as that of an IV contrast material reaction, and many failed to recognize the urgency of the patient's clinical status. One responder even sent the patient back to the hospital inpatient floor. Only 68% of the residents actually activated the code team, with many others calling for an attending radiologist or fellow instead. The time to activate the code team ranged from 9 seconds to almost 3.5 minutes. The study also demonstrated that only 1 of 19 residents performed the appropriate sequence of interventions (i.e., call code, give oxygen, give epinephrine). Such elements of effective resuscitation are difficult to observe or evaluate in daily practice but easy to identify in a simulated environment.

In this study, the use of resuscitation aids in some scenarios resulted in more accurate epinephrine dosing, rising from 23% of those residents without resuscitation aids available to 54% of those who had aids available.[18] Also, epinephrine was ordered faster when aids were available.[18] Residents showed a learning effect between scenarios, with faster responses to call a code team and administer epinephrine. A second phase of the study made available an interactive computer-based resuscitation tool that resulted in less medication dosing errors and a higher likelihood to call for the code team.[13] Another study has shown a learning effect, with improved performance in resuscitation management after just one training session involving both combined didactic and SBT activity.[11]

Although many of these resuscitation skills can be taught didactically or through basic life support (BLS) or pediatric advanced life support (PALS) courses, SBT bridges the gap between didactic teaching and real-life application of resuscitation skills in the clinical setting. Part of the effectiveness of SBT is a temporary suspension of disbelief by the participant immersed in the simulated scenario. For example, participants feel as though they are in the real environment and that their actions have similar consequences to reality.[15] The realism experienced is partly affected by the fidelity of the mannequin, as well as by the environment. Most simulation centers aim to reproduce the typical working environment (i.e., the trauma room, operating room suite, delivery room, or CT room), depending on the specialty. Participants act on environmental cues that can potentially create stressful situations,[15] but overall these training sessions are well-received and are considered worthwhile educational experiences.[11]

Although critical care, emergency, and pediatric residents participating in a high-fidelity SBT exercise would be required to run the full code scenario, including advanced drug administration and intubation, scenarios for radiology residents undergoing such SBT at the Hospital for Sick Children are more limited, with a particular focus placed on crisis management during the first few minutes of the code, before the arrival of the code team. Research has shown that patient survival has been linked to physician preparedness in the first few minutes of a contrast reaction.[19] Key learning features include early oxygen delivery, rapid cardiopulmonary assessment and cardiopulmonary resuscitation (CPR), and recognition of potential harm (e.g., shutting off IV antibiotic drips during an anaphylactic scenario or considering radiation hazards while entering a CT room). Furthermore, the participant would be expected to be familiar with the location of the crash cart, proper medication dose and delivery, and when and how to activate the hospital-wide code team.

USING SIMULATION FOR TEAM-BASED TRAINING: ENHANCING NONTECHNICAL SKILLS

As with most specialties in medicine, during a patient crisis, the radiologist is required to work in a team with other health care providers. Usually, this team consists of the radiologist, the nurse, the radiation technologist, and/or the respiratory therapist. During the transition of care to the code team, the team can expand to include other physicians and hospital personnel. Communication has been identified as a key factor for an effectively functioning team. The Hunt et al[4] study of cardiopulmonary arrest management in a pediatric hospital, however, revealed the presence of a communication error in 100% of mock code training exercises. In this study, an error in communication was defined as anything leading to a delay in treatment or negatively impacting decision-making, such as a doctor calling for a third fluid bolus but not observing that the nurse had not yet administered the first two boluses. Additional errors in communication noted in this study included failure to exemplify leadership or to communicate critical changes in patient status to the team, such as the patient becoming apneic.

In addition to effective communication, team leadership is critical for effective team function. Characteristics of a good team leader include clear self-identification as a leader, role assignment, cross-monitoring of the quality of care administered (e.g., adequate ventilations and compressions), effective communication, and consistent follow-up to ensure orders are performed.[20] In fact, poor team function resulting in more errors and delays arises when team leaders participate in resuscitations in a hands-on method (i.e., they perform technical tasks, such as placement of an endotracheal tube).[21]

Along with the aforementioned communication and leadership skills, SBT scenarios permit development of other important NTS required for effective teamwork, such as sharing information, asking questions of team members, maintaining a professional demeanor, and defusing conflict. Simulation-based training also highlights the importance of situation awareness, resource management (i.e., knowledge of the environment), critical decision-making, calling early for help, and asserting an opinion about management in a respectful manner during stressful times.[6,15,22–24] Focused debriefing sessions with participants discussing these NTS following a mock scenario has been shown to improve significantly NTS of anesthesia residents undergoing SBT.[25] Several obstacles to teamwork have been identified through SBT, including participant complacency; target fixation, in which participants have an overly narrowed focus and miss the big picture around them; and hazardous attitudes.[26]

Post-action debriefing of participants following a mock code is a tool used to explore and understand the personal roles and team dynamics that occurred during the SBT. It is based on maintaining a nonconfrontational, open dialogue and promoting group reflection to learn from one's mistakes without punishment or humiliation. Usually, debriefing sessions are staggered between the scenarios, so that participants have the opportunity to apply learned skills and try a new method of interaction.[23]

Another important benefit of conducting team-based simulated scenario exercises has been the identification of safety issues. In fact, the latent conditions that often underlie the safety issues are more efficiently identified and remedied when discovered in a mock scenario than from an incident report or e-mail.[26] For example, one study revealed that SBT uncovered that the medication dose was not printed or was incorrectly printed in a code manual.[26] Additionally, it revealed that the labeling on the defibrillation device was incorrect and that Adult Cardiac Life Support (ACLS) guidelines were not available.[26] Another study demonstrated that only 55% of radiographic rooms have a chart displayed for contrast reaction management.[12] In addition, the SBT revealed simple oversights, such as only 45% of team members knowing the correct emergency telephone number to use when calling for help.[12]

THE USE OF SIMULATION IN ASSESSMENT OF COMPETENCY

Simulation-based training has been widely accepted as an educational tool in medical education, particularly in critical care, emergency medicine, and anesthesia. Radiologists are now showing a growing interest in its use. With the increasing pressure from the public to reduce medical errors and improve patient safety, the use of simulation has begun to expand beyond the more low-stakes formative assessment role in training to the high-stakes summative assessment of competency.[27] In fact, a form of simulation is now used as part of the board examination for anesthesiologists in Israel and for vascular surgeons in the United States.[28] Also, the Accreditation Council for Graduate Medical Education (ACGME) recognizes the use of simulation as a desirable assessment method and recommends its implementation for testing competency.[29]

Objective assessment of skills necessitates a valid and reliable tool. Although many assessment tools have been generated, few have been well validated. One such tool developed for assessing pediatric resident resuscitation competency demonstrated good interrater reliability.[30] It also had good preliminary construct validity, with a trend toward better scores with higher levels of training.

The use of simulation for high-stakes summative assessment has reached serious levels of discussion for incorporation into future recertification in some specialties such as anesthesia and surgery.[26] Currently, the use of simulation for assessment in radiology is more limited, focusing more on providing a means of formative feedback. Some early discussion, however, has started regarding using simulated scenarios for residents to demonstrate competency prior to being allowed to start on-call duties.[31]

SIMULATION-BASED TRAINING AND PEDIATRIC CONSCIOUS SEDATION

It is common practice when attempting to image children to rely upon conscious sedation to acquire a study of appropriate diagnostic quality. This has become the standard in children who are uncooperative due to young age or developmental delay. Conscious sedation offers a shorter recovery time compared to general anesthesia.[32] Since it can be performed outside of an operating room setting, it is a common practice due to a rising demand and may be performed by nonanesthetists who have received nonuniform training.[33]

In contrast to adults, pediatric patients undergoing moderate conscious sedation represent a higher risk category, often needing deeper sedation and having the lowest tolerance for error.[34] Fortunately, recent data from the Pediatric Sedation Research Consortium describe critical adverse events related to pediatric sedation (such as cardiac arrest) as rare, being reported in only 1 of more than 30,000 cases. On the other hand, potentially critical events such as stridor, laryngospasm, wheezing, or apnea are fairly common, occurring in up to 1 in 44 procedures.[35] One in 1,500 sedations results in an unplanned admission due to complications.[35] Other studies suggest that hypoxia and vomiting are the most common sedation-related complications in pediatric patients undergoing imaging studies.[36] The most at-risk group experiencing the highest number of adverse events in one study were neonates, followed by infants aged 1 to 12 months old.[37] Thus, it is critical that those practicing any form of conscious sedation outside the operating room demonstrate competency in performing the procedure, monitoring, and responding to complications.[38]

A number of ways exist to improve patient safety related to conscious sedation, including strict adherence to published management guidelines, administration and supervision of drugs by fully trained staff, and accurate knowledge of medications.[34] Several studies have shown that improvement in these areas, as well as in technical skills related to administering conscious sedation, can be achieved through SBT. Farnsworth et al[39] used an anesthesia simulator to teach nurses sedation and analgesia skills, improving their test scores significantly. Shavit et al[33] showed significant differences in patient safety performance in those pediatricians and pediatric gastroenterologists who underwent SBT. The participants were part of a workshop that included a didactic component. In the simulated exercises, the participants were able to practice skills to avoid sedation complications, improve monitoring skills, and practice management of adverse events. Feedback was immediate through participant post-action debriefing sessions.[33]

SIMULATION-BASED TRAINING FOR ACQUISITION OF TECHNICAL SKILLS SPECIFIC TO PEDIATRIC RADIOLOGY

Intussusception Reduction

Intussusception is a relatively rare event, occurring in approximately 0.5–2.3 cases per 1,000 live births in the United States.[40] The limited incidence of this entity results in limited opportunity for residents and fellows to develop technical skills needed to reduce it. A recent survey of resident experiences demonstrated that 22% had no experience in reducing intussusception, whereas 21% had been involved in just one case throughout residency.[41] It has been suggested that radiologists require a minimum of four reductions to be considered competent and skilled in this practice.[42]

Intussusception is currently generally treated with a pneumatic reduction performed by the radiologist. A successful reduction starts with proper tube placement and cuff inflation, followed by proper positioning of the patient. Air is pumped into the bowel under carefully controlled pressure, while coordinating appropriate fluoroscopic guidance to monitor progression of the reduction. If the radiologist is unsuccessful, surgical reduction is the next step in management. In addition to knowing the proper steps for pneumatic reduction, the radiologist needs to be familiar with potential complications related to the procedure, such as bowel perforation. Finally, he or she has to have an awareness of radiation exposure and how to perform the study in a radiation-safe manner.

Stein-Wexler et al[43] have taken a novel approach to intussusception education with the development and use of an interactive teaching model. The baby doll has a tube with a bulb insufflator attached to an inner chamber, which essentially transmits pressure data to a computer program. Thus, both technical feedback and instructor feedback can be given to assist the trainee with the steps of intussusception reduction or recurrence during an attempted reduction, simulate complications, and monitor fluoroscopy time. The program is equipped with a library of captured images from actual clinical cases of intussusception reduction.

This model duplicates the necessary multiple technical and cognitive skills needed for a successful intussusception reduction, such as controlling the insufflator, maintaining a tight grip on the patient buttocks, monitoring pressure or air leaks, interpreting images, monitoring radiation delivery, and instituting appropriate management measures if complications arise.[43] Such a system may help trainees to build confidence and gain experience in performance of a relatively uncommon technique.

Radiation Dose Reduction

Strategies to minimize radiation dose have received a great deal of attention within the radiology community, as well as in the public media. Simulation-based techniques have been used to improve outcome without increasing patient dose. In part, this push has arisen from the rapid increase in the number of CT scan studies performed in recent years. Although concerns regarding radiation exposure are important for adults, several significant additional concerns exist in the pediatric patient. With radiation exposure, the major long-term side effect is that of radiation-induced cancer. Children have many more potential years to develop cancer and have rapidly dividing cells that are more radiosensitive.[44,45] Furthermore, organ doses are relatively larger in children than in adults.[46] On a societal scale, a significant public health concern is generated, considering that an estimated 11% of all CT studies in the United States are performed on children. A small individual risk is therefore amplified in such a large overall number of children exposed to a potential long-term health problem.[47] The current strategy is to follow the *as low as reasonably achievable* (ALARA) principle as closely as possible, such as promoted by the Image Gently campaign. It is estimated that, since the 1980s, there has been up to an 800% increase of CT scans performed in children.[48] As a result, many campaigns and guidelines have been published with the aim of tailoring the study parameters and the radiation dose to the child.

When attempting to investigate methods to reduce radiation dose in children and still obtain a quality diagnostic scan, several challenges arise. Ethical considerations limit performing full diagnostic scans at multiple doses upon the same patient in order to investigate which dose would allow for adequate structure visualization. Although this method would allow for direct comparison of diagnostic quality while limiting confounding parameters, the overall radiation dose would be impossible to justify, and repeat scans may vary in section position or motion artefact.[49] Furthermore, with administration of IV contrast, the phase of enhancement at the time of imaging would differ upon subsequent images.

Mayo et al[49] devised a method to circumvent these issues with the use of a computer-simulated dose reduction model. The raw data from a conventional chest CT was modified by increasing a controlled amount of random noise to simulate images obtained at various lower tube currents (100 mAs and 40 mAs). Lowering the tube current results in a directly proportional radiation dose reduction for the patient. The recognized tradeoff of lowering tube current is increased image noise.[44,50,51] The acceptable amount of dose reduction within children, however, has not yet been established and is a balance of diagnostic image quality and radiation dose.[49]

In this study, standard diagnostic CT scans were first performed using 200 milliampere seconds (mAs) followed by two sections at two designated levels with reduced current settings (100 and 40 mAs). These images were designated as "real-reduced" tube current images. Simulated reduced tube current images were directly compared to the real-reduced images for image quality and radiographic findings. No significant difference was found between the two groups. In fact, when asked to identify which study was real and which was simulated, the correct response was only obtained 50% of the time. This study provided support for the ability of computer simulation to accurately mimic various radiation dose reduction appearances without exposing a patient to increased radiation.[49]

Another difficulty in studying radiation dose strategy arises when attempting to divide children into experimental and control groups for their diagnostic scans. In this scenario, the experimental group may potentially receive a suboptimal study resulting in a missed diagnosis or a repeat study at the control dose, thus markedly increasing overall radiation exposure above levels in the control group.[52] Also, controlling for study parameters would be challenging and necessitate a large study population based on differences in pathology, indication, anatomy, and the range of patient size between infancy to adolescence. Although animal studies could be performed, other logistical factors are introduced, as well as their questionable applicability to the pediatric patient.[52]

An early clinical investigation[53] concluded that significant dose reduction was achievable for pelvic CT with preservation of diagnostic quality. Patients were divided into groups receiving a higher (240 mAs) and lower dose (80 mAs) imaging study. Specific indications were not controlled between the groups. The difficulty of controlling for patient size variation in the pediatric population was also highlighted as a trend for decline in diagnostic confidence and image quality as patient size and age increased.

Notable differences arise in radiation requirements to achieve quality diagnostic images depending on the imaged body part and specifically the indication for which the study was performed. For instance, a high contrast resolution region such as the lungs would require a lower radiation dose than an intrinsically low contrast resolution area such as the abdomen. Thus, a clinical study performed on one region of the body would not be directly applicable to another region.

Furthermore, even within a general area such as the abdomen, high- and low-visibility structures have been described,[52] thus necessitating consideration of dose based on clinical indication. A simulated technique has been validated and has permitted assessment in this area. Frush et al[52] utilized a technique similar to that of Mayo et al[49] to generate computer-simulated dose-reduced images by adding noise to mimic current reduction. The technique was validated using a water phantom model imaged at five different mAs settings. Upon comparison of the actual scans with simulated scans at the same mAs levels, no statistical differences were detected. In this study, done to investigate the potential for dose reduction, the original patient scans were all performed with 120 mAs, but the simulation scans were created at 100, 80, 60, and 40 mAs for each patient in the study. High-visibility structures, such as fat in the intrahepatic course of the falciform ligament and adrenal glands, were seen equally well in both simulated and real scans. Low-visibility structures, however, such as the extraparenchymal course of the hepatic artery, the common bile duct, and the intraparenchymal hepatic vessels, demonstrated decreased detection in scans with simulated mAs of 80 or lower. The findings would support accepting a certain degree of image noise generated with lowering tube current based on specific indications, as well as in follow-up studies with specific consideration based on patient size.[52] Support in the literature and media exists for tailoring CT parameters based on the clinical indication in an effort to reduce radiation exposure in children.

Although there are many recognized and well-understood parameters that can be adjusted to reduce radiation dose from CT scans, simulation-based techniques can be used to provide validation and scientific evaluation of these methods while providing assurance that diagnostic quality is maintained for optimal patient care.

SIMULATION-BASED TRAINING FOR THE PEDIATRIC PATIENT

The scope of medical SBT has moved beyond that of the health practitioner to now include the pediatric patient. This new emerging role of SBT is best exemplified in its proposed role for adequate preparation of the pediatric patient prior to undergoing an MRI study.

The advantages of MRI are well known. Detailed images provide excellent spatial and temporal resolution without subjecting the child to the ionizing effects of radiation.[54] The challenge, however, arises in overcoming common patient-related barriers to obtaining images of sufficient diagnostic quality. These barriers include patient anxiety and fear of the physical challenges associated with the MRI scanner. Several anxiety-provoking factors have been identified that limit a child's ability to cope and, thus, not be able to tolerate the study. These factors include the experience of lying in a confined space, being subjected to loud noises, the need to lie still for the relatively lengthy duration of the study, physical discomfort from surface coils, and the prospect of needle insertion for IV contrast.[55]

Traditionally, in such circumstances, children are required to undergo a degree of conscious sedation or submit to general anesthesia after a risk–benefit evaluation concludes that a scan is necessary. Both general anesthesia and conscious sedation pose additional risks to the pediatric patient. Use of sedation has been shown to have a higher failure rate compared to general anesthesia. Although complications are rare, general anesthesia has greater risks, including respiratory depression with oversedation, possibly compromising the ability to maintain an airway, aspiration, hypotension, arrhythmia, and cardiac arrest.[37] Also, the resources required for anesthetic intervention are costly secondary to the requirement of extra anesthesia and nursing staff, MR-compatible monitoring equipment, the possibility for hospital admission, and increased time within the scanner.

Children aged 3 to 8 years constitute the most challenging group, with the most to gain from nonpharmacologic methods. Younger children may be managed by altering feed and sleep schedules, or they may require anesthesia. Older children typically do not require more than explanation and direction. The methods employed during patient SBT are directed at improving patient and family understanding of the procedure in an attempt to reduce anxiety.

Simulation-based training of patients to acclimate to the MRI environment at its basic level may take the form of play therapy. In a study by Pressdee et al,[56] a specially trained play therapist met with the child and family prior to a scheduled MRI and described the technique in age-appropriate terms. The use of photos and interaction with a small-scale MRI model was encouraged. The model included the scanner, sliding table, and light, and had figures representing the child patient, family, and health

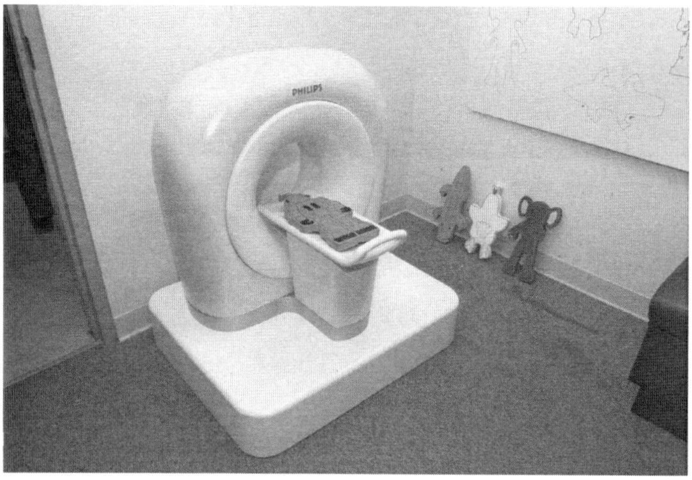

FIGURE 24.2 Small-scale magnetic resonance imaging (MRI) shell with a doll on the gantry. This allows children to familiarize themselves with the MRI procedure through play prior to their own scan.

care workers who would be present. Prerecorded noises commonly heard in MRI were played as well.

In playing with such a model, children establish an understanding of the environment, can ask questions, and can become familiar with expectations during the scan. Observed interaction also allows for correction of patient or family misconceptions. Families have subjectively reported less fear and anxiety surrounding the study and have responded favorably to the simulation-based experience. The study of Pressdee et al[56] described a higher rate of successful adherence to the MRI examination without necessitating conversion to a study requiring sedation or anesthesia. At the Hospital for Sick Children, a similar small-scale scanner model is used to help children understand how the MRI examination is performed, and has had many successes in anxiety reduction (Figure 24.2).

In another study, young children were given the opportunity to acquire the skills needed to complete successfully an MRI scan. Hallowell et al[57] described a full-scale 1.5T MRI shell scanner without a magnet in which the child was placed as a trial before the actual scan. An educational play therapist was involved in the process, while the child was taken through every step of the study from entering the room, positioning on the gantry, use of surface coils, and hearing tape-recorded noises of the unit. Children practiced lying still with breath-holding and were introduced to coping strategies, including relaxation, breathing, and visualization techniques. A clinically diagnostic scan without general anesthesia or sedation was achieved in 96% of those children who had either passed or were borderline pass in the simulated practice scenario.

A similar process was described by Carter et al,[58] who utilized a strategy of having children pass a mock MRI scan prior to a clinical study without anesthesia. A retrospective comparison of the number of MRI studies requiring general anesthesia performed prior to and after implementation of the simulated mock MRI training experience revealed a significant decline in frequency of the use of general anesthesia. In particular, there was a 16.8% reduction in the rate of general anesthesia in the mock MRI group compared to a non-mock MRI group in the 3- to 8-year-old range.

Thus, patient-centered SBT has shown benefits specific to the patient, with decreased anxiety and better compliance with the clinical MRI study, as well as a reduction in the frequency of the use of general anesthesia to obtain diagnostic studies.

CONCLUSION

Simulation-based training is particularly advantageous in pediatric imaging given the wide spectrum of patient ages and sizes (ranging from the very tiny premature neonate to the adult-sized adolescent) and frequent rarity of the underlying diseases encountered. Simulation-based training has been beneficial in radiology team-based early crisis intervention, before the arrival of the code team. Low-frequency, high-risk adverse events such as severe IV contrast medium reactions, difficult airway management, cardiopulmonary resuscitation, and sedation complications of hypoxia and vomiting require frequent management practice and immediate skilled care for successful outcomes in pediatric patients. SBT is useful in assuring that all necessary pediatric radiologic studies are done with constant attention to minimal radiation dose. Play therapy with a simulated CT or MRI gantry before the actual scan is done may assist the younger patient to cope with imaging tests, reducing the need for sedation or anesthesia for some young children. SBT is definitely beneficial in improving interventional procedure skills. Pre-procedure SBT for technically difficult and high risk interventional procedures can assist in optimizing patient safety.

REFERENCES

1. Overly FL, Sudikoff SN, Shapiro MJ. High-fidelity medical simulation as an assessment tool for pediatric residents' airway management skills. *Pediatric Emergency Care.* 2007; 23:11–15.

2. Shoenfeld PS, Baker MD. Management of cardiopulmonary and trauma resuscitation in the pediatric emergency department. *Pediatrics.* 1993;91:726–729.

3. White JR, Shugerman R, Brownlee C, et al. Performance of advanced resuscitation skills by pediatric housestaff. *Arch Pediatr Adolesc Med.*1998;152:1232–1235.

4. Hunt EA, Heine M, Hohenhaus SM, et al. Simulated pediatric trauma team management: assessment of an educational intervention. *Pediatr Emerg Care.* 2007;11:796–804.

5. O'Donnell CP, Kamlin CO, Davis PG, et al. Endotracheal intubation attempts during neonatal resuscitation: success rates, duration, and adverse effects. *Pediatrics.* 2006;117:e16–e21.

6. Eppich WJ, Adler MD, McGaghie WC. Emergency and critical care pediatrics: use of medical simulation in training in acute pediatric emergencies. *Curr Opin Pediatr.* 2006;18:266–271.

7. Shah AN, Frush K, Luo X, et al. Effect of an intervention standardization system on pediatric dosing and equipment size determination: a crossover trial involving simulated resuscitation events. *Arch Pediatr Adolesc Med.* 2003;157:229–236.

8. Cochran ST, Bomyea K, Sayre JW. Trends in adverse events after IV administration of contrast media. *AJR Am J Roentgenol.* 2001;176:1385–1388.

9. Mortele KJ, Oliva MR, Ondategui S, et al. Universal use of non-ionic iodinated contrast medium for CT: evaluation of safety in a large urban teaching hospital. *AJR Am J Roentgenol.* 2005;184:31–34.

10. Cohen MD, Smith JA. Intravenous use of ionic and non-ionic contrast agents in children. *Radiology.* 1994;191:793–794.

11. Sica GT, Barron DM, Blum R, et al. Computerized realistic simulation: a teaching module for crisis management in radiology. *AJR*;1999;172:301–304.

12. Bartlett MJ, Bynevelt M. Acute contrast reaction management by radiologists: a local audit study. *Australasian Radiology.* 2003;47:363–367.

13. Gaca AM, Lerner CB, Frush DP. The radiology perspective: needs and tools for management of life-threatening events. *Pediatric Radiology.* 2008;38(Suppl 4):S714-S719.

14. Donoghue AJ, Durbin DR, Nadel FM, et al. Perception of realism during mock resuscitations by pediatric housestaff: the impact of simulated physical features. *Simulation in Healthcare.* 2010;5:16–20.

15. Halamek LP, Kaegi DM, Gaba DM, et al. Time for a new paradigm in pediatric medical education: teaching neonatal resuscitation in a simulated delivery room environment. *Pediatrics.* 2000;106:e45.

16. Hunt EA, Hohenhaus SM, Luo X, et al. Simulation of pediatric trauma stabilization in 35 North Carolina emergency departments: identification of targets for performance improvement. *Pediatrics.* 2006;117:641–648.

17. Becker GJ. Simulation and the coming transformation of medical education and training. *Radiology.* 2007;245:7–9.

18. Gaca AM, Frush DP, Hohenhaus SM, et al. Enhancing pediatric safety: using simulation to assess radiology resident preparedness for anaphylaxis from intravenous contrast media. *Radiology.* 2007;245: 236–244.

19. American Academy of Pediatrics. *Pediatric Advanced Life Support Manual.* Dallas: American Heart Association, Dallas; 2002:1–39.

20. Hunt EA, Walker AR, Shaffner DH, et al. Simulation of in-hospital pediatric medical emergencies and cardiopulmonary arrests: highlighting the importance of the first 5 minutes. *Pediatrics.* 2008;121:e34–e43.

21. Cooper S, Wakelam A. Leadership of resuscitation teams: "lighthouse leadership." *Resuscitation.* 1999;42:27–45.

22. Thomas EJ, Sexton JB, Helmreich RL. Translating teamwork behaviours from aviation to healthcare: development of behavioural markers for neonatal resuscitation. *Qual Saf Health Care.* 2004;13(S1):57–64.

23. Zirkle M, Blum R, Raemer DB, et al. Teaching emergency airway management using medical simulation: a pilot program. *The Laryngoscope.* 2005;115:495–500.

24. Small DS, Wuerz RC, Simon R, et al. Demonstration of high-fidelity simulation team training for emergency medicine. *Academic Emergency Medicine.*1999;6:312–323.

25. Yee B, Naik VN, Joo HS, et al. Nontechnical skills in anesthesia crisis management with repeated exposure to simulation-based education. *Anesthesiology.* 2005;103:241–248.

26. Ruddy RM, Patterson D. Medical simulation: a tool for recognition of and response to risk. *Pediatric Radiology.* 2008;38(Suppl 4):S700–S706.

27. Weinberg ER, Auerbach MA, Shah NB. The use of simulation for pediatric training and assessment. *Current Opinion in Pediatrics.* 2009;21:282–287.

28. Berkenstadt H, Ziv A, Gafni N, et al. Incorporating simulation-based objective structured clinical examination into the Israeli National Board Examination in anaesthesiology. *Anesth Analg.* 2006;102:853–858.

29. Accreditation Council for Graduate Medical Education. *ACGME Bulletin.* December, 2005. Accessed at www.acgme.org

30. Brett-Fleegler MB, Vinci RJ, Weiner DL, et al. A simulator-based tool that assesses pediatric resident resuscitation competency. *Pediatrics.* 2008;121:e597–e603.

31. Monsky WL, Levine D, Mehta TS, et al. Using a sonographic simulator to assess residents before overnight call. *AJR.* 2002;178:35–39.

32. Keeter S, Benator RM, Weinberg SM, et al. Sedation in Pediatric CT: national survey of current practice. *Radiology.* 1990;175:745–752.

33. Shavit I, Keidan I, Hoffman Y, et al. Enhancing patient safety during pediatric sedation. *Arch Pediatr Adolesc Med.* 2007;161:740–743.

34. Horton ER. Adverse events in pediatric sedation. *US Pharmacist.* 2008;33:HS2–HS8.

35. Cravero JP, Blike GT, Beach M, et al. Pediatric Sedation Research Consortium. Incidence and nature of adverse events during pediatric sedation/anesthesia for procedures outside the operating room: report from the Pediatric Sedation Research Consortium. *Pediatrics.* 2006;118:1087–1096.

36. Sanborn PA, Michna E, Zurakowski D, et al. Adverse cardiovascular and respiratory events during sedation of pediatric patients for imaging examinations. *Radiology.* 2005;237:288–294.

37. Malviya S, Voepel-Lewis T, Tait AR. Adverse events and risk factors associated with the sedation of children by nonanesthesiologists. *Anesth Analg.*1997;85:1207–1213.

38. Chen MI, Edler A, Wald S, et al. Scenario and checklist for airway rescue during pediatric sedation. *Simulation in Healthcare.* 2007;2:194–198.

39. Farsworth ST, Egan TD, Johnson SE, et al. Teaching sedation and analgesia with simulation. *J Clin Monit.* 2000;16:273–285.

40. Bruce J, Huh YS, Cooney DR, et al. Intussusception: evolution of current management. *J Pediatr Gastroeneterol Nutr.* 1987;6:663–674.

41. Stein-Wexler R, Bateni C, Gorges SW, et al. Radiology residents' experience with intussusception reduction. *Pediatr Radiol.* 2010; 40:586–587, Abstract PA127.

42. Meyer JS, Dangman BC, Buonomo C, et al. Air and liquid contrast agents in the management of intussusception: a controlled randomized trial. *Radiology.* 1993;188: 507–511.

43. Stein-Wexler R, Sanchez T, Roper GE, et al. An interactive teaching device simulating intussusception reduction. *Pediatr Radiol.* 2010;40:1810-1815. Epub 2010, Jul 21.

44. Nievelstein RAJ, van Dam IM, van der Molen AJ. Multidetector CT in children: current concepts and dose reduction strategies. *Pediatric Radiology.* 2010;40:1324–1344.

45. Paterson A, Frush DP, Donnelly LF. Helical CT of the body: are settings adjusted for pediatric patients? *AJR.* 2001;176:297–301.

46. Pierce DA, Shimizu Y, Preston DL, et al. Studies of the mortality of atomic bomb survivors. Report 12, part I. Cancer: 1950–1990. *Radiat Res.*1996;146:1–27.

47. Brenner DJ, Elliston CD, Hall EJ, et al. Response to the statement by The Society for Pediatric Radiology on radiation risks from pediatric CT scans. *Pediatr Radiol.* 2001;31:389–391.

48. Goske MJ, Applegate KE, Boylan J, et al. The "Image Gently" campaign: increasing CT radiation dose awareness through a national education and awareness program. *Pediatr Radiol.* 2008;38: 265–269.

49. Mayo JR, Whittall KP, Leung AN, et al. Simulated dose reduction in conventional chest CT: validation study. *Radiology.* 1997;202:453–457.

50. Verdun FR, Gutierrez D, Schnyder PF, et al. CT dose optimization when changing to CT multi-detector row technology. *Curr Probl Diagn Radiol.* 2007;36:176–184.

51. Robinson AE, Hill EP, Harpen MD. Radiation dose reduction in pediatric CT. *Pediatr Radiol.* 1986;16:53–54.

52. Frush DP, Slack CC, Hollingsworth CL, et al. Computer-simulated radiation dose reduction for abdominal multidetector CT of pediatric patients. *AJR.* 2002;179:1107–1113.

53. Kamel IR, Ramiro JH, Martin JE, et al. Radiation dose reduction in CT of the pediatric pelvis. *Radiology.* 1994;190:683–687.

54. Rosenberg D, Sweeney J, Gillen J, et al. Magnetic resonance imaging of children without sedation: preparation with simulation. *J Amer Acad Child Adolesc Psychiatry.* 1997;36:853–859.

55. Marshall S, Smith M, Weinberger E. Perceived anxiety of pediatric patients to magnetic resonance. *Clin Pediatr (Phila).* 1995;34:59–60.

56. Pressdee D, May L, Eastman E, et al. The use of play therapy in the preparation of children undergoing MR imaging. *Clinical Radiology.* 1997;52:945–947.

57. Hallowell LM, Stewart SE, de Amorim e Silva CT, et al. Reviewing the process of preparing children for MRI. *Pediatr Radiol.* 2008;38: 271–279.

58. Carter AJ, Greer MLC, Gray SE, et al. Mock MRI: reducing the need for anaesthesia in children. *Pediatr Radiol.* 2010;40:1368–1374.

25

Simulation-Based Training for Ultrasound and Computed Tomography–Guided Interventional Procedures

MISHAL MENDIRATTA-LALA, JOHN BONNETT, AND TODD R. WILLIAMS

PERCUTANEOUS IMAGE-GUIDED procedures have become first-line interventions for performing biopsies in various locations within the superficial and deep cavities of the body, as well as for drainage of infected and noninfected fluid collections. Both ultrasound (US) and computed tomography (CT)-guided percutaneous biopsy are regarded as effective, safe, and high-yield methods for tissue diagnosis of solid organ abnormalities.[1–4] This trend toward less invasive diagnostic and therapeutic interventions is pervasive in all fields of medicine, including radiology. For example, some open surgical procedures have been replaced by laparoscopic, robotic, and even image-guided minimally invasive diagnostic or therapeutic equivalents. In fact, the performance of percutaneous biopsy or drainage is a major advance in the minimally invasive management of patients. When compared to more invasive techniques, such as excisional biopsy or incision and drainage, patient morbidity and mortality are not particularly different from the use of percutaneous procedures; however, percutaneous procedures should be the first line of treatment as they are less invasive and do not require general anesthesia.[5] Currently, most imaging-guided percutaneous interventional procedures are via US guidance or CT fluoroscopic guidance.

Ultrasound-guided localization is a basic radiological skill and is essential for many therapeutic and diagnostic procedures. Ultrasound-guided procedures are performed in many divisions of radiology, including mammography, body imaging, interventional radiology, and musculoskeletal imaging. The National Institute for Clinical Excellence has recommended that US be used during every elective central venous line insertion.[6] Ultrasound allows for real-time needle visualization during placement into a body cavity or vessel, thus allowing for precise lesion targeting.[6] Ultrasound imaging, however, is highly user dependent, and targeted needle placement requires good hand–eye coordination, as well as distinct operator-dependent psychomotor skills.[6]

Traditional Methods of Medical Training and Their Limitations

To attain proficiency in any aspect of medical care, especially technical procedures, practice is necessary. The traditional model of medical education, known as the Halsted model of education[7,8] uses patients as tools for teaching, with residents gaining an increased level of independence and responsibility through progression of training under the supervision of faculty.[7] Another term for this method of training is the "apprenticeship approach."[9,10]

Today, however, there are real inherent conflicts to this form of education. Changes in health care over the past few decades, such as the creation of federal mandates regarding duty hours compliance[11] and an emphasis on increased outpatient and minimally invasive procedures,[7] have negatively impacted medical education and training by reducing the number of training opportunities in the inpatient hospital setting. Increased patient education and awareness of contemporary medical practice and training has resulted in objection by some patients to resident trainees performing procedures, despite the assurance of experienced staff supervision.[12] Such increased public awareness was in part spurred by the Institute of Medicine's publication, in 1999, of the seminal report *To Err Is Human*, which revealed that medical errors were the eighth leading cause of death in the United States, exceeding motor vehicle fatalities; even more sobering was the fact that more than 50% of such deaths were deemed preventable.[13] Clearly, recent changes in the delivery of health care, combined with the current apprenticeship model of training, has the potential for increasing medical errors, negatively impacting patient safety, and warranting a more organized and systematic approach to medical education and resident training than the apprenticeship model. A proficiency-based model of simulation-based training (SBT) provides such an approach and can serve as a useful adjuvant to traditional training methods since it provides a format for learning a medical procedure based on a system of standard metrics that enable both formative and summative trainee assessment.[14]

Simulation-Based Methods of Medical Training

Simulation-based training has become an increasingly popular method of training in many fields of medicine, including laparoscopic surgery, gastrointestinal medicine (endoscopy), anesthesiology, and emergency medicine.[15–20] The use of simulation in radiology education and training is a developing and expanding field, especially in interventional radiological procedures. Ultrasound-guided SBT is particularly important, since US-guided percutaneous techniques are used frequently in radiology, as in the biopsy of masses and drainage of fluid collections in the abdominal and thoracic cavities (e.g., percutaneous cholecystostomy tube placement), core needle biopsy of masses in the breast, and joint aspiration throughout the body. Additionally, as percutaneous CT-guided procedures continue to increase in number, and as the complexity of equipment and procedures increase (e.g., radiofrequency ablation and cryotherapy of tumors), SBT will become indispensable in helping trainees attain proficiency in percutaneous interventions prior to actually attempting them on patients.

The utility and scope of US- and CT-guided SBT is extensive:

- Simulation-based training allows one to teach a trainee basic principles related to the use of US and CT equipment, including US- and CT-related physics.
- Simulation-based training can teach the trainee both the basic skills needed to perform US- and CT-guided procedures (e.g., biopsies, drainages, vascular access), as well as the necessary knowledge to do it safely (e.g., indications and contraindications of particular procedures).
- Simulation-based training provides an opportunity for giving trainees both formative and summative feedback related to their progress and technical skill development in a safe and controlled learning environment.
- Simulation-based training techniques provide an opportunity for trainees to progress at an individual pace as they master the skills and competencies needed for successful percutaneous US- and CT-guided performance of specific procedures (i.e., it allows for proficiency-based training).
- Simulation-based training has the potential for instilling public confidence related to physician and resident competence in performing invasive percutaneous procedures through documentation of its effectiveness and translation to clinical practice in the medical literature using valid and reliable assessment tools.
- A well-designed SBT curriculum can facilitate the acquisition of hard data related to its utility, which may in turn lead to its inclusion with other specified

criteria for specialty training certification, hospital physician credentialing, or specialty revalidation, which is now required annually by the American Board of Radiology for radiologists as part of the Maintenance of Certification.

CURRENT TYPES OF SIMULATION-BASED TRAINING AND THEIR UTILITY IN ULTRASOUND- AND COMPUTED TOMOGRAPHY–GUIDED INTERVENTIONAL TRAINING

Simulation-based training curricula for US- and CT-guided interventional procedures can incorporate several different types of models for teaching trainees (Table 25.1).

PART-TASK TRAINERS

Part-task trainers are simulation devices designed to mimic a specific system or item, such as a model of a specific body part.[11] These devices may focus on a particular task with only a few steps or a skill set to be acquired (e.g., central line insertion).[21] Part-task trainers are especially useful in US-guided SBT, ranging from homemade gelatin molds containing various targets to more sophisticated models such as Blue Phantom™ devices (Blue Phantom, Redmond, Washington) (Figures 25.1 and 25.2).

Part-task trainers are very useful for US SBT, as most US procedures focus on a specific body part and involve a specific task with a set number of steps (e.g., abscess drainage, organ biopsy, hip joint injection, venous or arterial puncture). Furthermore, the steps involved in needle or catheter placement and the skills required have many similarities, regardless of the specific organ or body part involved.

PHYSICAL MODEL SIMULATOR

A *physical model simulator* utilizes a mannequin with mechanical components. An example is the Human Patient Simulator™ (Medical Education Technologies, Inc., Sarasota, Florida), which is equipped with a transmitted voice, reactive eyes, chest movement, breath sounds, heart tones, and palpable pulses. Other similar mannequins exist. Typically, these are full-body, programmable mannequins capable of the full gamut of physiological responses. With them, realistic, immersive scenarios can be created that assist in teaching trainees how to manage and treat high-risk, low-frequency events (e.g., contrast medium allergic reactions or code blues in the radiology department). Although useful for some aspects of radiology training (i.e., contrast reactions), we have not used these simulators for US- or CT-guided SBT.

COMPUTER-BASED SIMULATION

Computer-based simulation (CBS) allows a user to interact with a virtual environment using devices that control the scene, much like popular computer games.[21] John et al[22] have designed a CBS for US- and CT-guided SBT by developing a virtual environment that detects needle guidance using patient-specific data and complex physics principles to detect the force applied. This system is being further developed by the Collaboration in Radiological Interventional Virtual Environments (CRaIVE)

Table 25.1 Types of simulators and utility in ultrasound-guided simulation-based training

TYPE OF SIMULATOR	UTILITY IN ULTRASOUND (US)-GUIDED SIMULATION-BASED TRAINING
Part-task trainer	Model of specific body part Acquire specific task with a set number of steps
Physical model simulator	Mannequins with mechanical components
Computer-based simulator	Computer games interact with a virtual environment US examination US-guided needle insertion
Hybrid simulator	Combines physical model with computer simulation US examination (probe insertion) US-guided needle insertion

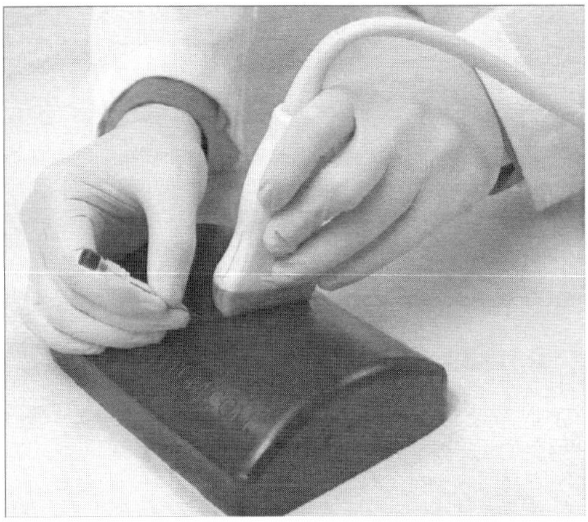

FIGURE 25.1 Image of needle insertion under ultrasound guidance into a Blue Phantom™ part-task trainer that has multiple inclusions within the mold to simulate real lesions.

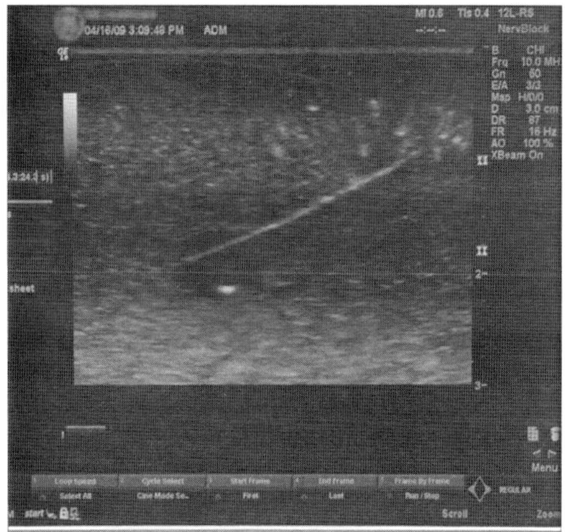

FIGURE 25.2 Real-time ultrasound image of needle within an anechoic target in the Blue Phantom™ part-task trainer.

consortium, a multidisciplinary group of clinicians, physicists, computer scientists, bioengineers, and psychologists who are working together to implement and validate sophisticated virtual environments for interventional radiology (IR) training.[22]

Forest et al[23] have created another CBS for US-guided examination and needle insertion. The simulated US images are mainly based on CT or magnetic resonance imaging (MRI) images. This CBS model differs from real-time US since the needle is simulated by adopting a 3 degrees of freedom (DOF) force feedback device that does not provide resistance torque force to maintain the original path of needle insertion, and consequently the haptic feedback is less realistic.[23] The CRaIVE Website (www.CRaIVE.org.uk) is an excellent source of information on simulation for interventional radiology.

HYBRID SIMULATORS

Hybrid simulators combine a physical model with CBS. This form of simulation may prove to be the most useful for US-guided procedural SBT.[21] Numerous such models already exist, including the UltraSim® sonographic simulator (MedSim Inc., Fort Lauderdale, Florida), which resembles a generic sonographic scanner and includes a monitor, transducers, and image quality controls with measurement, image storage, and printing capabilities.[24] Real-time scanning is performed on an included mannequin. Probe positioning is detected via a high-resolution 6 DOF electromagnetic sensing mechanism. Additionally, there are commercially available compact discs (CDs) for teaching purposes to demonstrate hybrid simulation.[24] They contain three-dimensional sonographic datasets from real patients and exercises for scanning anatomy and relevant abnormalities both transabdominally and transvaginally. Reference libraries for each case are included for trainees, providing gold standard images to use for simulation comparisons.[24] Additional hybrid simulation systems specific for US-guided procedures were created by Zhu et al[6] and Magee et al[25] using plastic mannequins and CBS systems to assist with scanning and needle identification. Finally, Ni et al[26] have created a predominantly computer-based hybrid simulation model that uses different US volumes calibrated from a phantom.

Current Ultrasound Simulation Models Used for Training

Currently, limited data exist on the utility of SBT for teaching residents to achieve proficiency in US-related interventional procedures. The use of US SBT for helping trainees understand anatomy and utilize the US equipment properly has been reported. In one study, 45 residents participated in a SBT involving an ectopic pregnancy scenario utilizing a hybrid model in which residents were required to manipulate an endovaginal US probe within a part-task trainer while examining real-time computerized images. These residents were compared to a similar group that used only a mannequin while examining static photo images. The study results showed that the hybrid simulation model improved not only the residents' educational experience, but also improved the faculty supervisors' ability to evaluate the residents' clinical and US skills.[27] The predictive validity of the SBT model (i.e., its ability to predict the future performance in the clinical realm), however, was not defined.

Another simulation study evaluating US skills in residents using a hybrid model demonstrated that sonographic SBT allowed for the objective assessment and identification of flaws in resident skills. Such faults could then be addressed with resultant improvement, thus enhancing resident education and providing the presumed benefit of improved patient care.[24] Although this study did not directly evaluate the utility of SBT to achieve proficiency in US-guided interventions, it did show that SBT of US skills is useful in resident education.

A study that investigated the utility of US-guided SBT for peripherally inserted central catheter (PICC) line placement demonstrated even more convincing results. Residents were divided into two groups: one group trained to perform US-guided PICC lines with SBT, and another group taught using the traditional apprenticeship models of training. The study results showed that those residents who underwent SBT for US-guided line placement had a significantly better transfer of skills to clinical practice, better performance on the procedure-specific tasks, and a higher success rate in ultimate PICC line placement compared to those trained via the traditional apprenticeship models.[28]

Another study used lightly embalmed cadavers as a "physical model" simulator, in which trained physicians with an average of 10.5 years of clinical experience practiced US-guided femoral venous puncture to evaluate the realism of the cadaveric SBT. The study included the evaluation of key psychomotor elements of performing a US-guided procedure, in order to ensure the effectiveness of the training. These elements included ultrasonographic imaging of vascular elements, needle penetration of the skin, needle penetration of a vein, US image of the needle penetrating the vein, passage of a dilator into the vein, US image of catheter insertion into the vein, and overall psychomotor feedback of the simulated procedure compared to the evaluators' assessment of actual patient procedural experience. Based on ratings using a 5-point Likert scale, the cadaveric model was found to resemble closely real-time clinical tasks.[29] The results of this study suggest that the use of US-guided SBT can augment standard methods of training, since certain simulation models are able to mimic realistically key aspects of the actual clinical performance of the procedure on patients.

Several studies have also demonstrated the benefit of US-guided SBT in skill acquisition. Lee et al[30] demonstrated improvement in resident technical skills, procedural competence, and confidence using US guidance for SBT placement of a central venous line. Mendiratta-Lala et al utilized a Blue Phantom™ part-task trainer to demonstrate improvements in resident performance of US-guided procedure. Additionally, they demonstrated a trend toward improvement in the technical skills required to perform US-guided procedures.[14]

Despite the positive results of all of these studies using simulation-based methods of training, the predictive validation of the assessment tools used to evaluate participants is lacking. Since simulations are designed to closely resemble real-life experiences and allow trainees to learn in a controlled environment at an individual pace, it is likely that future studies will succeed in demonstrating the effectiveness of such SBT on translation to actual clinical practice.

Image Guidance

Computed tomography and ultrasonography are two main imaging guidance modalities utilized for percutaneous interventional procedures. X-ray C-arm fluoroscopy is frequently used for spine pain interventional procedures. The choice of which modality to use for an individual case varies based on operator preference, equipment availability, the type of procedure being performed, and both the site and size of the target area.[31] Each modality has its advantages and disadvantages (Table 25.2).

In general, CT-guided interventional procedures are ideal for deep-seated lesions, lung-based lesions, and lesions close to osseous structures, whereas US-guided interventions are useful for more superficial soft tissue lesions.

To ensure accurate and successful outcomes, the interventional radiologist must keep in mind several key points when performing any US-guided procedure. In addition to having a complete understanding of the US equipment, including probe mechanics and the physics of the technology, the interventionalist must accurately identify the target region and select the appropriate needle trajectory. The overall goal of any interventional procedure is to reach the target tissue in the safest way possible via the shortest path. Sterile technique must be practiced at all times. The probe

Table 25.2 Advantages and disadvantages of ultrasound- and computed tomography-guided interventions

MODALITY	ADVANTAGES	DISADVANTAGES
Ultrasound	Low cost Portability Lack of ionizing radiation Real-time visualization of needle Faster time	Long learning curve Operator dependence Difficulty localizing deep tissue lesions Inability to track through air-filled or bony structures Limited field of view
Computed tomography	Ability to track through air-filled structures Wide field of view (i.e., ability to identify adjacent structures and landmarks) Localization of deep tissue lesions and lesions behind osseus structures	Ionizing radiation Imaging constraints secondary to gantry imaging plane "Snap shot" visualization of needle (i.e., lack of real-time imaging of needle)

and machine must be placed in sterile covers. The interventionalist must scrub properly and wear appropriate attire (i.e., sterile gown and gloves, face mask, and cap). The skin site must be properly prepared with antiseptic solution and sterilely draped. Once the procedure has begun, the interventionalist must provide adequate patient sedation and local anesthesia. The appropriate needle/catheter must be selected. Finally, the probe must be kept in a correct plane to visualize continuously the needle as it passes through the tissue en route to the target region. Simulation-based training is ideal for assisting trainees in practicing each of these critical steps in US-guided interventions.

Currently, no specific medical literature exists regarding SBT for CT-guided interventional procedures. As with US-guided interventional procedures, CT-guided procedures require an interventional radiologist to be cognizant of a variety of important factors. The safest and shortest target route must initially be selected after localizing the optimal view of the target area using limited CT scanning. As in US-guided procedure, the interventionalist must practice sterile technique, appropriately sedate the patient, provide adequate local anesthesia, and choose the proper needle/catheter for performing the procedure. Unlike US-guided procedures, the interventionalist must be able to guide the trajectory of the needle by intermittent CT "snap shots" of its progress through the tissues. Simulation-based training is an ideal format for practicing all these aspects of CT-guided interventions, especially since minimum benchmark criteria can be developed to train individuals to proficiency.

Simulation-Based Training for Ultrasound-Guided Interventional Procedures at Henry Ford Hospital

The scope of US-guided procedures in radiology is wide. Ultrasound guidance is used to biopsy tissue or drain fluid collections in the breast, thorax, and abdomen. Additionally, it can be used to assist with tumor ablation, vascular access, and joint aspiration. Fortunately, since the knowledge and skills required to perform successfully such a wide array of US-guided interventions are similar, an SBT curriculum focusing on them can be developed based on whatever interventional US-guided modality is convenient. At Henry Ford Hospital (Wayne State University, Detroit, Michigan), the authors have created a proficiency-based curriculum for performing US-guided procedures. The baseline knowledge of the residents is first assessed using a 20-question pre-test regarding all aspects of a procedure, including technique, indications, contraindications, and patient care (Table 25.3).

The residents then view an online web-based module that goes through all steps of a particular procedure.

Table 25.3 Sample pre-test and post-test questions (multiple choice).

1. Which needle is used for fine needle aspiration?
2. Which needle is used for core biopsy?
3. What is the Seldinger technique?
4. What is the trochar technique?
5. Regarding core biopsy procedures, which of the following is false?
6. Which of the following is true regarding a coaxial system?
7. All of the following are true regarding FNA, except?
8. All of the following are true regarding core biopsies, except?
9. If too much fluid is removed during a thoracentesis, what is the potential complication?
10. All of the following are true regarding coagulation/bleeding complications, except?
11. Which of the following is not an indication for ultrasound (US)-guided thoracentesis/paracentesis?
12. The proper needle entrance into a breast lesion under US guidance is:
13. Which of the following can be safely crossed when performing a percutaneous procedure?
14. Advantages of US-guided procedures over computed tomography (CT)-guided procedures include all but which of the following?
15. Visualization of needle tip can be improved by all of the following except?

These steps include turning on the US equipment, finding the target with the proper probe, advancing a needle into the target under continuous visualization, post-procedure care of the patient, and proper handling and labeling of biopsy specimens. The web-based module contains a short teaching video demonstrating the performance of an US-guided procedure. This didactic module is then followed by formal hands-on training in small groups, each mentored by an interventional radiologist. Each resident in the group is required to perform the procedure multiple times, with tutoring to ensure proper technique (Figure 25.3).

The residents are then allowed to return to the simulation center and practice the procedure at their

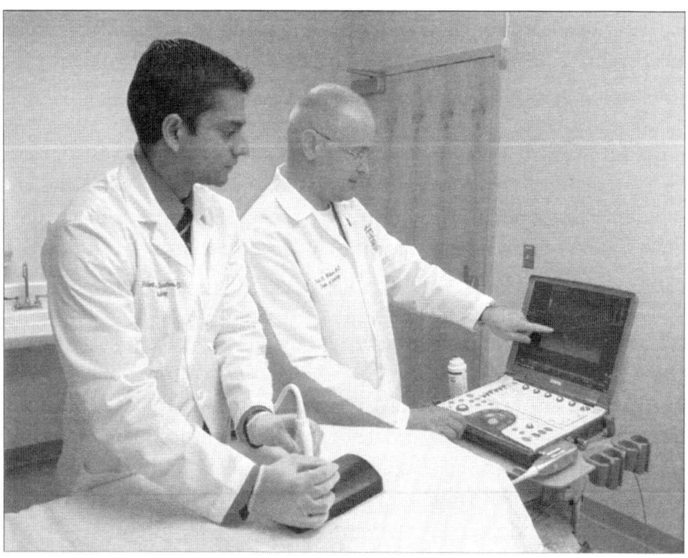

FIGURE 25.3 Resident with faculty member during ultrasound (US)-guided simulation-based training session. The US screen demonstrates the needle approaching a target.

Table 25.4 Ultrasound-guided procedures checklist

1. Checked coagulation factors/allergies
2. Consent obtained
3. Washed hands
4. Performed a "time out"
5. Appropriately turned on ultrasound device
6. Accurately identified the target lesion
7. Prepped area in sterile fashion/placed a sterile field
8. Used proper sterile technique (mask, sterile gown, sterile gloves)
9. Demonstrated technique for local anesthetic
10. Demonstrated sterile technique when using the probe sheath
11. Inserted needle at the appropriate distance from the transducer at an appropriate angle to the lesion
12. Needle tip is visualized throughout the course of the procedure
13. Needle tip is accurately placed within the lesion
14. Demonstrates technique for applying sterile dressing
15. Sharps (e.g., needles) management post-procedure
16. Fills out postprocedural forms accurately (biopsy/drainage); fills out procedure note

own convenience over the next 6 months. After this time period, the residents complete a written post-test assessing a knowledge base similar in content and scope to the pre-test. They then must complete a practical examination in which each one must perform an US-guided procedure in a simulated environment while being audio and video recorded. The procedure is monitored by a staff interventional radiologist. Resident performance is evaluated using an expert-derived checklist of specific steps considered essential for successful performance of an US-guided procedure (Table 25.4).

This checklist focuses on the general skills needed to perform US-guided interventions in any subspecialty of radiology. Checklist items include obtaining patient informed consent, employing proper handwashing technique, completing site and side marking, employing a "time-out" for patient data information review, demonstration of an understanding of the US equipment, proper use of sterile technique, accurate target localization, proper needle placement with continuous US visualization of the needle tip, and proper post-procedure sharps management, biopsy specimen handling/delivery, and patient care and orders.

Residents are required to begin this SBT for US-guided interventions on the first day of their second body imaging rotation. This timing ensures SBT of the entire process of performing an US-guided procedure prior to the procedure performance on actual patients. Initial results of the SBT at this time show significant improvement from pre-test to post-test scores. Additionally, an improvement in the overall performance of the procedure from the initial demonstration to the post-test practical examination has been demonstrated, as evaluated by the checklist instrument. Furthermore, the authors have found, over the course of the training, an improvement in such technical skills as skillful handling of the US probe, sonographic localization of the target lesion, correct technique for lidocaine local anesthetic administration, appropriate insertion of the needle through the simulated skin surface, continuous visualization of the needle throughout the procedure, and correct identification of the needle in the center of the target lesion.

Currently, only first-year radiology residents are required to complete SBT of US-guided procedures. It is likely, however, that all residents will soon be required to continue practicing the US-guided simulations throughout residency, taking the practical examination at the end of each year of training. Additionally, this SBT curriculum is available for staff radiologists to practice, improve, or acquire skills needed for US-guided interventional procedures.

Henry Ford Hospital is fortunate to have a well-funded, large simulation center supported by the hospital for all departments to utilize, but options for SBT at smaller programs lacking dedicated simulation facilities do exist. For example, Blue Phantom™ has a commercially available mold for performing US-guided simulations. Furthermore, inexpensive gelatin molds with internal targets can be created and utilized directly in the radiology department. A simulation-based training curriculum similar to what has been described above could then be employed using these models. Residents would still have the opportunity to practice needle placement into a target under US guidance within a safe, controlled learning environment with faculty supervision.

Simulation-Based Training for Computed Tomography-Guided Interventional Procedures

The development of CT fluoroscopy has opened a fast, safe, and minimally invasive avenue for the performance of percutaneous procedures, including abscess drainage,[31] fluid aspiration and tissue biopsy, and neurointerventional pain procedures. Although real-time CT scanning is limited when compared with US techniques, CT fluoroscopy allows for near real-time instant cross-sectional images at the needle site, as well as images directly cranial and caudal to the needle. The benefits of CT-guided procedures include visualization of adjacent organs, excellent needle visualization, and a shorter learning curve than for US guidance. Additionally, more complex angled procedures can be performed using an angled gantry technique. These skills can be mastered relatively easily, and SBT of CT-guided procedures is ideally suited to augment experience gained in the CT fluoroscopy suite, especially with the increasing demand for more complex percutaneous procedures, such as cryoablation or radiofrequency ablation (RFA).

At Henry Ford Hospital, we have developed an SBT curriculum for CT-guided procedures using a phantom, which allows for proficiency-based training of junior residents in basic percutaneous procedures. Such training is evaluated using a checklist similar to that used for US-guided SBT. In addition, it enables SBT of senior residents and staff in more complex CT-guided procedures. For example, the angled gantry technique can be taught in a simulated environment to help avoid injuring the lung or diaphragm when performing biopsy of the adrenal gland.

Simulation-based training in CT-guided interventional procedures provides an opportunity for instruction in radiation safety. *As low as reasonably achievable* (ALARA) fluoroscopy time, as well as distance and shielding principles are reviewed. All participants wear radiation badges and lead aprons. Procedures are performed with very low CT dose (20 mAs). Radiation safety metrics that are evaluated during the CT SBT include total radiation exposure during the procedure and the number of fluoroscopic images required by the trainee to complete the task. As expected, experienced staff instructors can perform the simulated procedure using very little fluoroscopic time, thus helping to minimize the radiation dose to the patient during an actual procedure. This efficient technique is demonstrated for the trainees on the CT phantom.

Our homemade CT phantom is constructed from an open cell urethane-ether foam commonly used for noise reduction or packaging. The phantom was cut in an arc shape to simulate the normal body contour. Small radiopaque 1 cm pieces of wooden dowel rod, used to simulate nodules, were cut and inserted into the phantom through small slits cut in the foam; they are easily visualized as hyperdense nodules on CT fluoroscopy (Figure 25.4).

The nodule provides some tactile feedback to the resident when the needle contacts the surface of the simulated mass (Figure 25.5).

This phantom is inexpensive and easy to replace. Trainees are walked through the process in a stepwise fashion, including hands-on participation with a staff mentor. Each trainee is then asked to perform the same procedure alone, while the mentor observes and offers guidance and formative feedback (Figure 25.6).

The number of images and the fluoroscopic time required to complete the task provided are logged to document resident improvement over time.

Currently, the SBT curriculum for CT-guided procedures is similar to that of the previously described SBT curriculum for US-guided procedures. Resident trainees complete a written pre-test and watch a short web-based video about training on the CT equipment and basic techniques for performing a CT-guided interventional procedure. The resident then undergoes tutored training with a staff interventional radiologist. This training begins on the first day of the body imaging rotation. At the completion of the first day of the rotation, the resident will have performed the simulated procedure. Assessment includes completion of the abovementioned checklist by the faculty observer, as well as logging of the total fluoroscopy time, radiation

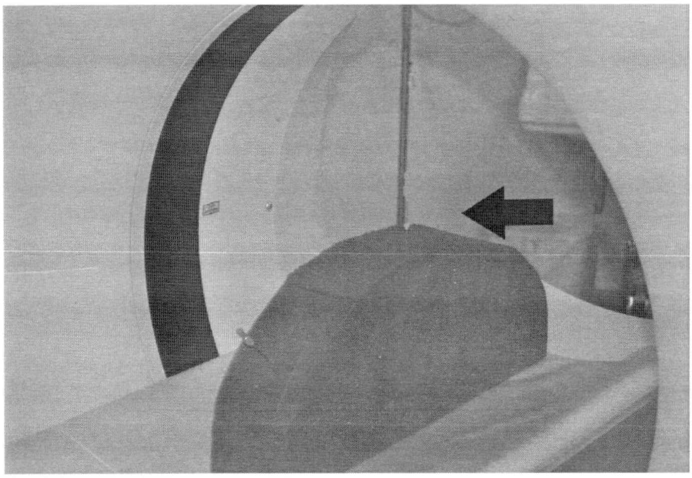

FIGURE 25.4 Image of the arc-shaped homemade part-task trainer for computed tomography fluoroscopic-guided simulation based training. A needle-catheter system placed by trochar technique is seen within the phantom (*arrow*).

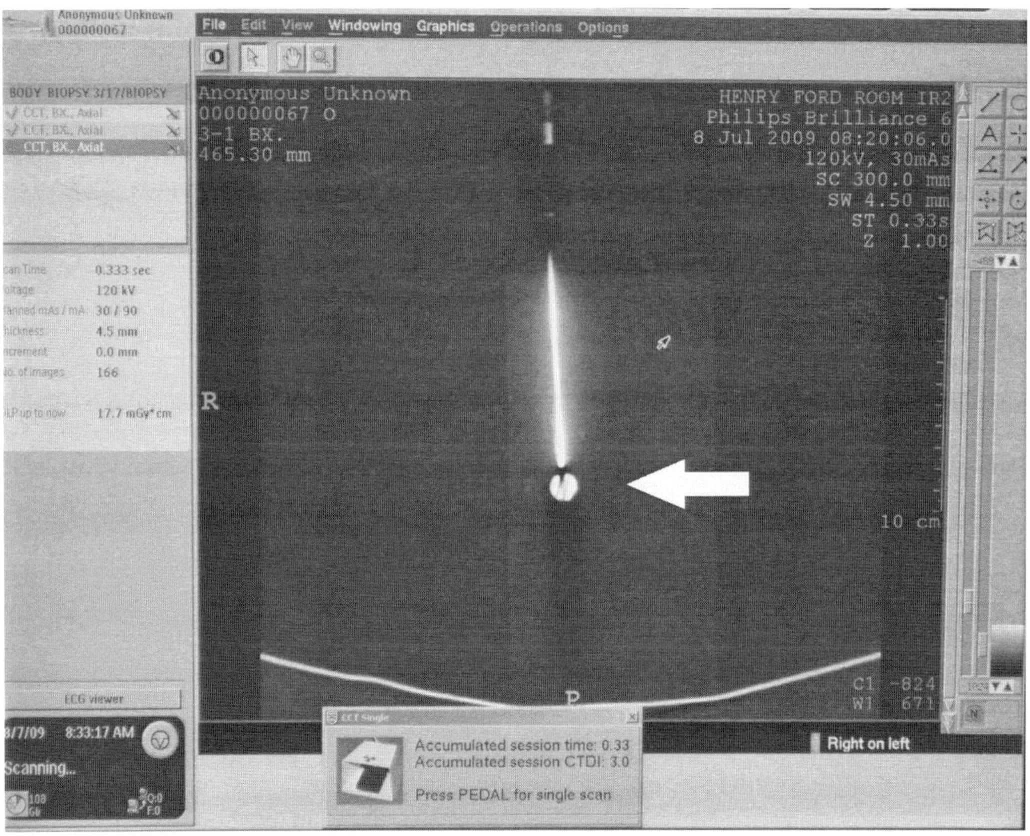

FIGURE 25.5 Image of a screenshot from a Philips eight-slice computed tomography fluoroscopic unit with a needle abutting a wood target within the phantom (*arrow*).

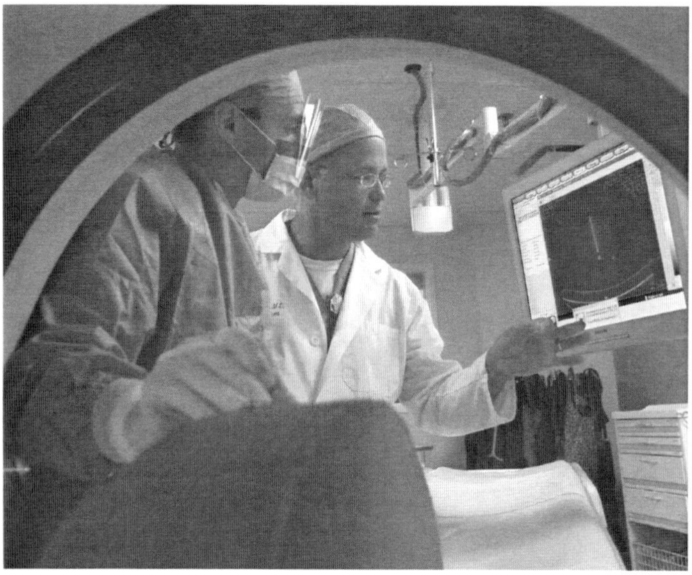

FIGURE 25.6 Image of interventional radiologist reviewing computed tomography fluoroscopy techniques with a resident utilizing a part-task trainer.

dose, and the number of saved images. The resident is expected to practice CT-guided techniques using the CT phantom device over the course of the month-long rotation. At the end of this period, the resident performs a practical examination on the CT phantom device. Improvement is measured by comparing pre- and post-rotation scores.

Simulation-based training using the CT phantom has been undertaken by radiology staff looking to improve their skills using angled gantry technique, in which the gantry is angled either cranially or caudally to allow visualization of the entire needle, despite a nonaxial needle course. The simulator has proved useful in orienting radiologists who are new to this technique.

CONCLUSION

Simulation-based training is currently utilized in many fields of medicine including laparoscopic surgery, emergency medicine, and even gastrointestinal endoscopy. Preliminary studies suggest that such training can be widely applicable in radiology.[14,27,28] The field of interventional radiology has witnessed a rapid development of technology and an increase in demand for increasingly complex percutaneous interventional procedures. Due to changes in training and federal mandates on resident hours, residents have fewer opportunities for learning in the hospital. Alternative approaches to training must be sought, therefore, in order to produce proficient and skilled physicians. Simulation-based training may well be a key tool to advance radiology training, especially through proficiency-based training of procedures. Ultrasound-guided procedures are utilized in most subspecialties of radiology, and, although the procedures differ, the basic skills and techniques are similar. Simulation-based training of US-guided techniques, therefore, is beneficial to all radiology residents. The use of CT fluoroscopic equipment continues to grow in technical sophistication, and CT-guided procedures have become increasingly complex. With limited opportunity for trainee practice in the clinical environment, SBT will likely become the standard for teaching knowledge and skills related to imaging-guided techniques to radiology residents in the future.

REFERENCES

1. Hatfield MK, Beres RA, Sane SS, et al. Percutaneous imaging-guided solid organ core needle biopsy: coaxial versus noncoaxial method. *AJR*. 2008;190:413–417.

2. Holm HH, Pederson JF, Kristensen JK, et al. Ultrasonically guided percutaneous puncture. *Radiol Clin North Am*. 1975;13:493–503.

3. Ferrucci JT, Jr, Wittenberg J. CT biopsy of abdominal tumors: aids for lesion localization. *Radiology*. 1978;129:739–744.

4. Lees WR, Hall-Craggs MA, Manhire A. Five years' experience of fine-needle aspiration biopsy: 454 consecutive cases. *Clin Radiol.* 1985;36:517–520.

5. Hemming A, Davis NL, Robins RE. Surgical versus percutaneous drainage of intra-abdominal abscesses. *Am J Surg.* 1991;161:593–595.

6. Magee D, Zhu Y, Ratnalingam R, et al. An augmented reality simulator for ultrasound guided needle placement training. *Med Biol Eng Comput.* 2007;45:957–967.

7. Long DM. Competency-based residency training: the next advance in graduate medical education. *Acad Med.* 2000;75:1178–1183.

8. Dawson, S. Procedural simulation: a primer. *Radiology.* 2006;241:17–25.

9. Rosendahl K, Aasland OG, Aslaksen A, et al. How is the specialist training in radiology? *Tidsskr Nor Laegeforen.* 2000;120:2289–2292.

10. Wang Y, Chui C, Lim H, et al. Real-time interactive simulator for percutaneous coronary revascularization procedures. *Comput Aided Surg.* 1998;3:211–227.

11. Desser TS. Simulation-based training: the next revolution in radiology education? *J Am Coll Radiol.* 2007;4:816–824.

12. Okuda Y, Bryson EO, DeMaria S, Jr, et al. The utility of simulation in medical education: what is the evidence? *Mt Sinai J Med.* 2009;76:330–343.

13. Mendiratta-Lala M, Brook OR, Midkiff BD, et al. Quality initiatives: strategies for anticipating and reducing complications and treatment failures in hepatic radiofrequency ablation. *Radiographics.* 2010;30:1107–1122.

14. Mendiratta-Lala M, Williams T, de Quadros N, et al. The use of a simulation center to improve resident proficiency in performing ultrasound-guided procedures. *Acad Radiol.* 2010;17:535–540.

15. Sedlack RE, Kolars JC. Computer simulator training enhances the competency of gastroenterology fellows at colonoscopy: results of a pilot study. *Am J Gastroenterol.* 2004;99:33–37.

16. Rowe R, Cohen RA. An evaluation of a virtual reality airway simulator. *Anesth Analg.* 2002;95: 62–66.

17. Seymour NE, Gallagher AG, Roman SA, et al. Virtual reality training improves operating room performance: results of a randomized, double-blinded study. *Ann Surg.* 2002;236:458–463. [Discussion 463]

18. Bloom MB, Rawn CL, Salzberg AD, et al. Virtual reality applied to procedural testing: the next era. *Ann Surg.* 2003;237:442–448.

19. Binstadt ES, Walls RM, White BA, et al. A comprehensive medical simulation education curriculum for emergency medicine residents. *Ann Emerg Med.* 2007;49:495–504.

20. Bond WF, Spillane L. The use of simulation for emergency medicine resident assessment. *Acad Emerg Med.* 2002;9:1295–1299.

21. Patel AA, Gould DA. Simulators in interventional radiology training and evaluation: a paradigm shift is on the horizon. *J Vasc Interv Radiol.* 2006;17(11 Pt 2):S163–S173.

22. John NW, Luboz V, Bello F, et al. Physics-based virtual environment for training core skills in vascular interventional radiological procedures. *Stud Health Technol Inform.* 2008;132:195–197.

23. Forest C, Comas O, Vaysiere C, et al. Ultrasound and needle insertion simulators built on real patient-based data. *Stud Health Technol Inform.* 2007;125:136–139.

24. Monsky WL, Levine D, Mehta TS, et al. Using a sonographic simulator to assess residents before overnight call. *AJR.* 2002;178:35–39.

25. Zhu Y, Magee D, Ratnalinam R, et al. A training system for ultrasound-guided needle insertion procedures. *Med Image Comput Assist Interv.* 2007;10(Pt 1):566–574.

26. Ni D, Chan WY, Qin J, et al. An ultrasound-guided organ biopsy simulation with 6DOF haptic feedback. *Med Image Comput Comput Assist Interv.* 2008;11(Pt 2):551–559.

27. Girzadas DV, Jr, Antonis MS, Zerth H, et al. Hybrid simulation combining a high fidelity scenario with a pelvic ultrasound task trainer enhances the training and evaluation of endovaginal ultrasound skills. *Acad Emerg Med.* 2009;16:429–435.

28. Andreatta P, Chen Y, Marsh M, et al. Simulation-based training improves applied clinical placement of ultrasound-guided PICCs. *Support Care Cancer* 2011; 19:539–543. doi 10.1007/s00520-010-0849-2

29. Wadman MC, Lomneth CS, Hoffman LH, et al. Assessment of a new model for femoral ultrasound-guided central venous access procedural training: a pilot study. *Acad Emerg Med.* 2010;17:88–92.

30. Lee AC, Thompson C, Frank J, et al. Effectiveness of a novel training program for emergency medicine residents in ultrasound-guided insertion of central venous catheters. *Canadian journal of emergency medicine.* 2009;11:343–348.

31. Hemming A, Davis NL, Robins RE. Surgical versus percutaneous drainage of intra-abdominal abscesses. *The American Journal of Surgery.* 1991;161:593–595.

26

Simulation in Nuclear Medicine Education

FREDERICK D. GRANT AND S. TED TREVES

NUCLEAR MEDICINE presents particular challenges in developing simulation-based educational curricula. Given its reliance on medical physics, radiopharmacy, and radiation biology, the typical simulation-based training (SBT) experiences that focus on procedural skills or patient-based encounters do not adequately address the knowledge, skills, and attitudes (KSAs) most pertinent to the field. Most nuclear medicine KSAs might be more appropriately taught and assessed using forms of cognitive simulation.[1,2] Although it may have few demands for specialized hardware or surrogate patients, the challenge is to make it an experiential learning experience for the student. Even image-based teaching files can be considered a basic type of cognitive simulation. Nuclear medicine, however, provides opportunities for more advanced cognitive SBT. Software simulation of clinical cases with integration of images, clinical material, and workflow can be used for both learning and student assessment. Another approach is to use existing clinical hardware, such as scanners and image phantoms, for medical physics and image processing education. Training in radiopharmacy procedures and dosimetric calculations for open-source radiotherapy can use existing websites and software packages. In addition, nuclear medicine physicians can play an important role in the institutional response to a radiation disaster, and they should participate in the planning, teaching, and implementation of simulated radiation events.

CLINICAL NUCLEAR MEDICINE EDUCATION

Although they are a common method of enriching medical education, teaching case files are hardly recognized as a form of simulation-based education. One advantage of teaching files is that teaching and assessment is not dependent on the particular patient mix that occurs when any particular trainee is in the reading room. Another advantage is that teaching files allow trainees to pursue clinical learning away from the distractions of clinical workflow. Nuclear medicine teaching files typically have included static clinical images accompanied by brief clinical information. However, with the increasing availability of digital image files and clinical information, more clinically realistic teaching files can be created.

Electronic Learning Resources

In nuclear medicine, clinical training occurs in the reading room, where trainees learn from cases that they interpret for clinical needs. Over the typical period of training, trainees are expected to see a sufficient number and diversity of cases to gain clinical competency.[3] However, unusual cases may be seen rarely or not at all. In addition, the availability and timing of cases may not provide an ideal pedagogical context for trainees to learn. The use of teaching cases allows both exposure to cases rarely seen in the reading room and goal-directed learning with more common studies. Goal-directed learning can be based on a series of cases—for example, lung perfusion scans—that encourages the trainee to directly compare a variety of pathologies and imaging findings.

Traditional teaching files presented cases on film or other hard media. With the widespread availability of computers and introduction of picture archiving and communication systems (PACS), nearly all teaching files are now in digital formats. This allows a variety of presentation formats and gives the trainees flexibility in where and when they use the teaching files. With the availability of the Internet, electronic case-based teaching files can be accessed on the worldwide web.[4,5] Digital case files present new challenges for educators. Digital formats raise the expectations of trainees that cases will be presented clearly, logically, and linked to other information. The transition from film to PACS provides users a wider variety of cases, the use of realistic images, the availability of correlative imaging, and learner-directed access of cases away from the departmental library.

Digital case files have been developed in a wide variety of formats and with varying degrees of sophistication. Towbin et al[6] suggested five key components of an electronic teaching case file. These include simulation of the appearance of the images in a PACS system (preferably the same PACS as used in the trainee's home department), availability of the entire study as acquired, so that images can be manipulated in a realistic manner; ability to use digital imaging and communication in medicine (DICOM) image files, easy case entry and retrieval, and the capability to provide feedback to users. Although this might be possible on the hospital PACS, the limitations of some PACS may require the use of a stand-alone system to accomplish these goals. However, one limitation of typical teaching cases is that they have been chosen to demonstrate a particular finding or make a specific educational point and are not always presented in a realistic clinical context. The most effective teaching files allow the trainee to access imaging studies from the PACS and clinical information from the electronic medical record, so that clinical correlation is possible. Digital case files then can be used by trainees for independent study, used for case-based teaching in the reading room, and incorporated into lectures.

Ease of use encourages use of teaching files. In our department, we have incorporated a teaching file list into our nuclear medicine dashboard. Cases are categorized by organ and disease type using the content manual of the American Board of Nuclear Medicine (www.abnm.org) as a guide. When a trainee selects a case from a digital case list, the dashboard launches both the departmental PACS and the hospital electronic medical record. Interesting or illustrative cases can be easily identified and annotated. The flexibility of this system allows cases to be identified and stored in real time. This system is easily accessed by nuclear medicine and radiology trainees while sitting at any reading station in the reading room. New cases entered into the teaching file remain "open" until clinical or pathological follow-up is entered and the case is "closed." The process of periodically updating and closing the open cases is assigned to trainees during their nuclear medicine rotation. This process of clinical follow-up can provide structure for trainees to use the cases for independent study and peer teaching.

Security and patient privacy must be addressed when clinical material is used for teaching. Both can be maintained by providing appropriate clinical privileges and limiting access to clinical trainees with legitimate access to the PACS and the electronic medical record. Alternatively, cases could be rendered anonymous and loaded onto a freestanding PACS simulator or web-based teaching file.[7] However, this approach limits easy clinical and pathological correlation, which is essential for adequate simulation.

When using teaching case files, feedback can be provided in a number of ways. In the simplest form of self-directed learning, individual teaching cases will stimulate trainees to use additional resources, including textbooks, clinical literature, and the Internet, to assess and supplement their understanding of a particular case. Similarly, faculty can provide feedback and assess competence while reviewing teaching case files with a trainee. Training files can be used as an examination that requires trainees to answer specific questions about each case. For example, trainees may be required to demonstrate a minimal level of knowledge or competency before being allowed to take call.[8,9] Similarly, case files can be used to develop more sophisticated simulation-based assessment tools.

Objective Structured Clinical Examination

The Objective Structured Clinical Examination (or Exercise), better known as the OSCE, is commonly used in medical education to reinforce and assess clinical skills. The OSCE is used by most medical schools[10] and now is part of the series of the United States Medical Licensing Examinations (USMLE). Whereas clinical OSCEs use patients or actors to provide a realistic simulation of the clinical environment, a diagnostic imaging OSCE is built around radiology and nuclear medicine images. However, in addition to image interpretation, a nuclear medicine OSCE should require a trainee to interpret a study in the context of realistic clinical and laboratory information, correlate findings with prior studies and other imaging, and produce a well-crafted, accurate, and informative report that integrates all available information. Therefore, examinees are able to demonstrate not only competent interpretation of an imaging finding, but the ability to perform many of the other functions necessary to the clinical practice of nuclear medicine or radiology.

An OSCE differs from a typical written exam in that the trainee can be presented with both a complete set of images and extensive clinical information from which to synthesize an interpretation. It differs from an oral board exam in that it can accurately simulate the work environment of the reading room, thus forcing the trainee to produce the final product of a written report. An OSCE offers several advantages over assessing trainee performance during day-to-day reading room activity. First, the choice of cases is not dependent on the clinical schedule, but can be chosen to represent the broader range of the practice of nuclear medicine. Second, the OSCE also can introduce equity into the examination process, since all examinees are tested with the same cases, and their performance on these standardized cases can be evaluated by multiple graders.

Success in clinical practice may depend as much upon the proper performance of the full spectrum of reading room activities as on medical knowledge alone. Our early experience[11] suggests that there is little association between performance on a nuclear medicine OSCE and performance on the American Board of Nuclear Medicine (ABNM) in-training examination. This finding supports the hypothesis that an OSCE tests different skills than a typical knowledge-based written or oral examination. One limitation of the OSCE is that, due to the time commitment required from both trainees and faculty, only a small number of cases can realistically be used for an examination. Therefore, many knowledge-based topics will not be evaluated, and other complementary testing methods, such as written examinations, may better assess a trainee's breadth of knowledge across a wider range of topics.

The greatest logistical limitations to an OSCE appear to be computer capability and the time of trainees and faculty. Most hospital-wide simulation centers are not yet equipped to provide realistic PACS and report dictation systems.[12] Conversely, the hospital PACS system may not have the flexibility to present simulated cases that are segregated from the electronic medical record. The use of freestanding software or reading stations may be a solution, but this arrangement frequently complicates administration of a simulation exercise if examinees require training in the use of an unfamiliar PACS application. Also, it may be more difficult to correlate with clinical information on a freestanding workstation. Depending on the configuration of the dictation system, if examinees are not be able to use a dictation/report creation system for nonclinical work, the creation of each report will seem a laborious and time-consuming process to the examinee. Evaluation of the examinees' resulting reports also takes many hours of effort, thus placing further time pressures on faculty evaluators. Cases developed for an OSCE also can be used for teaching with a case-based approach. Simulation cases can be used for online tutorials, with or without faculty participation, which allow trainees to receive rapid feedback while performance is monitored. With proper case selection of simulated cases, trainees can learn and practice the appropriate use of pharmaceutical intervention in renal and hepatobiliary imaging. Finally, faculty can incorporate preexisting simulation cases into didactic cases to engage the audience in active learning.

NUCLEAR MEDICINE PHYSICS EDUCATION

Nuclear medicine physicists use imaging phantoms for a wide variety of quality assurance procedures, including acceptance testing of new cameras, routine quality control procedures, troubleshooting when image quality is degraded, and estimating dosimetry.[13] The development of nuclear medicine phantoms has been incremental, and the most primitive phantoms remain simple flasks that are imaged after they are filled with a solution of radiotracer. More sophisticated phantoms contain an arrangement of multiple structures or chambers that can be filled with radioactive or nonradioactive solutions.[14] Other phantoms have been developed to specifically assess imaging of certain regions of the body, such as the head.[15] More recently, anthropometric phantoms have been developed for experimental determination of whole-body and organ-based dosimetry.[16]

Phantoms remain an underutilized resource for SBT of nuclear medicine trainees. Phantoms can be used in a variety of ways to provide trainees with an opportunity for active learning to gain insight into physical concepts involved in medical imaging. For example, they can be used to help trainees acquire hands-on experience with the routine procedures of quality control such as uniformity, spatial resolution, and contrast resolution. Additionally, they can be incorporated to help trainees mimic the process of acceptance testing of a single photon emission computed tomography (SPECT) or positron emission tomography (PET) camera. Such exercises help trainees become familiar with a particular model of camera and understand the quality control procedures that are needed in any nuclear medicine department. Trainees also can use phantoms to perform the procedures needed to participate in an imaging accreditation program.[17] As with quality control procedures, such an experience can serve as a "dry run" for a trainee whose future job might make him or her the clinician responsible for ensuring accreditation of a nuclear medicine program. A drawback to such use of a phantom is that clinical trainees may consider some of these exercises to be tedious and time-consuming, without providing much useful conceptual learning. A more fruitful application of the phantom may be in laboratory exercises, in which trainees experimentally demonstrate the effects of camera manipulation on image quality with either a gamma camera or PET scanner. For example, the phantom can be used to demonstrate the effect of the distance of an object from the gamma camera on resolution and sensitivity. With PET, an external source can be used to experimentally demonstrate the effects of an out-of-field hot object on image acquisition.

Few phantoms have been developed primarily for education and training. Simulated thyroid glands have been used for many years for teaching nuclear medicine imaging of the thyroid. In one recently described thyroid phantom,[18] solid acrylic fillers are placed in the phantom to create photopenic thyroid nodules of different sizes on the simulated thyroid scan. With such a model, trainees have the opportunity to hone their recognition of "cold" nodules prior to entering the actual clinical environment.

Recently developed anthropomorphic phantoms provide the greatest opportunity for enhancing simulation-based teaching in nuclear medicine. Many of these phantoms were developed as reference standards for estimating dosimetry in patients exposed to radioactive fallout or for use in trauma or military-medicine simulated exercises. They typically are made of synthetic material with radiation-absorbing properties similar to body tissue and contain an inert high-density skeleton that can be made more or less realistic. Radioactive solution or plugs can be placed in individual organs, and varying degrees of soft-tissue attenuation can be simulated with additional layers of "soft-tissue" plates. In addition to whole-body phantoms, organ-specific phantoms also are available. These include a brain or head phantom that allows radioactive solution to be placed in specific regions of the basal ganglia, and a heart phantom that can be used for optimizing myocardial perfusion imaging. Although originally marketed for the development and fine-tuning of imaging protocols, these phantoms now also are marketed as training devices, with a particular focus on training nuclear medicine technologists in techniques of image acquisition and processing and for simulating radiation therapy procedures. In addition to static phantoms, dynamic anthropomorphic phantoms have been developed for specific research applications,[19] but, to date, there have been no reports in the literature describing the use of these dynamic phantoms for teaching nuclear medicine trainees.

Using phantoms for SBT provides a far richer learning experience than can be provided by the occasional "physics" case that may be identified in the reading room. Even simulated training, however, has its limitations. Few opportunities exist to use a phantom for educational purposes when the camera is not working properly. Consequently, a functioning camera is a prerequisite before any SBT can take place. This limitation may be balanced by the ability of the trainees to manipulate and experiment with the phantom. A greater limitation to the use of phantoms for education may be the availability of the necessary imaging camera. In most busy nuclear medicine departments, camera time may be fully scheduled with patient imaging and routine quality control activities. Therefore, simulation-based physics training may need to be relegated to after-hours use or use on a research-based gamma camera or PET scanner.

An alternative to whole-body or organ-based phantoms is the use of software to create standardized images. The advantage of a phantom is that the abnormality is known to the creator, but even the most realistic phantom is unlikely to produce an image that exactly replicates the appearance of a clinical scan. On the other hand, when clinical scans are used for teaching, the only gold standard may be the interpretation of the scan by the teacher or another expert. Software can be used to insert standard lesions into clinical images. This lesion can function as a gold standard for an abnormality when images are used to assess the quality of image processing procedures or to compare the performance of different readers. Earlier attempts to accomplish this were limited by the unrealistic appearance of the synthesized abnormalities. Recent methods, using lesions digitally extracted from other studies, allow realistic-appearing abnormalities to be introduced into the background of an otherwise normal study. The process of digital insertion of a realistic-appearing artificial lesion, however, remains technically difficult.[20] Similar methods could be used for site validation in multi-institutional research studies and will surely have a future role in education and testing.

RADIOPHARMACY AND RADIOTHERAPY

Safe handling of radioactive materials is critical for nuclear medicine professionals. Physicians, technologists, and radiopharmacists must be competent and safe in drawing up, preparing, aliquoting, and administering radiopharmaceuticals without radioactive or biological contamination. Training in these skills has become even more important with the recent revision of chapter 797 of the U.S. Pharmacopeia (USP), which mandates specific sterile procedures when handling radiopharmaceuticals.[21] Mastery of the skills necessary to comply with these regulations is made more challenging by the need to use syringe shields and perform procedures behind lead glass shields or in chemical safety hoods that are required for radiation protection. Trainees need hands-on training to be able to accomplish these skills.

Although radiotracers can be very sensitive detectors of contamination, dye may be a good substitute for novice trainees, who can practice using a syringe to draw up, measure, and aliquot nonradioactive liquid that has been colored with a food dye. After demonstrating competence with the basic procedures, a syringe shield can be added, and then the procedure can be performed behind a shield and in a hood. With dye, there is no safety concern about spread of contamination. An alternative to colored dye is a fluorescent dye, such as fluorescein, which can be detected by ultraviolet light after the procedures are completed.[22] Fluorescent dye provides increased sensitivity for detecting contamination, but gives less visual feedback to the trainee during the actual performance of the procedure. As part of training to meet the requirements of chapter 797 of the USP, trainees need to demonstrate an ability to transfer radiopharmaceuticals while maintaining sterility. Procedures like the media fill test can confirm adequate sterile transfer techniques.[23] These hands-on nonradioactive methods, therefore, are an excellent simulated model for trainees to learn and gain competence in the skills of handling and administering radiopharmaceuticals.

Another approach for radiopharmacy teaching is computer-based simulation. For example, the Virtual Radiopharmacy (www.virrad.eu.org) is an online resource that includes an interactive virtual three-dimensional radiopharmacy. Using an avatar, trainees can interactively navigate through a virtual radiopharmacy, where they can simulate the use of radiopharmacy equipment and perform typical radiopharmacy procedures.

Administration of open-source radiotherapy is one of the core competencies of nuclear medicine. This includes estimation of the effective dose and organ-specific dose that will result from this therapy. Software packages[24,25] have been developed to assist clinicians and physicists with these calculations. Although designed for clinical management, these software packages also can serve an educational function. After being presented with simulated patients, trainees can be asked to determine the clinically appropriate radiopharmaceutical dose and then to calculate the estimated effective dose and critical organ dose. Such SBT exercises can supplement a trainee's clinical experience, especially at an institution with a limited radiotherapy program.

RESPONSE TO RADIATION EVENTS

The institutional response to a radiation disaster will depend, in part, on the participation of professionals trained in radiation safety and protection. A lead role should be taken by the institutional radiation safety officer. Although the radiation safety officer may be specifically trained in radiation hygiene or may be primarily trained as a clinical specialist, individuals with training in nuclear medicine, medical physics, radiology, radiation oncology, radiopharmacy, and radiology and nuclear medicine technology all may be part of the response team. Ideally, these individuals have been identified and their respective roles defined before an incident occurs. During an event, these individuals may have a wide variety of roles. These include evaluation of patients for potential contamination, assisting treating clinicians in understanding the significance of any detected contamination, and monitoring contamination procedures.[26] They also may be called upon to communicate with public health authorities and the media.[26] To be effective members of the response team, radiation professionals must be involved in the planning, training, and implementation of radiation event drills.[27]

Because the disaster response team will include individuals from a wide range of disciplines with varying levels of familiarity with radiation safety, one of the roles of the radiation professionals is to assist in training other members of the team in the fundamentals of radiation protection.[28] However, clinical training for specialties in nuclear medicine or radiology typically does not include extensive training in radiation event management. Therefore, specialists in radiation-related fields who may participate in a radiation disaster response team must be trained, so that they become the local experts in the response to a radiation disaster, can train other members of the team, and can be functional members of the larger disaster response team.

Schleipman et al[29] describe the role of nuclear medicine staff at one large hospital during a citywide, multiagency radiation event exercise in Boston. Within the emergency department, nuclear medicine and health physics staff acted as radiation control officers. These individuals were assigned to a triage or treatment team, in order to monitor patients and staff for contamination, direct radioactive decontamination, and monitor staff radiation protection. Within the nuclear medicine department, nuclear medicine technologists were responsible for identification of radiation contamination in clothing, surface swabs, and blood and urine samples. In addition, they were responsible for identifying radionuclides by γ-spectroscopy using a well counter. Nuclear medicine and health physics staff were actively involved in the planning and implementation of the drill. Prior to the drill, the health physics staff had provided extensive didactic and hands-on radiation protection training for emergency department and operating room staff. This pretraining included didactic teaching and detection of simulated radioactive contamination, using manikins and sealed radiation sources. In addition to basic training in radiation protection, some institutions[30] have utilized a high-fidelity simulation center to provide realistic training in providing patient care while using personal protective devices. However, more research is needed to determine the optimal approaches for effectively preparing a diverse group of clinicians for a potential radiation emergency.[31]

CONCLUSION

In nuclear medicine, computer-based or web-based simulation is relatively easy to implement. For example, numerous websites exist that include nuclear medicine teaching files. Additionally, other websites can be accessed for learning radiopharmacy procedures or performing dosimetry calculations for simulated open-source radiotherapy. Although useful, such websites fail to recreate the work environment of the reading room, thus limiting their realism.

More realistic simulation-based methods may utilize existing institutional resources. For example, the departmental PACS and hospital electronic medical record can be used to develop realistic teaching files. Existing phantoms and cameras in the nuclear medicine department can be used as models in SBT to teach medical physics. If institutional or workflow issues limit this use of clinical equipment, then freestanding nuclear medicine workstations can be used for teaching files or for development of a nuclear medicine OSCE. To promote the most effective simulation-based educational and/or evaluative experience, teaching files should replicate the appearance of the departmental PACS, with access to both correlative imaging and the clinical record. The nuclear medicine OSCE is such an example.

Nuclear medicine physicians and other specialists in radiation-related fields may participate in a radiation disaster response team and in large-scale simulations. These individuals must be trained to become the local experts in the response to a radiation disaster, train other members of the team, and participate as functional members of the larger disaster response team. To be effective members of the response team they must be involved in the planning and implementation of radiation event simulation exercises.

Nuclear medicine education can be enhanced using SBT. Such SBT may range from computer-based exercises to hands-on physics and radiopharmacy training to participation in large-scale disaster drills. The most effective simulation methods for clinical nuclear medicine education likely will be those that faithfully replicate the environment of the reading room or imaging room, and that require the trainee to integrate nuclear medicine images, prior studies, medical physics, and clinical information. As SBT becomes more incorporated into medical education, an opportunity exists to develop more realistic and more effective simulated learning experiences for teaching the practice of nuclear medicine.

REFERENCES

1. Eden C, Smithin T, Wiltshire J. Cognition simulation and learning. *J Exper Learn Simul.* 1980;2:131–143.
2. Nirenburg S, McShane M, Beale S, et al. Cognitive simulation in virtual patients. In: *Proceedings of the 19th International FLAIRS Conference 2006*; Melbourne Beach, FL.
3. Alavi A, Blahd WH, DeNardo SJ, et al. Components of professional competence for nuclear medicine physicians. *J Nucl Med.* 2003;44:988–990.
4. Parker JA, Wallis JW, Halama JR, et al. Collaboration using internet for the development of case-based teaching files: report of the computer and instrumentation council internet focus group. *J Nucl Med.* 1996;37:178–184.
5. Wallis JW, Parker JA. Use of the internet for teaching in nuclear medicine. *Semin Nucl Med.* 1998;28:165–176.
6. Towbin AJ, Paterson BE, Chang PJ. Computer-based simulator for radiology: an educational tool. *RadioGraphics.* 2008;28:309–316.
7. Weinberger E, Jakobovits R, Halsted M. MyPACS.net: a web-based teaching file authoring tool. *Am J Roentgenol.* 2002;179:579–582.
8. Talanow R. Radiology teacher: a free, internet-based radiology teaching file server. *J Am Coll Radiol.* 2009;6:871–875.
9. Ganguli S, Camacho M, Yam CS, et al. Preparing first-year radiology residents and assessing their readiness for on-call responsibilities: results over 5 years. *Am J Roentgenol.* 2009;192:539–544.
10. Brzansky B, Etzel SI. Educational programs in US medical schools, 2003–2004. *JAMA.* 2004;292:1025–1031.
11. Grant FD, Treves ST. Development of a computerized objective structured clinical examination for nuclear medicine trainees [abstract]. Presented at: The Annual Meeting of the Association of University Radiologists; 2010; San Diego.
12. Taylor T. How to create a clinical data station for use in a high fidelity medical simulation lab. *Simul Healthc.* 2008;3:128–130.
13. Daube-Witherspoon ME, Karp JS, Casey ME, et al. PET performance measurements using the NEMA NU 2-2001 standard. *J Nucl Med.* 2002;43:1398–1409.
14. Fahey FH, Kinahan PE, Doot RK, et al. Variability in PET quantification within a multicenter consortium. *Med Phys.* 2010;37:3660–3666.
15. Koch W, Radau PE, Munzing W, et al. Cross-camera comparison of SPECT measurements of a 3-D anthropomorphic basal ganglia phantom. *Eur J Nucl Med Mol Imaging.* 2006;33:495–502.
16. He B, Du Y, Segars P, et al. Evaluation of quantitative imaging methods for organ activity and residence time estimation using a population of phantoms having realistic variations in anatomy and uptake. *Med Phys.* 2009;36:612–619.
17. Scheuerman JS, Saffer JR, Karp JS, et al. Qualification of PET scanners for use in multicenter cancer clinical trials: the American College of Radiology Imaging Network experience. *J Nucl Med.* 2009;50:1187–1193.
18. Ferreira FCL, Peixoto JA, Maciel MF, et al. Development of a simulator with thyroid nodules for nuclear medicine. *Scientia Plena.* 2009;5:109902.
19. Idoine JD, Holman BL, Jones AG, et al. Quantification of flow in a dynamic phantom using ^{81}Rb-^{81m}Kr, and a NaI detector. *J Nucl Med.* 1977;18:570–578.
20. Zhu Y, Magee D, Ratnalingam R, et al. A physics based method for combining multiple anatomy models with application to

medical simulation. *Stud Health Technol Inform.* 2009;142:465–467.

21. Norenberg JP, Petry NA, Schwarz S. Operation of a radiopharmacy for a clinical trial. *Semin Nucl Med.* 2010;40:347–356.

22. Mosman EA, Peterson LJ, Hung JC, et al. Practical methods for reducing radioactive contamination incidents in the nuclear cardiology laboratory. *J Nucl Med Technol.* 1999;27:287–289.

23. Isanhart CM, McCall KL, Kretschmer D, et al. Parenteral laboratory course to reduce microbial contamination rates in media fill tests performed by pharmacy students. *Am J Pharm Educ.* 2008;72:27.

24. Stabin MG, Sparks RB, Crowe E. OLINDA/EXM: the second generation personal computer software for internal dose assessment in nuclear medicine. *J Nucl Med.* 2005;46:1023–1027.

25. Visser E, Postema E, Boerman O, et al. Software package for integrated data processing for internal dose assessment in nuclear medicine (SPRIND). *Eur J Nucl Med Mol Imaging.* 2007;34:413–421.

26. Miller CW, Whitcomb RC, Ansair A, et al. The roles of medical health physicists in a medical radiation emergency. *Health Phys.* 2007;93:S187–S190.

27. Miller K, Erdman M. Health physics considerations in medical radiation emergencies. *Health Phys.* 2004;87:S19–S24.

28. McCurley MC, Miller CW, Tucker FE, et al. Educating medical staff about responding to a radiological or nuclear emergency. *Health Phys.* 2009;96:S50–S54.

29. Schleipman AR, Gerbaudo VH, Castronovo FP. Radiation disaster response: preparation and simulation experience at an academic medical center. *J Nucl Med Technol.* 2004;32:22–27.

30. Summerhill EM, Matthew MC, Stipho S, et al. A simulation-based biodefense and disaster preparedness curriculum for internal medicine residents. *Med Teach.* 2008;30:e145–e151.

31. Hsu EB, Jenckes MW, Catlett CL, et al. Effectiveness of hospital staff mass-casualty incident training methods: a systematic literature review. *Prehosp Disast Med.* 2004;19:191–199.

Index